TEACHING IN NURSING AND ROLE OF THE EDUCATOR

Marilyn H. Oermann, PhD, RN, ANEF, FAAN, is professor and director of Evaluation and Educational Research at Duke University School of Nursing, Durham, North Carolina. She is the author/coauthor of 15 nursing education books and many articles on teaching and evaluation in nursing, and on writing for publication. She is the editor of the *Journal of Nursing Care Quality* and *Nurse Author & Editor* and is past editor of the *Annual Review of Nursing Education*. Dr. Oermann received the National League for Nursing Award for Excellence in Nursing Education Research and the Sigma Theta Tau International Elizabeth Russell Belford Award for Excellence in Education.

TEACHING IN NURSING AND ROLE OF THE EDUCATOR

THE COMPLETE GUIDE TO BEST PRACTICE IN TEACHING, EVALUATION, AND CURRICULUM DEVELOPMENT

MARILYN H. OERMANN, PhD, RN, ANEF, FAAN

EDITOR

SPRINGER PUBLISHING COMPANY

NEW YORK

Springer Publishing Company, LLC
11 West 42nd Street
New York, NY 10036
www.springerpub.com

Acquisitions Editor: Margaret Zuccarini
Composition: diacriTech

ISBN: 978-0-8261-9553-1
e-book ISBN: 978-0-8261-9561-6
Instructors' PowerPoints: 978-0-8261-2003-8
Instructors' Manual: 978-0-8261-2002-1

**Instructors' Materials: Instructors may request supplements by emailing
*textbook@springerpub.com***

14 15 16 17 / 5 4 3 2 1

The author and the publisher of this Work have made every effort to use sources believed to be reliable to provide information that is accurate and compatible with the standards generally accepted at the time of publication. The author and publisher shall not be liable for any special, consequential, or exemplary damages resulting, in whole or in part, from the readers' use of, or reliance on, the information contained in this book. The publisher has no responsibility for the persistence or accuracy of URLs for external or third-party Internet websites referred to in this publication and does not guarantee that any content on such websites is, or will remain, accurate or appropriate.

Library of Congress Cataloging-in-Publication Data

Teaching in nursing : the guide to best practice / [edited by] Marilyn H. Oermann.
    pages ; cm
 Includes bibliographical references and index.
 ISBN 978-0-8261-9553-1 — ISBN 978-0-8261-9561-6 (e-book)
 I. Oermann, Marilyn H., editor of compilation.
 [DNLM: 1. Education, Nursing—methods. 2. Faculty, Nursing. 3. Teaching—methods. WY 18]
 RT90
 610.73071'1—dc23
                                        2013034827

Printed in the United States of America by Bradford & Bigelow.

*To nurse educators and students preparing for a
future role as a teacher in nursing*

Contents

Contributors

Katie Anne Adamson, PhD, RN
Assistant Professor
Nursing and Healthcare Leadership
    Programs
University of Washington Tacoma
Tacoma, Washington

Diane S. Aschenbrenner, MS, RN
Undergraduate Course Coordinator
Faculty Coordinator of the Nursing
    Simulation and Practice Labs
School of Nursing
Johns Hopkins University
Baltimore, Maryland

Darlene E. Baker, MSN, RN, CNE
Assistant Director, Education-
    Innovation-Simulation Learning
    Environment
School of Nursing
University of North Carolina at Chapel
    Hill
Chapel Hill, North Carolina

Donna L. Boland, PhD, RN, ANEF
Associate Professor Emeritus
School of Nursing
Indiana University
Indianapolis, Indiana

Helen B. Connors, PhD, RN, FAAN
E. Jean M. Hill Endowed Professor
Associate Dean, Integrated Technologies
Executive Director of Kansas University
    Center for Health Informatics
The University of Kansas
Kansas City, Kansas

**Kristina Thomas Dreifuerst, PhD, RN,
    ACNS-BC, CNE**
Assistant Professor
School of Nursing
Indiana University
Indianapolis, Indiana

Carol F. Durham, EdD, RN, ANEF
Clinical Professor
Director, Education-Innovation-
    Simulation Learning Environment
School of Nursing
University of North Carolina at Chapel
    Hill
Chapel Hill, North Carolina

Katherine Foss, MSN, RN
Clinical Placement Coordinator
University of Colorado College of
    Nursing
University of Colorado Hospital
Aurora, Colorado

Betsy Frank, PhD, RN, ANEF
Professor Emerita
College of Nursing, Health, and Human
    Services
Indiana State University
Terre Haute, Indiana

**Kathleen B. Gaberson, PhD, RN,
    CNOR, CNE, ANEF**
Owner and Nursing Education
    Consultant
OWK Consulting
Pittsburgh, Pennsylvania

Debra Hagler, PhD, RN, ACNS-BC,
CNE, CHSE, ANEF, FAAN
Clinical Professor
College of Nursing and Health
    Innovation
Arizona State University
Phoenix, Arizona

Pamela R. Jeffries, PhD, RN, ANEF,
FAAN
Professor and Associate Dean for
    Academic Affairs
School of Nursing
Johns Hopkins University
Baltimore, Maryland

Sarah B. Keating, EdD, RN, FAAN
Endowed Professor
Orvis School of Nursing
University of Nevada Reno
Reno, Nevada

Brenda C. Morris, EdD, RN, CNE
Associate Dean for Academics
Clinical Associate Professor
College of Nursing and Health
    Innovation
Arizona State University
Phoenix, Arizona

Marilyn H. Oermann, PhD, RN, ANEF,
FAAN
Professor and Director of Evaluation and
    Educational Research
Duke University School of Nursing
Durham, North Carolina

Carol O'Neil, PhD, RN, CNE
Associate Professor
Co-Director of Institute for Educators in
    Nursing and Health Professions
School of Nursing
University of Maryland
Baltimore, Maryland

Amy C. Pettigrew, PhD, RN, CNE,
ANEF
Dean, Benjamín León School of Nursing
Medical Campus
Miami Dade College
Miami, Florida

Gayle Preheim, EdD, RN, CENP, CNE
Professor and Director of Baccalaureate
    Nursing Program
College of Nursing
University of Colorado
Aurora, Colorado

Andrea Parsons Schram, DNP, CRNP,
FNP-BC
Assistant Professor
School of Nursing
Johns Hopkins University
Baltimore, Maryland

Kathy Tally, MS
Director of Instructional Systems
    Design
Saint Luke's College of Health
    Sciences
Kansas City, Missouri

Lisa K. Woodley, MSN, RN
Clinical Assistant Professor
School of Nursing
University of North Carolina at Chapel
    Hill
Chapel Hill, North Carolina

Preface

There is a critical need to prepare nurses for roles as educators in schools of nursing and health care settings. This book was written to meet that need: it is a comprehensive text that provides, under one cover, essential concepts for effective teaching in nursing and carrying out other dimensions of the educator role. The book examines the role of a faculty member in a school of nursing and nurse educator in other settings; theories of learning; teaching methods, including integrating technology in teaching; teaching in online environments, simulation, learning laboratories, and clinical settings; and developing partnerships with clinical agencies. Nurse educators also need to assess learning and performance, and for this reason the book includes chapters on assessment, testing, and clinical evaluation. Teachers in nursing should understand the curriculum and how it is developed and evaluated, also explained in this book. It is important in nursing education that teachers use evidence to guide their educational practices and develop their scholarship; those areas are addressed in the last section of the book. Chapters are written by leading experts who integrate research findings and other evidence in their chapters.

The book was written for students in master's, DNP, and PhD nursing programs who are preparing themselves for a teaching role; nurses in clinical settings who are transitioning into nurse educator roles or are teaching students in addition to their practice positions; students and nurses learning about nursing education through continuing education and certificate programs; and novice and experienced teachers who want to expand their knowledge about teaching and gain new ideas for their courses. If students are taking only one or two nursing education courses in their graduate program, this book will be of particular value because of its comprehensiveness. One of the goals was to prepare a scholarly book on teaching in nursing that is also practical, and the chapters are written with that goal in mind.

Nurse educators are employed in academic institutions and a variety of health care agencies. They educate nursing students at all levels, and in health care agencies they are responsible for providing nurses and other health care professionals' continuing education and training. Chapter 1 discusses trends supporting careers in nursing education, educational preparation for employment as a faculty member in a school of nursing, and preparation for educator roles in service settings. Competencies and responsibilities of the nurse educator, transition to the educator role, balancing roles, and faculty development are examined in the chapter.

Understanding how students learn is essential to effective teaching. It is also important for the nurse educator to recognize that no two students will have the same background, previous experiences, and preferences for teaching methods, and these differences have a potential effect on their learning. Chapter 2 examines theories of learning;

the diverse learning needs of students, including culture and ethnicity, learning styles, and other characteristics; motivation to learn; and teacher–student relationships.

The most important question to ask about any teaching method is whether it is a good fit for the specific learning objectives, learners, teachers, and available resources. Chapter 3 describes a variety of teaching methods and offers guidance in selecting methods to fit the intended outcomes, learner characteristics, and available resources. Teaching methods are considered in relation to supporting learner development in the cognitive, affective, and psychomotor learning domains. Strategies are described for incorporating active learning and for promoting critical thinking.

The rapid advances and constant pace of change in technology create challenges and opportunities for teaching and learning. Successful integration of technology in the nursing curriculum requires a paradigm shift and new competencies for the teacher as the technology continues to evolve. Chapter 4 focuses on technology integration that supports achievement of learning outcomes with attention to curriculum and classroom alignment. The chapter guides nurse educators in exploring and embracing technology tools that support good teaching practices.

Traditionally, simulations have been used to provide opportunities for students to practice patient care in a "'safe'" environment before going into the clinical setting. However, in the current environment of increasing patient acuity and limited clinical placements, simulation may serve a broader role as an adjunct or replacement for traditional clinical experiences. Chapter 5 provides an overview of types of clinical simulations in nursing and how to integrate them into a nursing curriculum. Debriefing approaches, evaluation processes to use when developing and implementing clinical simulations, and evidence on the use of clinical simulations are discussed in this chapter.

Teaching online is not the same as teaching in a classroom. Chapter 6 focuses on the differences between teaching in the traditional classroom and teaching online. The roles of the facilitator and the student are discussed in relation to pedagogy, course content, teaching strategies, reconceptualizing and designing online learning environments, interacting online, and using technology to teach and learn.

Skills acquisition is an important component of nursing education, beginning early in the curriculum and continuing throughout the nursing program. Learning laboratories provide a safe environment for initial psychomotor skills acquisition while offering opportunities to socialize students into the professional role of a nurse. Chapter 7 examines phases of skill development, deliberate practice, and development of professional confidence; roles of the teacher, staff, mentors, and others in the learning laboratory; expectations for learners; types of learning laboratories and their integration into the curriculum; competency evaluations; and other important topics. The chapter is comprehensive and also describes laboratory organization and management.

The clinical teacher plays a pivotal role in shaping the learning for nursing students in the clinical setting. Because of this, it is essential that clinical teachers exhibit effective teaching behaviors, use best practices in teaching nursing, and inspire students. Chapter 8 explains why effective clinical teaching is so critical and the process of clinical teaching. Specific teaching strategies, such as how to create a learning climate that is inviting and supportive to students, how to foster effective relationships in the clinical setting, how to design an effective and inspirational clinical orientation, and how to choose the best patient assignments for students are discussed.

Academic-practice partnerships exist at several levels for the purpose of preparing the nursing workforce to meet nursing practice realities and contemporary health care challenges. Chapter 9 provides guidelines for establishing and sustaining meaningful partnerships between education and practice to stimulate collaborative models of clinical nursing education. Nurse educator roles and responsibilities are explored. Specific examples are provided to illustrate concepts and strategies to improve the educational preparation of nurses and ultimately the quality and safety of patient care.

Through the process of assessment, the teacher collects information about student learning and performance. With this information, the teacher can determine further learning needs, plan learning activities to meet those needs, and confirm the outcomes and competencies met by the students. Chapter 10 explains assessment, evaluation, and grading in nursing education. Methods are described for assessing learning, and examples are provided of many of these methods.

Tests are a common assessment method used in nursing education, and varied types of test items are described in Chapter 11. A test must produce relevant and consistent results to form the basis for sound inferences about what learners know and can do. Good planning, careful test construction, proper administration, accurate scoring, and sound interpretation of scores are essential for producing useful test results. This chapter describes the process of planning, constructing, administering, scoring, and analyzing tests. Various types of test items are presented with examples of each item.

As students learn about nursing, they develop their knowledge base, higher level thinking skills, and a wide range of practice competencies essential for patient care. Learning concepts in a classroom or an online environment is not sufficient: students need to apply those concepts and other knowledge to clinical situations and be proficient in carrying out care. Teachers guide student learning in the clinical setting and evaluate their performance in practice. Chapter 12 describes the clinical evaluation process, the importance of giving prompt and specific feedback to students as they are learning, principles that are important when observing and rating performance, and grading clinical practice.

It is vital that nurse educators take into account the context in which teaching takes place. Often, both new and experienced teachers focus on the specific content of the classes or sessions they teach and lose sight of the objectives and how they relate to the overall program. Chapter 13 describes the processes for curriculum development or revision for schools of nursing and for educational programs in health care settings. The chapter reviews the factors that influence educational programs and curricula and provides guidelines for collecting and analyzing data to make informed decisions about revising or developing curricula.

Evaluation provides decision makers with information about the institution's or program's aims, purpose, and goals and how well it is functioning in relation to these intentions. Chapter 14 focuses on various theories and theoretical frameworks that underpin program evaluation efforts and discusses evaluation models and their use in approaching evaluation systematically. The chapter also examines research methodologies for generating useful evaluative information, especially within the context of nursing programs, connections between accountability and accreditation, and approaches to developing and implementing program evaluation meaningful to nursing programs.

Evidence-based teaching is the use of research findings and other evidence to guide educational decisions and practices. Available evidence should be used when developing the curriculum and courses, selecting teaching methods and approaches to use with students, planning clinical learning activities, and assessing students' learning and performance. Chapter 15 describes evidence-based teaching in nursing, the need for better research in nursing education, and a process for engaging in evidence-based teaching.

The role of the nurse educator includes more than teaching, assessing learning, and developing courses: it also includes scholarship and contributing to the development of nursing education as a science. Scholars in nursing education question and search for new ideas; they debate and think beyond how it has always been done. For the teacher's work to be considered as scholarship, it needs to be public, peer-reviewed and critiqued, and shared with others so they can build on that work. The last chapter in the book, Chapter 16, examines scholarship in nursing education and developing one's role as a scholar. Because of the importance of dissemination to scholarship, the chapter includes a description of the process of writing for publication and other strategies for dissemination. Assessment of teaching, by students and peers, and the scholarship of teaching also are discussed, including development of a teaching portfolio to document teaching excellence and scholarship. This chapter builds on the first chapter, which examines career development as a nurse educator.

In addition to this book, I have provided an *Instructor's Manual* that includes a sample course syllabus; chapter-based PowerPoint presentations; and materials for an online course (with chapter summaries, student learning activities, discussion questions, online resources, and assessment strategies). **To obtain your electronic copy of these materials, faculty should contact Springer Publishing Company at textbook@springerpub.com**. Margaret Zuccarini, my editor at Springer, deserves a special acknowledgment for her continued support and enthusiasm and for asking me to write this book. I also thank Springer Publishing Company for its support of nursing education and for publishing my books for many years.

Marilyn H. Oermann

1

The Process of Becoming a Nurse Educator

BETSY FRANK

Several recent reports have highlighted the need for more nurse educators. Nurse educators are found in academic institutions and in a variety of health care agencies. They educate nursing students at all levels, from certified nursing assistants to doctorally prepared current and future nurse educators, clinicians, and researchers. Staff educators in health care agencies are responsible for providing nurses and other health care professionals continuing education and training.

TRENDS SUPPORTING CAREERS IN NURSING EDUCATION

Although the nursing shortage has abated somewhat because of economic trends that led to older nurses staying longer in the workforce, a nursing shortage is expected in the long run. According to Buerhaus and others, by 2025 at least 260,000 more registered nurses (RNs) will be needed in the United States (Buerhaus, Auerbach, & Staiger, 2009). Though the number of nurses under age 30 has increased due to an upsurge in persons choosing careers in nursing, a 2013 report from the Health Resources and Services Administration (HRSA) has stated that one-third of nurses are over the age of 50. Furthermore, health care reform, as enacted through the Patient Protection and Affordable Care Act, will increase the demand for all health care services.

Despite an increase in nurses who have passed the National Council Licensure Examination for Registered Nurses (NCLEX-RN®) since 2011 (HRSA, 2013), greater demand for health care will require even more nurses to deliver those needed services. As a result, more faculty in academic and service settings will be needed to educate nursing personnel to fulfill current and future roles within the health care system.

Aside from the fact that more nurses will be needed, the nursing faculty workforce is aging and will need replacing. A 2007 report by the Robert Wood Johnson Foundation (RWJF) reported that 63% of nursing faculty were over the age of 45, with 9% over 61. The National League for Nursing's (NLN) data have also reinforced the aging faculty trend. A recent survey from the NLN has shown that 93% of full-time educators are over the age of 45 (NLN, 2010). Not only are nursing faculty aging, but an overall nursing faculty shortage exists. In 2012, the American Association of Colleges of Nursing (AACN) reported that 1,181 faculty positions were vacant in colleges and universities offering baccalaureate and graduate degrees in nursing.

Academic nurse educators (ANEs) are not the only educators needed to meet the needs of the health care delivery system. Clinical educators in the service setting are also vital. A rapidly changing health care delivery system requires those in the workforce to keep abreast of changing standards of practice, skill competency, and regulatory requirements. Educators in health care agencies play a key role in helping nursing and other staff members in keeping up to date in their job requirements.

As one can see, prospects of long-term employment for nurse educators across all education and service settings are excellent. By choosing a career as a nurse educator, one has the opportunity to be a role model, coach, and mentor for the current and next generation of nurses (Yoder-Wise & Kowalski, 2012).

ROLE PREPARATION

EDUCATIONAL PREPARATION FOR ACADEMIC EMPLOYMENT

Nursing education occurs across the spectrum of educational settings. In the United States, preparation for the NCLEX-RN occurs in community colleges at the associate degree level, the diploma level in hospital schools of nursing, and in colleges and universities that award bachelor's, master's, and doctoral degrees. The RNs from these programs work across a range of health care institutions. Increasingly, however, health care agencies are requiring their staff to be baccalaureate prepared or working on a baccalaureate degree. The requirement for a baccalaureate degree is found particularly in job descriptions at Magnet® hospitals (Perez-Pena, 2012). In fact, a recent report sponsored by the RWJF (2011) has called for 80% of the nursing workforce to be prepared at the baccalaureate degree level or higher by the year 2020.

Most Practical Nursing programs and some Certified Nursing Assistant programs also take place in community college settings. Many of these occur in career ladder education programs leading to an associate degree in nursing.

Academic credentials for nurse educators employed in postsecondary institutions are set by state Boards of Nursing and accreditation agencies. For example, the Collegiate Commission on Nursing Education (CCNE), an agency that accredits baccalaureate and higher degree programs, requires faculty have a graduate degree (CCNE, 2009). The National League for Nursing Accrediting Commission (NLNAC; now called the Accreditation Commission for Education in Nursing) criteria for baccalaureate programs state that full- and part-time faculty must have a graduate degree in nursing, with 25% of full-time faculty holding doctoral degrees or enrolled in doctoral programs (NLNAC, 2013b). For master's programs, the NLNAC requires both full- and part-time faculty have at a minimum a graduate degree and appropriate expertise and certification. Furthermore, 50% of all full- and part-time faculty must have a doctoral degree or be enrolled in a doctoral program (NLNAC, 2013e). For Clinical Doctorate programs, 75% of all faculty must have a doctorate or be enrolled in a doctoral program (NLNAC, 2013c).

The NLNAC also accredits associate degree, diploma, and practical nursing programs. Accreditation criteria for both associate and diploma programs require full-time faculty to have a graduate degree in nursing, and 50% of the part-time faculty must hold a graduate degree in nursing (NLNAC, 2013a, 2013d). Each practical nursing program must have 50% of its faculty prepared at the master's level in nursing (NLNAC, 2013f).

Graduate programs in nursing often have nurse educator tracks based on the NLN's *The Scope of Practice for Academic Nurse Educators* (National League for Nursing Certification Commission Certification Test Development Committee, 2012). Nurse educator tracks include theoretical content related to nursing education, as well as a practice teaching practicum. These tracks are found in master's and Doctorate of Nursing

Practice (DNP) programs. At the Doctor of Philosophy (PhD) level, role development may include educator tracks as well, with a research focus in the science of nursing education. Many PhD programs, however, focus on clinical and nursing systems research. Graduates from PhD programs often have career goals that include teaching in prelicensure and graduate nursing programs, as well as becoming nurse researchers in academic or health care agencies.

Given the recommendation for a primarily baccalaureate-prepared nursing workforce, more nurse educators will need to be prepared at the doctoral level to meet the educational needs of future nurses. A master's degree with a major in nursing education could be considered a stepping stone for future doctoral study.

The educational path one chooses depends on the type of nursing program in which one wishes to teach. Colleges and universities have specific degree requirements for employment. For example, some universities require a terminal degree (doctorate) for tenure track positions or positions with some guarantee of permanency, provided certain requirements are met. For universities with a Carnegie Classification of Very High Research Activity (Carnegie Foundation for the Advancement of Teaching, n.d.), a PhD is required for a tenure track position. However, such universities may have clinical tracks, which have different requirements for tenure, yearly, or multiyear contracts. These appointments in Very High Research Activity universities are for faculty who wish to teach and focus their scholarship on teaching, practice, and community engagement. Full-time clinical appointments may also require a PhD, DNP, or a master's degree in nursing. Universities that do not have high research missions may have tenure track appointments that require only a master's degree. However, these appointments are becoming rarer. Full- or part-time clinical teaching appointments, or those teaching appointments that involve clinical supervision of students, will require the master's degree. Community colleges generally do not have tenure track positions. Nevertheless, master's degrees will be required to teach full- and part-time in those settings.

When interviewing for employment in an academic institution, it is important to clarify what the job description is and what the expectations are for role performance (Halstead & Frank, 2011). By clarifying these criteria, one can better match career goals to institutional expectations. For example, if a prospective faculty member has expertise in nursing education research, that person should know whether the institution values this type of research when considering promotion and retention. Table 1.1 summarizes the types of academic appointments and the educational preparation required.

TABLE 1.1 Summary of Educational Requirements for Nurse Educator Employment

Employment Setting	Education Required
Hospitals and other health care agencies	BSN or MSN
Community colleges: Practical Nursing and CNA programs	BSN or MSN
Community colleges: Associate degree programs	MSN
Colleges and universities: Baccalaureate and Master's programs	MSN with doctorate preferred
Colleges and universities: Doctoral programs	Doctorate

BSN, bachelor's of science in nursing; CNA, certified nursing assistant; MSN, master's of science in nursing.

EDUCATIONAL PREPARATION FOR EMPLOYMENT IN SERVICE SETTINGS

Some staff educator positions in service settings may require less than a master's degree. However, having a master's degree in nursing education, or a clinically focused master's degree with elective courses in nursing education, will enhance one's ability to carry out the responsibilities of the job. Clinical educators have a wide range of responsibilities, which require knowledge and skills related to the principles of adult education.

NURSE EDUCATOR COMPETENCIES

In 2005, the NLN published *The Scope and Practice for Academic Nurse Educators*. This document has served as the guiding force in setting the expectations for the NLN certification as an ANE (NLN, 2012), and it has been published in a revised edition in 2012. Although the competencies have been directed at ANEs, educators in service settings have similar competency expectations (Bradley & Benedict, 2010).

The NLN competencies are as follows:

- Facilitate learning
- Facilitate learner development and socialization
- Use assessment and evaluation strategies
- Participate in curriculum design and evaluation of programs
- Function as a change agent and leader
- Pursue continuous quality improvement in the nurse educator role
- Engage in scholarship
- Function within the educational environment (NLN, 2012, pp. 14–22)

RESPONSIBILITIES OF NURSE EDUCATORS

ACADEMIC NURSE EDUCATORS

Responsibilities of nurse educators differ according to institutional type and whether one teaches primarily at the prelicensure or graduate level. Prior to deciding on a career in nursing education, job shadowing a nurse educator can provide a realistic picture of the demands of the role (Culleiton & Shellenbarger, 2007).

Academic institutions require faculty to teach, have some form of scholarly activity, and perform service to the institution and the profession. How one's overall duties are allotted depends on the institutional type. Those who are employed in community colleges will spend most of their time teaching in the classroom, laboratories, and clinical area, with some time allotted for service and scholarship. Those who teach in undergraduate and graduate programs in colleges and universities will also teach, but will have greater expectations for scholarly productivity, including supporting research through funded grants.

When considering employment in an academic setting, one should be clear about the job expectations. Is the position tenure track, or with a renewable yearly or multi-year contract? If the position is part-time and involves only clinical teaching, how much grading of assignments is involved, and is the grading time paid for? If the position is full-time, but on the clinical track, what kind of scholarship is expected? In some academic institutions, those on the clinical track have opportunities for promotion and tenure, but teaching loads are generally higher than for those on the regular tenure track, and the nature of scholarship expected might be different (Lee, Kim, Young, Shin, & Kim, 2007).

Teaching Responsibilities

Teaching involves more than transmitting knowledge through lectures and supervising students in clinical practice. Faculty must have evidence-based knowledge of student learning styles, methods of content delivery, and methods for evaluating student learning. Facilitating students' assimilation of theory into practice is key. In fact, Benner, Sutphen, Leonard, and Day (2010) have advocated a closer integration of the clinical and classroom components of a student's education to promote effective clinical decision making. Some nursing education programs employ full-time clinical faculty, whose primary role is supervision in the clinical laboratory, hospitals, and other health care settings. All full- and part-time clinical faculty teaching in the classroom, online, and in the clinical area need to have intimate knowledge of the curriculum and expected learning outcomes. This knowledge helps them facilitate the students' integration of theory with clinical practice. Sometimes, as previously noted, full-time clinical faculty have responsibilities similar to those of regular tenure-track faculty, with some modification in the type of scholarship required for promotion and retention (Lee et al., 2007).

Aside from the actual classroom, online, and clinical teaching, faculty also have the responsibility of formulating the curriculum that not only meets contemporary standards of practice, but also prepares students for future nursing roles. Curriculum is not static, but constantly needs revision to meet changing licensure examination expectations, societal changes, and changes in the health care delivery system. For example, the RWJF *Future of Nursing* report has recommended expanded roles for nurses in the health care system (RWJF, 2011). This recommendation will, no doubt, necessitate curriculum revision at both the undergraduate and graduate levels. Participation in the curriculum revision process requires faculty to function as change agents and leaders in order to enact the needed revisions (Tartavoulle, Manning, & Fowler, 2011). Providing leadership and promoting curriculum change involves ensuring the curriculum is based on the most current educational standards and competencies including those delineated by the Quality and Safety Education for Nurses (QSEN) project. Based on the Institute of Medicine (IOM; 2003) report, these competencies are:

- Patient-centered care
- Teamwork and collaboration
- Evidence-based practice
- Quality improvement
- Safety
- Informatics (QSEN, n.d.)

Committee work will be essential to the process, including leading taskforces within the nursing program and perhaps in the larger institution in order to shepherd the revised curriculum through the approval process.

Scholarship Responsibilities

Halstead and Frank (2011) have pointed out that all teachers are scholars. In fact, the various accreditation criteria have expectations for scholarship for faculty at all levels of nursing education. These expectations include teachers at all levels of postsecondary education and in service settings. For example, the NLNAC accreditation criteria for associate degree programs states that "faculty (full- and part-time) maintain expertise in their areas of responsibility, and their performance reflects scholarship and evidence-based teaching and clinical practices" (NLNAC, 2013a, p. 86).

Scholarship is more than only traditional research, presenting at professional conferences, and publishing in academic journals. Obtaining grant funding for research has also been included in the traditional definition. Scholarship, however, is also a "spirit of inquiry" to find support for the practice of teaching (Halstead & Frank, 2011, p. 122). A spirit of inquiry involves the ability to search the literature for evidence, and working with colleagues to understand their practices in the classroom, online, and in clinical settings.

This view of scholarship grows out of Boyer's 1990 seminal work, *Scholarship Reconsidered: Priorities of the Professoriate,* which broadened the definition of scholarship. The original work included the scholarship of teaching, discovery, application, and integration. In 1996, Boyer added the scholarship of engagement, which for nurse educators could include clinical practice. The AACN (1999) has outlined definitions of categories of scholarship based on the Boyer model. Table 1.2 lists the forms of scholarship and their definitions, based on the AACN definitions, and specific examples of each form of scholarship.

TABLE 1.2 Summary of Boyer's Categories of Scholarship as Adapted for Nursing by the American Association of Colleges of Nursing (1999)

Type of Scholarship	Definition	Evidence
Scholarship of Discovery	Various forms of research including empirical, historical, methodological, and theory development	Grants, peer-reviewed publications, presentations
Scholarship of Teaching	Teaching innovations, program development and evaluation, role modeling	Accreditation reports, peer-reviewed publications, grants, presentations, authoring textbooks
Scholarship of Practice (Application)	Development of clinical knowledge, self-improvement of clinical competency, application of research skills. Includes service to profession and aspects of scholarship of engagement	Consultations, peer reviews of manuscripts, patents, presentations about practice, program grants
Scholarship of Integration	Synthesis and analysis of other's writings. Integrates in new ways and may include knowledge from nonnursing disciplines	Peer-reviewed publications of research, policy papers; books, interdisciplinary efforts

Service Responsibilities

Service responsibilities contribute to the functioning of the organization. No matter the academic setting, all full-time faculty will be expected to participate in nursing program committees and committees of the larger institution. Committees include those concerned with faculty issues; student admission, progression, and retention issues; curriculum development; and program evaluation.

Professional service includes leadership within professional organizations and such activities as reviewing manuscripts for prospective publication. Other forms of professional service may include committee work in service settings or providing consultation for staff nurses who are preparing presentations for professional meetings (Ashton, 2012). Faculty expertise may also be needed to facilitate research in service settings or to assist with quality assurance activities (Halstead & Frank, 2011).

CLINICAL STAFF EDUCATORS

Clinical staff educators also have teaching, scholarship, and service responsibilities. Though typically the curriculum process is thought of as occurring in the academic setting, educators in health care settings must also formulate, implement, and evaluate curriculum. For example, clinical educators in the service setting design and evaluate nurse residency and orientation programs, as well as programs for the purpose of ensuring continuing competency of staff. Knowledge of standards of practice, including the IOM (2003) competencies, is critical for the staff educator. For example, patient-centered care, an IOM (2003) competency, can be promoted through staff development programs (Okougha, 2013). Staff educators also have a crucial role in promoting evidence-based practice in the service setting (Bradley & Benedict, 2010). Moreover, staff educators can promote another IOM (2003) competency, interprofessional collaboration (Gordon et al., 2013; Slater, Lawton, Armitage, Bibby, & Wright, 2012; Turner, 2012).

Staff educators working collaboratively with clinical specialists may function as change agents by advocating for changes in the larger health care delivery system (Bradley & Benedict, 2010; Gerard, 2010). Educators can promote increased access to health care through their community and professional service efforts, such as volunteering in a free clinic or taking a leadership role in a professional organization.

In addition to having job responsibilities in the service setting, some clinical educators might also function as part-time clinical faculty in nursing programs. In serving as part-time faculty, clinical educators have an important role in developing future nursing professionals (Adelman-Mullally et al., 2013).

Although much scholarship takes place in academic settings, staff educators also participate in and facilitate scholarship activities. According to the American Nurses Credentialing Center (2008), Magnet Hospitals have the obligation to create new knowledge through practice innovations, evidence-based practice, and quality improvement. Staff educators play a key role in creating programs that help staff nurses engage in these important ventures. Exhibit 1.1 suggests some questions related to all aspects of role performance when considering full- or part-time employment as a nurse educator in service and academe.

**EXHIBIT 1.1 Questions to Consider Prior to Seeking Employment
as a Nurse Educator**

1. Do I want to work in an academic environment or service setting?
2. What are the academic credentials needed for employment?
3. What kind of flexibility do I want and need in setting my work hours?
4. Do I want to work full- or part-time in an academic or service setting?
5. Do I want to combine academic and service setting responsibilities?
6. In my career do I want to spend the majority of my time teaching or combining research and teaching?
7. What service activities are expected?
8. If I seek employment in an academic setting, what level of students do I wish to teach?
9. If I work in an academic setting, do I wish to maintain some practice as a staff nurse, nurse practitioner, or clinical specialist?

TRANSITION TO THE EDUCATOR ROLE

Clinicians who transition to the clinical role go through stages similar to the novice-to-expert trajectory that Benner (1984) described for those in clinical roles (Ramsburg & Childress, 2012). Moreover, Schoening (2013) found clinicians go through four phases, which are: anticipation/expectation, disorientation, information seeking, and identity formation. According to Schoening's Nurse Educator Transition model, successful transition results in "feeling and thinking like a teacher" (p. 170).

As novice nurse educators transition into the educator role, not only must they learn skills related to classroom and clinical teaching, but they must also learn how to function within an academic setting, be it a staff development office or a community college or university. Included in this transition is learning how to balance the requirements of the job. The nurse educator in academic settings typically does not function on a day-to-day basis within a particular work shift such as 7 a.m. to 7 p.m., even if the educator is in a staff development role. Planning for class presentations and grading may take place outside of the formal work setting. If one is transitioning to an ANE role, balancing teaching, scholarship, and service expectations may cause role stress if the scholarship expectations are much higher than what was required when employed in the service setting.

Although staff educators who have been full-time clinicians have no doubt become familiar with a health care agency's culture and role expectations, becoming socialized to higher education presents additional challenges. As previously noted, expectations vary by academic environment. Furthermore, understanding institutional culture is an important factor in acclimating to the values and norms of the academic setting. These cultural values and norms, then, get incorporated into a new role identity (Anderson, 2009). Academic preparation for the educator role and having a good mentor can ease the transition process (Duphily, 2011).

Good communication skills are important for adjustment. For example, a clinical nurse educator in a school of nursing must communicate with nursing staff to make appropriate clinical assignments for students (Mitchell & King-Jones, 2012). Committee work in the academic and service setting requires good communication skills to facilitate effective committee functioning.

Orientation to a role can also ease the transition from clinician to educator (Gilbert & Womack, 2012). Orientation is critical for all educator roles, but particularly for the part-time clinical educator role in a school of nursing. This educator can feel isolated from the larger academic program. Therefore, knowing expectations and how the clinical practice fits into the curriculum can ease feelings of isolation. Orientation should include not only information on the overall curriculum, but also clinical teaching expectations, including the nature of clinical assignments and how to evaluate student performance (Hewitt & Lewallen, 2010). Full-time faculty will need orientation to the academic environment, including the curriculum and information regarding the university's promotion, retention, and tenure criteria (Clark, Alcala-Van Houten, & Perea-Ryan, 2010).

BALANCING ROLE RESPONSIBILITIES

Part of the transition to becoming a nurse educator is balancing all dimensions of the role. Whereas the staff educator has some autonomy in how to organize responsibilities, the educator in a health care agency will generally have more regular work hours as compared to the educator in academe. Aside from assigned class and clinical times and posted office hours, most academic educators can decide when and where work is done. Those with caregiving responsibilities are free to prepare classes and do some scholarship activities from home. Some faculty might prefer, however, to keep work and family time separate (Poronsky, Doering, Mkandawire-Valmu, & Rice, 2012).

Clinical instruction is essential for a practice profession (Dahlke, Baumbusch, Affleck, & Kown, 2012), and faculty members need to be clinically competent if their clinical education is to be effective. Faculty who need to maintain some clinical practice to maintain specialty certification have special challenges. Beck and Ruth-Sahd (2013) found that faculty want to remain clinically competent to enhance their teaching. Therefore, finding a dedicated time for clinical practice is one way to maintain clinical competence. This dedicated time could occur during the academic year or in the summer, if faculty are not on 12-month contracts. Based on their research, Beck and Ruth-Sahd (2013) have advocated including clinical practice within the Boyer (1990) model of scholarship. They have also recommended the inclusion of clinical practice, in some way, in tenure and promotion criteria.

On the other hand, some faculty members may wish or need to focus more of their time on research (Roberts & Glod, 2013). If faculty focus more on research, their teaching could become divorced from the realities of clinical practice, unless they find other ways to keep abreast of current practice. Working with clinical partners in research efforts or on health care agency committees are ways to keep clinically grounded.

FACULTY DEVELOPMENT

Transition to the nurse educator role doesn't end with orientation. All full- and part-time faculty in the academic setting, and staff educators in health care agencies, need continuing education to maintain competency. Although continuing education related to one's clinical specialty is important, so too is continuing education related to the educator competencies. For example, the NLN and AACN hold meetings for faculty development. Health care agency staff educators can attend the Association for Nursing Professional Development annual convention. Like any specialty, nursing education changes with regard to expectations for role performance and standards of practice. Attending professional meetings helps one to stay abreast of new trends and best practices. A list of websites of selected professional organizations that offer continuing education for educators is found in Table 1.3.

TABLE 1.3 Websites of Interest for Nurse Educators

Name of Organization	Mission of Organization Stated on Website	Web Address
National League for Nursing (NLN)	"The National League for Nursing promotes excellence in nursing education to build a strong and diverse nursing workforce to advance the nation's health."	www.nln.org
American Association of Colleges of Nursing (AACN)	"The American Association of Colleges of Nursing (AACN), a unique asset for the nation, serves the public interest by setting standards, providing resources, and developing the leadership capacity of member schools to advance nursing education, research, and practice."	www.aacn.nche.edu
National Association for Associate Degree Nursing (NOADN)	"The National Organization for Associate Degree Nursing promotes Associate Degree Nursing through collaboration, advocacy, and education to ensure excellence in the future of health care and professional nursing practice."	www.noadn.org
Association for Nursing Professional Development (ANPD)	"The Association for Nursing Professional Development (ANPD) advances the specialty practice of nursing professional development for the enhancement of health care outcomes. Professional development as a specialty of nursing practice is defined by standards, based on research, and critical to quality patient and organizational outcomes."	anpd.site-ym.com/?page=about
Accreditation Commission for Education in Nursing (ACEN)	The Accreditation Commission for Education in Nursing (ACEN), formerly the National League for Nursing Accrediting Commission (NLNAC), is responsible for the specialized accreditation of nursing education programs (Clinical Doctorate, Master's, Baccalaureate, Associate, Diploma, and Practical programs).	http://acenursing.org
Commission on Collegiate Nursing Education (CCNE)	"The Commission on Collegiate Nursing Education (CCNE) is an autonomous accrediting agency, contributing to the improvement of the public's health. The Commission ensures the quality and integrity of baccalaureate, graduate, and residency programs in nursing."	http://www.aacn.nche.edu/ccne-accreditation/about/mission-values-history

SUMMARY

Choosing a career as a nurse educator provides many rewards and presents a few obstacles. One thing that is certain is that nurse educators in academic and service settings can have a profound influence on how the current and next generation of nurses function within the health care system. Staff educators promote continuing professional development (Ashton, 2012). Through their research, ANEs advance the science of nursing education. In partnership with practitioners, their clinical research improves patient care and strengthens the connection between education, practice, and research. Moreover, no matter the setting, all nurse educators function as change agents and leaders (Adelman-Mullally et al., 2013).

Rewards always come with a few stumbling blocks. Balancing one's responsibilities is a challenge. Transitioning to a new role is always stressful and has been described by some as "dancing as fast as I can" (Duphily, 2011, p. 126). Included in this balancing act is the ability to give attention to one's personal life. Flexible work hours can enhance the ability to use good time management skills to accomplish all that is expected. Furthermore, the adjustment to new responsibilities is enhanced with good mentors (NLN, 2006). One particular challenge for those in schools of nursing, however, is salary levels (MacDonald, 2010). Often nurses in practice have higher salaries (AACN, 2012). Although salaries might reflect working 9 or 10 months during the academic year, faculty often work uncompensated over the summers on their scholarly activities and class preparation. Some faculty, however, may use summers to keep current in their clinical skills and earn extra income.

Finally, making decisions regarding further education can also be daunting. If one's career choice is to teach full-time in a baccalaureate and higher degree program, a doctorate will more than likely be required for promotion, tenure, and retention. The type of doctorate chosen, research (PhD) or practice (DNP), depends on one's career goals, the type of scholarly trajectory desired, and the type of doctorate accepted for the tenure track. Nurse educators prepared at the DNP level are uniquely equipped to make the connection between education and practice through their clinical skills and programs of applied research, which translate research into practice (Bellini, McCauley, & Cusson, 2012; Danzey et al., 2011). These educators have strong clinical skills, which can be used to teach at the prelicensure level and in graduate programs that prepare advanced practice nurses. Those prepared at the PhD level may have more skills in generating new knowledge through more traditional forms of research. Such nurse faculty may teach at the undergraduate level as well, but they are often found teaching in graduate programs that focus on developing advanced research skills.

The nurse educator role is most certainly complex. Each succeeding chapter in this book presents an in-depth discussion of the specific role competencies that are necessary for functioning as a nurse educator across many settings. Understanding all the dimensions of the role will foster the all-important transition from clinician to nurse educator.

REFERENCES

Adelman-Mullally, T., Mulder, C. K., McCarter-Spalding, D. E., Hagler, D. A., Gaberson, K. B., Hanner, M. B., … Young, P. K. (2013). The clinical nurse educator as leader. *Nurse Education in Practice, 13*, 29–34. doi:http://dx.doi.org/10.1016/j.nepr.2012.07.006

American Association of Colleges of Nursing. (1999). *Defining scholarship for the discipline of Nursing.* Retrieved from http://www.aacn.nche.edu/publications/position/defining-Scholarship

American Association of Colleges of Nursing. (2012). *Nursing faculty shortage* [Fact sheet]. Retrieved from http://www.aacn.nche.edu/media-relations/fact-sheets/nursing-faculty-shortage

American Nurses Credentialing Center. (2008). *A new model for ANCC's Magnet recognition program.* Retrieved from http://www.nursecredentialing.org/Documents/Magnet/NewModel Brochure.pdf

Anderson, J. K. (2009). The work-role transition of expert clinician to novice academic educator. *Journal of Nursing Education, 46,* 203–208.

Ashton, K. S. (2012). Nurse educators and the future of nursing. *The Journal of Continuing Education in Nursing, 43,* 113–116. doi:10.3928/00220124-20120116-02

Beck, J., & Ruth-Sahd, L. (2013). The lived experience of seeking tenure while practicing clinically. *Dimensions of Critical Care Nursing, 32,* 37–45. doi:10.1097/DCC.0b013e31826bc6e9

Bellini, S., McCauley, P., & Cusson, R. M. (2012). The Doctor of Nursing Practice graduate as faculty member. *Nursing Clinics of North America, 47,* 547–556. doi:http://dx.doi.org/10.1016/j.cnur.2012.07.004

Benner, P. (1984). *From novice to expert: Excellence and power in clinical nursing practice.* Menlo Park, CA: Addison-Wesley.

Benner, P., Sutphen, M., Leonard, V., & Day, L. (2010). *Educating nurses: A call for radical transformation.* San Francisco, CA: Jossey-Bass.

Boyer, E. (1990). *Scholarship reconsidered: Priorities of the professoriate.* Princeton, NJ: The Carnegie Foundation for the Advancement of Teaching.

Boyer, E. L. (1996). The scholarship of engagement. *Journal of Public Service and Outreach, 1*(1), 11–20.

Bradley, D., & Benedict, M. B. (2010). *The ANA professional nursing development scope and standards, 2009: A continuing education perspective.* Retrieved from http://www.medscape.com/viewarticle/715465

Buerhaus, P. I., Auerbach, D. I., & Staiger, D. O. (2009). The recent surge in nurse employment: Causes and implications. *Health Affairs, 28,* w657–w658. doi:10.1377/hlthaff.28.4.w657

Carnegie Association for the Advancement of Teaching (n.d.). *Classification description.* Retrieved from http://classifications.carnegiefoundation.org/descriptions/basic.php

Clark, N. J., Alcala-Van Houten, L., & Perea-Ryan, M. (2010). Transitioning from clinical practice to academia: University expectations on the tenure track. *Nurse Educator, 35,* 105–109. doi:10.1097/NNE.0b013e3181d95069

Commission on Collegiate Nursing Education. (2009). *Standards for accreditation of baccalaureate and graduate degree nursing programs.* Retrieved from http://www.aacn.nche.edu/ccne-accreditation/standards-procedures-resources/baccalaureate-graduate/standards

Culleiton, A. L., & Shellenbarger, T. (2007). The transition of a bedside clinician to a nurse educator. *MEDSURG Nursing, 16,* 253–257.

Dahlke, S., Baumbusch, J., Affleck, F., & Kown, J. (2012). The clinical instructor role in nursing education: A structured literature review. *Journal of Nursing Education, 51,* 692–696. doi:10.3928/01484834-20121022-01

Danzey, I. M., Emerson, E., Fitzpatrick, J., Garbutt, S. J., Rafferty, M., & Zychowicz, M. E. (2011). The Doctor of Nursing Practice and nursing education: Highlights, potential, and promise. *Journal of Professional Nursing, 27,* 311–314. doi:10.1016/j.profnurs.2011.06.008

Duphily, N. H. (2011). The experience of novice nurse faculty in an associate degree program. *Teaching and Learning in Nursing, 6,* 124–130. doi:10.1016/j.teln.2011.01.002

Gerard, P. (2010). Reinventing the role of the clinical nurse specialist as practitioner-teacher to transform nursing education. *Clinical Nurse Specialist, 24,* 277–278. doi:10.1097/NUR.0b013e3181fac535

Gilbert, C., & Womack, B. (2012). Successful transition from expert nurse to novice educator? Expert educator: It's about you. *Teaching and Learning in Nursing, 7,* 100–102. doi:10.1016/j.teln.2012.01.004

Gordon, M., Uppal, E., Holt, K., Lythgoe, J., Mitchell, A., & Hollins-Martin, B. (2013). Application of the team objective structured clinical encounter (TOSCE) for continuing professional development amongst postgraduate health professionals. *Journal of Interprofessional Care, 27,* 191–193. doi:10.3109/13561820.2012.725232

Halstead, J. A., & Frank, B. (2011). *Pathways to a nursing education career*. New York, NY: Springer Publishing Company.

Hewitt, P., & Lewallen, L. P. (2010). Ready, set, teach! How to transform the clinical nurse expert into the part-time clinical nurse instructor. *The Journal of Continuing Education in Nursing*, 41, 403–407. doi:10.3928/00220124-20100503-10

Health Resources and Services Administration. (2013). *The U. S. nursing workforce: Trends and supply—Results in brief*. Retrieved from http://bhpr.hrsa.gov/healthworkforce/reports/nursingworkforce/nursingworkforcebrief.pdf

Institute of Medicine. (2003). *Health professions education: A bridge to quality*. Washington, DC: The National Academies Press.

Lee, W., Kim, C. J., Young, S. R., Shin, H., & Kim, M. J. (2007). Clinical track faculty: Merits and issues. *Journal of Professional Nursing*, 23, 5–12. doi:10.1016/j.profnurs.2006.12.003

MacDonald, P. J. (2010). Transitioning from clinical practice to nursing faculty: Lessons learned. *Journal of Nursing Education*, 49, 126–131. doi:10.3928/01484834-20091022-02

Mitchell, A., & King-Jones, M. (2012). Direct care nurses transitioning to clinical faculty. *Nursing*, 42(6), 58–60. doi:10.3928/01484834-20091022-02

National League for Nursing. (2006). *Position statement: Mentoring of nurse faculty*. Retrieved from http://www.nln.org/aboutnln/positionstatements/mentoring_3_21_06.pdf

National League for Nursing. (2010). *NLN nurse educator shortage fact sheet* [Fact sheet]. Retrieved from www.nln.org/governmentaffairs/pdf/nursefacultyshortage.pdf

National League for Nursing Accrediting Commission. (2013a). *NLNAC2013 standards and criteria Associate*. Retrieved from http://nlnac.org/manuals/SC2013_ASSOCIATE.pdf

National League for Nursing Accrediting Commission. (2013b). *NLNAC2013 standards and criteria Baccalaureate*. Retrieved from http://nlnac.org/manuals/SC2013_BACCALAUREATE.pdf

National League for Nursing Accrediting Commission. (2013c). *NLNAC2013 standards and criteria Clinical Doctorate*. Retrieved from http://nlnac.org/manuals/SC2013_DOCTORATE.pdf

National League for Nursing Accrediting Commission. (2013d). *NLNAC2013 standards and criteria Diploma*. Retrieved from http://nlnac.org/manuals/SC2013_DIPLOMA.pdf

National League for Nursing Accrediting Commission. (2013e). *NLNAC2013 standards and criteria Master's/Post-Master's certificate*. Retrieved from http://nlnac.org/manuals/SC2013_MASTERS.pdf

National League for Nursing Accrediting Commission. (2013f). *NLNAC2013 standards and criteria practical*. Retrieved from http://nlnac.org/manuals/SC2013_PRACTICAL.pdf

National League for Nursing Certification Commission Certification Test Development Committee. (2012). *The scope of practice for academic nurse educators: 2012 revision*. New York, NY: National League for Nursing.

Okougha, M. (2013). Promoting patient-centred care through staff development. *Nursing Standard*, 27(34), 42–46.

Perez-Pena, R. (2012). More stringent requirements send nurses back to school. *New York Times*. Retrieved from http://www.nytimes.com/2012/06/24/education/changing-requirements-send-nurses-back-to-school.html?pagewanted=all&_r=0

Poronsky, C. B., Doering, J. J., Mkandawire-Valmu, L., & Rice, E. I. (2012). Transition to the tenure track for nurse faculty with young children: A case study. *Nursing Education Perspectives*, 33, 255–259. doi:http://dx.doi.org/10.5480/1536-5026-33.4.255

QSEN Institute. (n.d.). Pre-licensure KSAs. Retrieved from http://qsen.org/competencies/pre-licensure-ksas

Ramsburg, L., & Childress, R. (2012). An initial investigation of the applicability of the Dreyfus Skill Acquisition Model to the professional development of nurse educators. *Nursing Education Perspectives*, 33, 312–316. doi:http://dx.doi.org/10.5480/1536-5026-33.5.312

Robert Wood Johnson Foundation. (2007). *Charting nursing's future—The nursing faculty shortage: Public and private partnerships address a growing need*. Retrieved from http://www.rwjf.org/content/dam/farm/reports/issue_briefs/2007/rwjf13911

Robert Wood Johnson Foundation. (2011). *Charting nursing's future—Implementing the IOM Future of Nursing Report—Part I*. Retrieved from http://www.rwjf.org/content/dam/farm/reports/issue_briefs/2011/rwjf70968

Roberts, S. J., & Glod, C. (2013). Faculty roles: Dilemmas for the future of nursing education. *Nursing Forum, 48*, 99–105. doi:10.1111/nuf.12018

Schoening, A. M. (2013). From bedside to classroom: The Nurse Educator Transition Model. *Nursing Education Perspectives, 34*, 167–172. doi:http://dx.doi.org/10.5480/1536-5026-34.3.167

Slater, B., Lawton, R., Armitage, G., Bibby, J., & Wright, J. (2012). Training and action for patient safety: Embedding interprofessional education for patient safety within an improvement methodology. *Journal of Continuing Education in the Health Professions, 32*, 80–89. doi:10.1002/chp

Tartavoulle, T., Manning, J., & Fowler, L. (2011). Smoothing the transition from bedside to classroom. *American Nurse Today, 6*(5), 45–46.

Turner, P. (2012). Implementation of TeamSTEPPS in the emergency department. *Critical Care Nursing Quarterly, 35*, 208–212. doi:10.1097/CNQ.0b013e3182542c6c

Yoder-Wise, P. S., & Kowalski, K. E. (2012). *Fast facts for the classroom nursing instructor: Classroom teaching in a nutshell*. New York, NY: Springer Publishing Company.

2

Learning and Students

AMY C. PETTIGREW

Nurse educators play a key role in the teaching and learning process. They must be effective teachers not only in the classroom but also in the nursing skills laboratory, in the simulation center, in the clinical area, and during student advising. Understanding how students learn in each of these settings is paramount to good instruction. It is also important for the nurse educator to understand that no two students have the same cultural heritage, ethnicity, age, social background, previous experience in health care, or preferences for teaching methods, all of which have a potential impact on learning. Like snowflakes, no two students bring identical needs to the classroom or clinical setting. Nurse educators, therefore, need to construct instruction that is based on the best evidence for teaching and learning.

Teaching and learning processes have been used for eons. At first children were taught by their parents how to look after basic needs. The first known writing about teaching and learning dates to 2100 BCE, in the Babylonian Code of Hammurabi, which briefly addressed teaching as an apprenticeship model, where learning was by practical experience (King, n.d.). The Greeks were well-known for using the question and answer method of teaching, primarily recognized as the Socratic Method, which dates back to 300 BCE. (Phillips, 2010). Until relatively recent times, learners were considered empty vessels, and the teacher's job was to fill the empty mind with information.

Over the past 150 years, scientists, lacking today's technology, developed theoretical and conceptual models that represented the learning process. How could they account for learning? The puzzle of short-term memory versus long-term memory was an enigma.

Current neuroscience research has changed forever the theory and practice of education. Now, as at no time in the past, we have the capability to see learning happen in the brain. Through the use of positron emission tomography scans and now via functional magnetic resonance imaging, one can actually see the components of the brain in action as information is processed. From this research has emerged the concept of brain plasticity, the idea that experience can actually change both the brain's anatomy and physiology (Chaney, 2006). Research related to neurotransmitters in the brain also contributes to insight into how to best structure learning processes.

WHAT IS LEARNING?

Learning is a core element of human existence, and teachers are a requisite for much of human learning. The puzzle of explaining how we learn, and therefore how to teach, has been in the forefront of thinking since the middle of the 19th century. Though there are many definitions of learning, the following discussion of learning theories is based on Schunk's definition: "Learning is an enduring change in behavior, or in the capacity to behave in a given fashion, which results from practice or other forms of experience" (Schunk, 2012, p. 3).

THEORIES OF LEARNING

Any model of teaching and learning theories needs to include the teacher, student, personal attributes of each, learning environment, learning content, and teaching strategies (Utley, 2011). Because it has been only in the past 10 years that we have actually seen learning happen in the brain, scientists were left to hypothesize how learning worked, as a means of creating a rationale for an event (learning) that they could not otherwise explain.

The major theories of learning can be categorized as: behaviorism, cognitivism, social cognitivism, humanism, constructivism, and brain-based learning. Early theories were based on direct observation and then elaborated on by further schools of thought. Table 2.1 provides a general overview of the schools of thought.

TABLE 2.1 Major Learning Theories

Schools of Thought	Major Tenets	Major Theorists and Contributors
Behaviorism	Learning is a change in behavior, shaped by an external environment.	Pavlov Skinner Thorndike
Cognitivism	Learning is an internal process.	Bruner Piaget Gagne
Social cognitivism	Role of social processes in addition to internal processes.	Vygotsky
Humanism	People intentionally act based on perceived needs.	Rogers Maslow
Constructivism	Learning is an internal process built on previous learning.	Dewey Piaget Kolb
Brain-based learning	Cognitive neuroscience has identified actual neural processes of learning. Teaching methods should focus on how the brain learns.	Sousa Jensen

Behaviorism

With no method to see inside the brain and watch learning happen, teachers and scientists were left to hypothesize how people learned. Beginning during the second half of the 19th century and continuing into the early 20th century, scientists looked at changing basic behavior. Behavioral theories defined learning as change in the method or frequency of a behavior due to some interaction with the outer environment.

Three well-known scientists, Pavlov, Thorndike, and Skinner, examined learning using a behaviorist perspective. Their work focused on learning as behavior change developed through external conditioning and reinforcement (Schunk, 2012).

Ivan Pavlov (1849–1936) is known for his work with *classical conditioning*, a multistep process that entailed introducing an unconditioned stimulus, which brings about an unconditioned response. For Pavlov, this entailed presenting a dog with meat, which in turn resulted in salivation. While he was training the dog, a metronome would be ticking in the background. Over time, the dog would become conditioned to the metronome and would start to salivate when the metronome ticked. "A stimulus that was neutral in and of itself had been superimposed upon the action of the inborn alimentary reflex" Pavlov wrote of the results. "We observed that, after several repetitions of the combined stimulation, the sounds of the metronome had acquired the property of stimulating salivary secretion" (Pavlov, 1927).

Edward Thorndike (1874–1949) is known for his work that focused on learning, individual differences, intelligence, and transfer of knowledge (Hilgard, 1996). Thorndike developed psychological *connectionism*. He hypothesized that learning is the formulation of connections between sensory stimuli and neural impulses that are identified through behavior. He also believed that learning often occurred by trial and error. Thorndike noted that teachers need to help students form good habits and that teaching should contextualize content for students to understand how to apply what they have learned. He also proposed that information should be presented when the student is ready to learn or just before the information can be used in a serviceable way (Thorndike & Gates, 1929).

B. F. Skinner (1904–1990) formulated the theory of *operant conditioning* in the 1930s. Based on the work of Thorndike, Skinner believed that the best way to understand behavior was to examine the causes of an action and its consequences. Skinner created the term *operant conditioning*, which is changing behavior using reinforcement that follows the desired response. Skinner identified three types of responses that can follow behavior: neutral operants or responses from the environment that neither increase nor decrease the probability of a behavior being repeated; reinforcers, which are responses from the environment that increase the probability of a behavior being repeated; and punishers or responses from the environment that decrease the likelihood of a behavior being repeated.

Positive reinforcement strengthens a behavior by providing a consequence an individual finds rewarding. The removal of an unpleasant reinforcer can also strengthen behavior. This is known as negative reinforcement because it is the removal of an adverse stimulus. Negative reinforcement strengthens behavior because it stops or removes an unpleasant experience (Skinner, 1953). Punishment inhibits behavior and is the opposite of reinforcement, as it is designed to eliminate a response. Like reinforcement, punishment occurs by directly applying an unpleasant stimulus after a response or by removing a potentially rewarding stimulus (McLeod, 2007).

Although popular through much of the 20th century, behaviorism is no longer a predominant educational perspective. However, the concepts of positive and negative reinforcement retain their usefulness today. Behavioral objectives, learning contracts, and programmed learning are based on behaviorism. Examples of teaching methods with this educational perspective are listed in Exhibit 2.1.

EXHIBIT 2.1 Examples of Teaching Methods Based on Behaviorism

- Guided practice
- Lecture without discussion
- Programmed learning and instruction
- Repetition
- Skill exercises

Cognitivism

Cognitivism comprises a group of theories that include the work of Bruner, Gagne, Vygotsky, and others. During the 1960s, cognitive aspects of learning were recognized, primarily because the behaviourist perspective could not explain why people organize and make sense of the information they learn. Cognitive theory defines learning as a semipermanent change in mental processes or associations. Cognitivists do not require an outward demonstration of learning but focus more on the internal processes and connections that take place during learning.

Cognitivists consider learning as mental structures that provide a base for organizing and building knowledge. Learning is not a change in behavior but a change in mental structures. Changes may be observed in behavior, but the behavior is due to a change in cognition. The locus of control for learning is in the learner, not in the environment (Utley, 2011).

Jerome Bruner (born 1915) proposed the *Cognitive Growth Theory* to examine intellectual growth of children. He proposed that, as children grow, they depend on a widening array of modes of understanding. Infants rely on enactive responses (action) to process and represent information, children 1 to 4 years of age rely on images to process information, and, finally, children over the age of 4 begin to use language to shape and augment information processing (Bruner, 1964).

A primary focus of cognitive psychology is on memory, a subject that has been studied for thousands of years. *Information Processing Theory* explains acquisition of knowledge in a step-wise manner. Information processing theorists such as **Robert Gagne** (1919–2002) are less concerned with external factors. They focus instead on the mental processes that come between stimulus and response (Schunk, 2012). These theorists hypothesize that people selectively pay attention to environmental details, transform data into information, and rehearse the information, relating the new information to that already known (Mayer, 1996).

Within the information processing model, Gagne (1985) described four processes: (1) encoding when environmental information is sensed or attended to (generation of neural impulses), (2) processing of information (filtering out of irrelevant information), (3) storage after encoding (may be short-term or long-term), and (4) retrieval, when the information is needed for a task (action). Examples of teaching methods based on cognitivism include use of problem-solving, reciprocal teaching (activities involving a dialogue between the teacher and students about segments of text to understand their meaning), and scaffolding (providing support such as resources and guides during the learning process to promote a deeper level of learning; Crutchshank, Metcalf, & Jenkins, 2011; Gagne, Wager, Golas, & Keller, 2005).

Social Cognitivism

Lev Vygotsky (1896–1934) expanded Piaget's basic developmental theory of cognitive abilities of the individual to include the concept of social–cultural cognition, the idea that all learning occurs in a cultural context and involves social interactions. He emphasized the role that culture and language play in developing students' thinking and the ways in which teachers and peers assist learners in developing new ideas and skills. Vygotsky proposed the concept of the zone of proximal development, which suggested that students best learn subjects just beyond their range of existing experience with assistance from the teacher or another classmate. Assistance from others bridges the distance from what students know or can do independently to what they can know or do with assistance (Schunk, 2012).

Social Learning Theory, based on the work of **Albert Bandura** (born 1925), focuses on the concept that much of human learning occurs in the environment (Schunk, 2012). Social Learning Theory is built on the importance of observational learning, imitation, and modeling. Bandura's theory hypothesizes that there is a continuous interaction among behaviors, cognitions, and the environment. The learner and environment are in a reciprocal relationship, where one influences the other, and human behavior is learned visually through modeling from observing others (Bandura, 1977, 1986). For a student to learn, three internal processes must occur: attention or observation, retention or processing in memory, and motivation or having a reason to replicate another's behavior. Exhibit 2.2 provides examples of teaching methods based on social cognitivism theory.

EXHIBIT 2.2 Examples of Teaching Methods Based on Social Cognitivism

- Demonstration/return demonstration
- Observational learning
- Role modeling
- Scaffolding

Humanism

Humanistic Theory, largely constructivist, emphasizes both cognitive and affective learning. Within this paradigm, learning is viewed as a personal act to fulfill one's potential (Schunk, 2012).

The *Hierarchy of Needs* theory, first discussed by **Abraham Maslow** in 1943, posits that all human actions are directed toward goal attainment. Most human actions are based on hierarchical needs, with lower order needs taking precedence over higher-order needs (Maslow, 1968). The lowest order needs are physiological needs such as food, air, and water. Safety needs become predominant when there are environmental threats. Love and belongingness needs become important once physiological and safety needs are met. Esteem needs are needs based on real capacity, achievement, and respect from others. The highest level is the need for self-actualization, which leads to self-fulfillment and personal growth (Maslow, 1943).

The first four needs are deprivation needs that motivate people to resolve them (Maslow, 1968). Self-actualization, according to Maslow (1943), can be reached only by an individual who has satisfied all lower level needs and who is then able to "become everything that one is capable of becoming" (Maslow, 1943, p. 382).

Carl Rogers (1902–1987) concurred with Maslow and extended Maslow's work by concluding that for people to grow, they need an environment that provides genuineness, acceptance, and empathy. Rogers believed that every person could achieve his or her goals, wishes, and desires in life; self-actualization took place when, or if, a person did achieve those goals (McLeod, 2012). Examples of teaching methods based on humanism include participatory and discovery methods, allowing students choices and opportunities for their learning, and providing resources and encouragement for learning (Schunk, 2012).

Constructivism

A reaction to didactic approaches such as behaviorism and programmed instruction, constructivism states that learning is an active, contextualized process of constructing knowledge through experiencing and reflecting on the experience rather than acquiring it. Knowledge is constructed based on personal experiences and hypotheses made of the environment. Learners continuously test these hypotheses through social interaction. Each person has a different interpretation and construction of knowledge process. The learner is not a blank slate, but brings past experiences and cultural factors to a situation (Bruning, Schraw, Norby, & Ronning, 2010)

John Dewey (1859–1952) was one of the 20th century's most influential educators. His ideas of experiential education placed an emphasis on meaningful activity in learning and participation in the classroom (Schunk, 2012). Unlike earlier models of teaching, which relied on a teacher-centered classroom and rote learning, Dewey's idea of progressive education asserted that students must be invested in what they were learning. He proposed that curricula should be relevant to students' lives. He viewed experiential learning of practical life skills as crucial to education (Schunk, 2012).

Jean Piaget (1896–1980) was the first to state that learning is a developmental process and that children create knowledge rather than learn from the teacher. He recognized that children construct knowledge based on practice, which is related to biological and developmental maturation. Piaget observed young children and mapped out four stages of growth: sensorimotor (birth to about 2 years), preoperational (ages 2–7), concrete operations (ages 7–14) and formal operations (beginning around age 11–12 and extending into adulthood). His work recognized the importance of some rote learning while also hypothesizing that other activities that support students' exploration are essential (Hilgard & Bower, 1975; Huitt & Hummel, 2003).

In the early 1970s, **David Kolb** and **Roger Fry** (1975) developed the Experiential Learning Model, composed of four elements: concrete experience, observation of and reflection on that experience, formation of abstract concepts based on the reflection, and testing the new concepts. These four elements are the basis of a cycle of learning that can begin with any one of the four elements, but that typically begins with a concrete experience. He named his model to emphasize its links to ideas from John Dewey, Jean Piaget, and other writers of the cognitivist paradigm. His model was developed predominantly for use with adult education, but it has had widespread pedagogical implications in higher education. Kolb (1984) created a graphic representation of his model using two perpendicular continua, one related to process and the other related to perception. Some examples of teaching methods based on constructivism are in Exhibit 2.3.

Brain-Based Learning

Based on the rapid influx of information from brain research over the past 20 years, a new paradigm has emerged that bridges research and education. Brain-based learning is "the active engagement of purposeful strategies based on principles derived from an understanding of the brain" (Jensen, 2008, p. 4).

According to cognitive neuroscientists, learning literally changes our brain. An increased rate of signaling by cortical neurons generates an increased number of branches in the neocortex, which in turn increases the density of cellular material and enhances connections with other neurons (creating more synapses). The changes happen only in the areas of the brain that are stimulated. The synapses increase because of the repeated firing of the particular neurons engaged in learning in the presence of

EXHIBIT 2.3 Examples of Teaching Methods Based on Constructivism

- Case studies
- Class discussions and debates
- Cooperative learning
- Field trips (allow students to put the concepts and ideas discussed in class in a real-world context)
- Guided experimentation (students individually perform an experiment and then come together as a group to discuss the results)
- Peer tutoring
- Problem-based learning
- Research projects
- Simulation
- Other methods that ensure learning outcomes are at a high level on Bloom's Taxonomy

From Petty (2004).

emotion chemicals such as adrenaline and serotonin around the neurons. The longevity of learning is in proportion to the number of neocortical areas engaged (Sousa, 2011). Exhibit 2.4 lists examples of teaching strategies based on concepts of brain-based learning.

EXHIBIT 2.4 Examples of Teaching Strategies Based on Brain-Based Learning

- Preexpose the learners to content and context a week before the lesson
- Teach less content and educate more in depth on important concepts
- Provide frequent, nonjudgmental feedback
- Provide some form of feedback to each student during the class
- Engage students socially and physically
- Empower learners by providing choices
- Set high standards
- Encourage peer support
- Ensure the classroom is safe for risk-taking
- Manage high levels of student stress
- Allow students time to practice prior to testing
- Maintain a variety of teaching methods that complement diverse learning styles
- Celebrate successes

From Jensen (2008).

DIVERSE LEARNING NEEDS OF STUDENTS

As stated in the introduction to this chapter, each student in the classroom is unique. The students may range in culture, ethnicity, learning style, age, gender, motivation, economic background, previous life experiences, and many other independent factors, all of which can have an influence on learning. Currently, the majority of students in nursing education programs are White, non-Hispanic (74%), female (85%), and under the age of 30 years (National League for Nursing [NLN], 2012). As the United States becomes more diverse, so must our nursing education programs.

Our increasingly global society brings with it a diversity never before experienced in higher education. One nursing faculty member recently disclosed that in her classroom of 50 students, students spoke 11 different native languages and had an age range from 20 to 62 years old (D. Walker, Personal communication, January 12, 2013).

CULTURE AND ETHNICITY

As more and more non-Western students from Latin America, Africa, Asia, and the Middle East attend nursing education program, it is important that faculty members have a general understanding of how cultures view learning and knowing (Merriam & Associates, 2007). The rising complexity of teaching to a diverse class requires that faculty members be attuned to the learning needs of each student, recognizing that effective teaching should incorporate multiple methods to meet the range of needs.

We are generally immersed in a Western perspective of learning and knowing. Western perspectives value the individual learner over the collective, promote autonomy and independence of thought and action, and emphasize scientific research (Merriam & Associates, 2007). In the 21st century we need to recognize our past ethnocentrism and develop courses with multicultural perspectives.

Faculty members can no longer assume that they are knowledgeable about students in their courses. One of the major cultural differences is communication (Svinicki & McKeachie, 2013). For example, looking away rather than establishing eye contact with a faculty member is indicative of careful attention rather than inattention in Asian and Native American cultures (Gudykunst, 2004). Nonparticipation, such as not answering questions as to the clarity of a concept or questioning the teacher, may be related to a cultural norm of showing respect to elders in certain cultures (Svinicki & McKeachie). In this situation, use of tools such as clickers may assist the students and give the faculty member more input as to student comprehension.

Another important cultural difference is related to collectivism (the better good of the whole) or individualism (focus on the individual). Our Western norms relate to individualism, but many cultures, such as Asian and certain African, Latin American, and Native American cultures, value the success of the whole more than individual success (Merriam & Associates, 2007). Small group projects and activities in the classroom may assist in achieving deeper learning for these groups. Study groups are also helpful for this population of students.

Students from other countries and cultures might have a lower level of verbal English fluency (Svinicki & McKeachie, 2013). Students whose native language is not English may have an easier time with reading and writing than with verbal communication. In this situation, having class sessions digitally archived in video and audio and available to students outside of class may be of help to students. Other strategies of value include having content available in written format and using activities such as simulation, which provide kinesthetic as well as auditory and visual cues. Examples of teaching strategies for use in multicultural classrooms are provided in Exhibit 2.5.

LEARNING STYLES

The concept of learning styles has been actively studied for more than 50 years. Simply put, *learning style* is the manner in which an individual approaches a learning situation that has implications for performance and learning outcomes. Do students learn and retain

EXHIBIT 2.5 Teaching Strategies for Inclusion in Multicultural Classrooms

- Become aware of your own cultural biases
- Treat each student as different from every other student in the classroom
- Maintain a culturally neutral classroom
- Recognize the complexity of diversity
- Foster intergroup relations
- Be concrete
- Monitor your use of idioms
- Be accessible
- Digitally archive videos or audio files of classes for students to review

From Adeniran and Smith-Glasgow (2010); Davis (2009); Suinn (2013).

more when teaching methods match their learning style? Does purposeful matching of teaching to learning style improve learning outcomes? Learning styles were developed to guide students' understanding of how they learn best. Learning style identification has been a useful tool to help students examine their own learning preferences, develop better study methods, and identify particular styles to improve their learning outcomes.

There are many models of learning styles (Davis, 2009). Popular theorists such as Kolb (1984) and Fleming and Mills (1992) have described learning styles and learner preferences, using different theoretical and physiological perspectives. Using the concepts of his Experiential Learning Model, Kolb hypothesized that each of the four quadrants of the perceiving and processing continua could be interpreted as four preferred learning preferences (Figure 2.1). *Divergers* (concrete and reflective) view concrete experiences from multiple perspectives and adapt by thinking rather than doing. *Convergers* (abstract and active) prefer the practical application of problem solving and technical tasks over personal issues. *Assimilators* (abstract and reflective) focus more on ideas than people and integrate multiple ideas into a conceptual whole. *Accommodators* (concrete and active) are comfortable with people and tend to use trial and error in problem-solving (Kolb).

FIGURE 2.1 Kolb's learning cycle and learning styles.

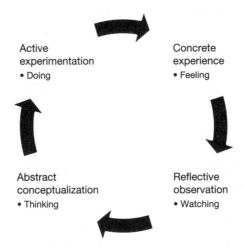

In 1992, **Fleming** and **Mills** introduced the VARK learning preference model, which introduces four learning style preferences, visual, auditory, read/write, and kinesthetic (VARK). They suggest that this learning preference relates to only one component of learning style—the preference for how to take in and give out information. This particular component of learning style is measured using the VARK tool (Fleming, 2012).

The four learning style modes are described as:

- A *visual* preference entails a preference for information in graphic formats, such as maps, charts, and flow charts, rather than in text format.
- An *aural/auditory* preference describes a preference for information that is language based (heard or spoken).
- A *read/write* style indicates a preference for information in text format.
- A *kinesthetic* learner prefers information that is concrete and experience-based.

Pashler, McDaniel, Rohrer, and Bjork (2008) undertook a comprehensive meta-analysis of the research supporting the concept of learning styles and application of learning styles to improve instruction. Their review found evidence that individuals, if asked, will express preferences for how material is presented to them. However, they found that there was no evidence to support the hypothesis that matching teaching methods to learning styles will lead to improved learning outcomes. There is little research on the validity and reliability of the commonly used measurement tools, and few studies have used methodologies capable of testing the validity of learning styles applied to education. Pashler et al. (2008) also report that there are several relatively well-structured studies that do not support the learning styles hypotheses. More research needs to be done.

No single assessment of learning style guarantees that a student's learning needs will be satisfied. The teacher should create learning environments that address the content using a multitude of methods rather than try to match instruction to each student's learning style preference. Being aware of one's own style assists the teacher to not impose one learning preference on the students. Using multiple approaches makes it easier for students to learn. This allows the teacher to meet the array of students' learning styles, which often do not match the teacher's own personal, preferred style (Sternberg, Grigorenko, & Zhang, 2008). Additionally, material presented with a variety of methods keeps the students engaged with the content. Exhibit 2.6 provides examples of teaching strategies for diverse learning styles.

EXHIBIT 2.6 Examples of Teaching Strategies for Diverse Learning Styles

- Vary teaching methods, assignments, and learning activities
- Include individual and group activities
- Use classroom discussion
- Use color, charts, and graphics in visual presentations
- Use role play and simulations
- Provide opportunities to learn by doing
- Provide opportunities for the diverse learning styles in the classroom
- Don't teach using solely your personal learning style preference

AGE

Over the past 60 years, the age makeup of the college student population has changed significantly. Starting with the returning veterans of World War II, college campuses have seen rapid increases in the number of adult learners. Currently, nontraditional or adult learners make up the majority of students on college campuses (American Association of Colleges and Universities, 2006). Research on learners has shown that adults come from a wide variety of backgrounds and bring many different perspectives to the classroom (Wlodkowski, 2010). Although adults as learners are often classified into one group, adult learners today comprise of Traditionalists, Baby Boomers, GenXers, and Millennials, based on birth date (Table 2.2). Much is published about learning styles, values, motivation, and preferences for delivery methods for each of these generations. However, there is little actual research other than general surveys to support these differences.

TABLE 2.2 Generations of Learners

Generation	Age Group	Values	Learning Motivation	Delivery Methods	Feedback
Traditionalists	Born before 1945	Conservative, respectful of authority, formal, structured environments with clear objectives	Leadership goals, public recognition	Classroom lectures, dislike games, and role play	Assume they are doing fine until receive constructive feedback
Baby boomers	1945–1964	Optimistic, involved, and hard workers	Public and peer recognition; relevant to career goals	Lecture, small group discussion	Well-documented feedback all at once
Gen xers	1965–1979	Informal, skeptical, self-reliant	Relevance to personal goals, recognition by faculty	On-the-job training, e-learning, active learning	Regular ongoing feedback
Millennials	1980 or later	Realists, confident, social networking	Fast track to success, structured assignments with tight deadlines	e-learning, blogs, wikis, podcasts, mobile apps, hands-on learning	Frequent feedback

Currently in nursing education, 44% of students in associate degree programs are over the age of 30, compared to 15% of baccalaureate students; 70% of registered nurse (RN)-BSN students, 70% of master's nursing students, and 91% of doctoral nursing students are over the age of 30 (NLN, 2012).

It is important to examine adult learners based on their unique learning needs. In 1973, Malcolm Knowles introduced the term *andragogy*, outlining differences between children and adult learners (Knowles, 1973). Andragogy focuses on learning needs of adult learners. Knowles identified six assumptions about adult learning:

1. Need to know: Adults prefer to know why they are learning particular content at the outset of learning. Teachers should assist adults to contextualize the learning to recognize its importance.
2. Learner's self-concept: Adult self-concept is dependent on progress toward self-direction. Adults need to be approached as capable and self-directed learners.

3. Role of the learner's experiences. Adults enter into education with prior experiences, which provide them with additional valuable resources. The richest resource for learning resides within; therefore, tapping into adults' experiences through active learning exercises is beneficial (Svinicki & McKeachie, 2013).
4. Readiness to learn. Adults become ready to learn to deal effectively with real-life situations or to perform a task. They want to learn what they can apply in the present.
5. Orientation to learning. Adults are life-centered (task-centered, problem-centered) in their orientation to learning. They want to learn what will help them perform tasks or deal with problems they confront in everyday situations and those presented in the context of application to real life.
6. Motivation. Adults are responsive to some external motivators (e.g., a better job and higher salaries), but the most potent motivators are internal (e.g., desire for increased job satisfaction and self-esteem; Knowles, Holton, & Swanson, 2011).

Nursing faculty members are faced with intergenerational classrooms and concurrently with the needs of traditional and adult learners. Well-organized classes, with introductions that contextualize the content (meeting the need to know and motivating learners), parallel to clinical experiences (readiness to learn and orientation to learning), and containing active learning exercises (role of the learner's experiences and the learner's self-concept) will meet the needs of both traditional and adult students.

In clinical situations, it is important to assist the nursing staff and preceptors to understand the differences in generation learners. As the average age of RNs continues to climb (Health Resources and Services Administration [HRSA], 2010), Baby Boomer and Gen X nurses will often be working with Gen X and Millennial students. For example, students may be embracing technology with nursing reference books accessible on cell phones, a behavior that the older nursing staff may interpret as texting and indifference on the part of the student. Exhibit 2.7 lists teaching strategies for use in multigenerational classrooms.

EXHIBIT 2.7 Examples of Teaching Strategies for Multigenerational Classrooms

- Clarify the essentials when preparing syllabus, assignments, and evaluation tools
- Contextualize the content
- Offer choices for assignments
- Create multigenerational team assignments
- Provide frequent feedback
- Use simulation activities and case studies
- Use web-enhanced (hybrid) classes

From Wilson and Gerber (2008).

GENDER

Nationally, 6.6% of the RN workforce is male (HRSA, 2010, p. A-10). However, in 2011, 15% of all students in basic nursing programs were male (NLN, 2012). Only 5% of full-time faculty teaching in baccalaureate and higher degree programs are men (Robert Wood Johnson Foundation, 2012). As more and more men enter nursing education programs, faculty members need to take into account gender differences in learning styles and expectations. Throughout recent history, nursing has been a career undertaken primarily by females. Our classrooms have been filled with female students with female faculty members. The word *nurse* generally has a female connotation. However, over the past 15 years the number of men in nursing education programs has increased, and creating a gender-neutral classroom is a necessity.

Through the 1990s, there was a flurry of research investigating how male and female students differed in the college classroom. Rocca (2010) conducted an analysis of literature on student participation in the general college classroom and found continued subtle gender biases. Male college students tend to participate and be more engaged in the college classroom, especially when the faculty member is male, and female students were more likely to participate with a female faculty member. Faculty members tend to ask male students more abstract questions and female students more factual questions. Male students speak more frequently and longer in class discussions. Female students receive less feedback on answers than do males (Rocca, 2010).

To promote a gender-neutral classroom, nursing faculty members should assess their own gender biases and create a classroom that addresses males and females equally. Language needs to remain gender neutral, not assuming that every nurse is a female, including on examinations. Exhibit 2.8 provides some strategies for nurse educators to use to create a gender-neutral teaching situation.

EXHIBIT 2.8 Teaching Strategies to Create a Gender-Neutral Learning Environment

- Treat all students equally, making no assumptions with regard to gender
- Observe for gender differences, and get to know how each student responds in the classroom
- If quiet, engage gently and encourage participation
- Protect those students who are interrupted or intimidated by others
- Develop openings for hesitant students
- Be sure to ask questions of all students
- Use small group activities that engage all students
- Give students time to answer questions
- Avoid interrupting student responses
- Allow quiet pauses
- Call on all students, not only those who are the most talkative
- Do not allow a few students to dominate discussion
- Do not exclude men (or women) as you call on students
- Be sure that examples include both male and female references
- Be consistent in addressing all students either by first or last names
- Ensure that male and female students are held to the same academic standards

From Derek Bok Center for Teaching and Learning (2007).

MOTIVATION AND ACADEMIC SELF-REGULATION

The interaction of evidence-based teaching strategies and students' strategic use of learning methods, motivation, and self-regulation leads to good learning outcomes (Weinstein, Acee, & Jung, 2010). Many students begin college without the specific skills needed to study a particular discipline. As students learn content, they also need to learn the skills to be successful in studying the discipline (Weinstein et al., 2013). Strategic learners are active learners, and they are persistent in reaching learning goals. They know when they do not understand content, and they seek out resources to help them understand it. They recognize that learning is under their own control (Schunk & Zimmerman, 2012).

Strategic learners are effective learners who set reasonable and attainable goals for learning, which motivate them to continue studying (Schunk, Pintrich, & Meece, 2008). Students who consciously set learning goals tend to be self-reflective, use metacognitive processes, be self-aware, and have higher levels of self-efficacy than other students (Kitsantas, Winsler, & Huie, 2008). They attribute success to effort, time management, and learning skills rather than to luck (Weinstein et al., 2010). Strategic learners are motivated learners who want to learn (Zimmerman, 2011). A final key component needed for strategic learning is self-regulation, the use of executive control functions (Weinstein et al., 2010; Zimmerman & Schunk, 2011).

MOTIVATION

Motivation is a key dimension of self-regulated learning and a prerequisite for meaningful learning (Ginsberg, 2005; Mayer, 2011). Motivation as a biological phenomenon is a process that mediates how much energy and attention the brain allocates to a given stimulus. Motivation as a social science phenomenon is an internal state that begins and sustains goal-directed behavior. Motivation is based on multiple factors, which include goal orientation, interest, self-efficacy, and causal attribution (Mayer, 2011; Zimmerman & Schunk, 2012).

Goal orientation can be learning- or performance-based. Research has shown that students with stronger learning goals use deep learning skills more frequently. They also recover from a poor grade and improve performance to a higher degree than students with a performance goal orientation (Zimmerman & Schunk, 2012).

Interest is another contributor to motivation and is a precursor to learning. Students will work harder to learn when the content is of interest to them, related to their career plans (individual), or of high personal value at the time (situational; Mayer, 2011; Zimmerman & Schunk, 2012).

Self-efficacy, the individual's self-assessed ability to complete tasks needed to achieve goals, is believed to be a strong element of motivation (Kitsantas et al., 2008; Wlodkowski, 2008). Self-efficacy is generally situation-based and future-oriented, but it is based on previous experience.

Causal attributions are a student's beliefs about the causation of academic outcomes. Perceptions rather than actual causes, attributions are influenced by preexisting factors such as self-efficacy and by external environmental factors such as rewards (Zimmerman & Schunk, 2012). Students who make effort-based attributions are likely to put forth effort during learning to be successful (Mayer, 2011). A number of strategies to increase motivation are presented in Exhibit 2.9.

SELF-REGULATION

Self-regulation is "the process by which learners personally activate and sustain cognitions, affects, and behaviors that are systematically oriented to the attainment of learning goals" (Schunk & Zimmerman, 2012, p. vii). Self-regulation is employed as students recognize that there might be improved ways to accomplish a goal and change their learning strategies (Winne & Hadwin, 2012). With self-regulated

EXHIBIT 2.9 Teaching Strategies to Increase Student Motivation

- Maintain a high level of enthusiasm for the content
- Maintain a cohesive course structure
- Keep content relevant to the intended outcome
- Maintain a positive learning environment
- Make the course personal
- Foster good lines of communication
- When needed, lighten the mood with humor
- Assist students to transfer previously achieved skills
- Connect learning to the real world
- Use lots of examples
- Use active learning strategies
- Hold students to high expectations
- Use appropriate assessment tools
- Focus class and assessments on conceptual understanding
- Provide many opportunities for graded assessments
- Use rubrics for grading
- Limit the use of high-stakes testing

From Nilson (2010).

learning, students are motivated to learn and can transform their cognitive abilities into improved academic performance.

Litchtinger and Kaplan (2011) suggested that self-regulation was a precursor to success in higher education and that motivation was a key component of the first component of self-regulation, forethought. When students set mastery goals, they are more likely to engage in self-regulation than if they set performance goals.

Current literature supports a model of self-regulated learning that has three main phases (Zimmerman, 2008; Zusho & Edwards, 2011). The first phase, forethought, includes the processes of goal setting and task-planning. The second phase is the action phase, which entails the processes of monitoring, controlling, and evaluating learning. The final phase of self-regulation is management, during which the student engages in reaction and reflection (Zusho & Edwards, 2011).

TEACHER-STUDENT RELATIONSHIPS

Student engagement, in both curricular and cocurricular activities, is a strong predictor of student success in higher education, and student contact with faculty is associated with the development of key relationships and better outcomes (National Survey of Student Engagement [NSSE], 2012). An excellent predictor of student satisfaction with college is the extent to which students believe that the campus environment is supportive of their curricular and cocurricular needs (NSSE, 2012). Nurse educators need to understand that one of the major hallmarks of the supportive learning environment is student-faculty interaction. Interaction includes discussing ideas from class, clinical practice, and other environments of learning with students both in and out of those settings; giving prompt feedback on student work; discussing grades; talking about career plans with students; working with students on activities other than coursework; and engaging students in their own research projects outside of course requirements (NSSE, 2012). Exhibit 2.10 includes other strategies to promote student engagement. Creasey, Jarvis, and Knapcik (2009) reported that students who had a strong sense of connection and nonthreatening associations with faculty members had less anxiety than their peers, who felt less connected.

EXHIBIT 2.10 Faculty-Driven Teaching Strategies to Promote Student Engagement

- Improve students' self-beliefs by giving them some control over learning processes
- Give students opportunities to work alone, cultivating intrinsic motivation
- Be approachable, sensitive to student needs, and well prepared
- Create learning experiences that include active and collaborative learning components
- Create challenging learning activities that push students to grow in academic abilities
- Ensure that your course (classroom, online, laboratory, simulation, clinical practice, other settings) is welcoming to diverse students

From Weimer (2012).

There is currently attention being placed on instructional immediacy, the behavior that brings the instructor and students closer together in terms of perceived distance (Mehrabian, 1971). Nonverbal immediacy includes behaviors such as smiling, gesturing, eye contact, and having relaxed body language. Verbal immediacy refers to calling the students by name, using humor, and encouraging student input and discussion. Both verbal immediacy and nonverbal immediacy have been found to have a positive effect on student motivation (Velez & Cano, 2009).

Cox and Orehovec (2007) identified five types of faculty-student interactions in a residential college designed to increase faculty–student interaction. Disengagement, where interaction did not occur, was a common finding. Incidental or unintentional interactions were perfunctory polite greetings or recognition. Functional interactions occurred for a specific purpose such as asking a question, which frequently led to more interaction. Personal interaction was often the outcome of functional interactions, and it was highly valued by students, often leading to the beginning of a relationship between teacher and student. Mentoring, a rare outcome of interaction, occurred when a faculty member provided direct assistance with professional development, emotional and psychosocial support, and role modeling (p. 356).

SUMMARY

For many years, parents, educators, psychologists, and more recently, cognitive neuroscientists have explored the concepts of teaching and learning. The science of teaching and learning, going back to Pavlov in the 19th century, has now evolved from theories based on observation to knowing which parts of the brain are activated by different stimuli. We now know that the brain is constantly learning by creating new connections. The question still remains, however, as to what is the ideal way to assist students in the learning process.

Nurse educators are in an ideal position to make a significant impact on students' learning. The diversity of our classrooms no longer allows a one-size-fits-all approach to learning. To effectively engage students in the learning process, nurse educators need to understand multiple factors. First, the teacher should assess the diversity of the students. Cultural heritage and ethnicity, age, gender, learning style, motivation, and ability to self-regulate are only a few of the significant differences among students. The teacher should also assess the content of the course. What is the goal of the learning? How best will most students in the course learn the concepts and other types of material? What do the students already know about the subject? How can you best connect the new content to the material the students have already learned? These are a few of the basic questions that should be answered as the teacher plans the course.

Nursing faculty members should also be aware of the need to teach students, how to learn, and how to be successful in their courses. What are the best ways to motivate the students to learn? What are the best ways to engage students in the classroom and online environment to encourage the deep understanding of material?

An engaged classroom, with students actively participating in the process of learning, is our challenge. Nurse educators must accept this challenge by finding new and different ways of teaching to reach all students and creating motivated, self-regulated nurses for the future.

REFERENCES

Adeniran, R., & Smith-Glasgow, M. (2010). Creating and promoting a positive learning environment among culturally diverse nurses and students. *Creative Nursing, 16*(2), 53–58.

American Association of Colleges and Universities. (2006). Addressing the needs of adult learners. *Policy Matters, 3*(2), 1–4.

Bandura, A. (1977). *Social learning theory.* New York, NY: General Learning Press.

Bandura, A. (1986). *Social foundations of thought and action: A social cognitive theory.* Englewood Cliffs, NJ: Prentice Hall.

Bruner, J. (1964). The course of cognitive growth. *American Psychologist, 19*, 1–15.

Bruning, R. H., Schraw, G. J., Norby, M. M., & Ronning, R. R. (2010). *Cognitive psychology and instruction* (5th ed.). Upper Saddle River, NJ: Pearson.

Chaney, W. (2006). *Workbook for a dynamic mind.* Las Vegas, NV: Houghton-Brace Publishing.

Cox, B., & Orehovec, E. (2007). Faculty-student interaction outside the classroom: A typology from a residential college. *The Review of Higher Education, 30*, 343–362.

Creasey, G., Jarvis, P., & Knapcik, E. (2009). A measure to assess student-instructor relationships. *International Journal for the Scholarship of Teaching and Learning, 3*(2), 1–10.

Crutchshank, D., Metcalf, K., & Jenkins, D. (2011). *The act of teaching.* San Francisco, CA: McGraw Hill Higher Education.

Davis, B. (2009). *Tools for teaching.* San Francisco, CA: Jossey Bass.

Derek Bok Center for Teaching and Learning. (2007). *Tips for teachers: Sensitivity to women in the contemporary classroom.* Cambridge, MA: Harvard University.

Fleming, N. (2012). VARK: A guide to learning styles. Retrieved from http://www.vark-learn.com/english/index.asp

Fleming, N., & Mills, C. (1992). Not another inventory, rather a catalyst for reflection. *To Improve the Academy, 11*, 137.

Gagne, R. M. (1985). *The conditions of learning and theory of instruction* (4th ed.). New York, NY: Holt, Rinehart, and Winston.

Gagne, R. M., Wager, W. W., Golas, F. C., & Keller, J. M. (2005). *Principles of instructional design* (5th ed.). Belmont, CA: Thomas/Wadsworth Publishing.

Ginsberg, M. B. (2005). Cultural diversity, motivation, and differentiation. *Theory Into Practice, 44*, 218–225.

Gudykunst, W. (2004). *Bridging differences: Effective intergroup communication* (4th ed.). Thousand Oaks, CA: Sage.

Health Resources and Services Administration. (2010). *The registered nurse population: Findings from the 2008 national sample survey of registered nurses.* Retrieved from http://bhpr.hrsa.gov/healthworkforce/rnsurveys/rnsurveyfinal.pdf

Hilgard, E. R. (1996). Perspectives on educational psychology. *Educational Psychology Review, 8,* 419–431.

Hilgard, E. R., & Bower, G. H. (1975). *Theories of learning.* Englewood Cliffs, NJ: Prentice-Hall.

Huitt, W., & Hummel, J. (2003). Piaget's theory of cognitive development. *Educational Psychology Interactive.* Valdosta, GA: Valdosta State University. Retrieved from http://www.edpsycinteractive.org/topics/cognition/piaget.html

Jensen, E. (2008). *Brain-based learning* (2nd ed.). Thousand Oaks, CA: Corwin Press.

King, L. (n.d.). Ancient history sourcebook: Code of Hammurabi. Retrieved from http://www.fordham.edu/halsall/ancient/hamcode.asp

Kitsantas, A., Winsler, A., & Huie, F. (2008). Self-regulation and ability predictors of academic success: A predictive validity study. *Journal of Advanced Academics, 20,* 42–68.

Knowles, M. S. (1973). *The adult learner: A neglected species.* Houston, TX: Gulf Publishing Company.

Knowles, M. S., Holton, E. F., & Swanson, R. A. (2011). *The adult learner: The definitive classic in adult education and human resource development* (7th ed.). London: Elsevier.

Kolb, D. (1984). *Experiential learning: Experience as the source of learning and development.* Englewood Cliffs, NJ: Prentice-Hall.

Kolb, D. A., & Fry, R. (1975). Toward an applied theory of experiential learning. In C. Cooper (Ed.), *Theories of group process.* London: John Wiley.

Litchtinger, E., & Kaplan, A. (2011). Purposes of engagement in academic self-regulation. In H. Bembenutty (Ed.), *Self-regulated learning. New directions for teaching and learning 126*(summer), 9–17. doi:10.1002/tl.440

Maslow, A. (1943). A theory of human motivation. *Psychological Review, 50,* 370–396.

Maslow, A. H. (1968). *Toward a psychology of being* (2nd ed.). New York, NY: Van Nostrand Reinhold.

Mayer, R. E. (2011). *Applying the science of learning.* Boston, MA: Pearson.

Mayer, R. W. (1996). Learners as information processors: Legacies and limitations of educational psychology's second metaphor. *Educational Psychologist, 31,* 151–161.

McLeod, S. A. (2007). *B.F. Skinner operant conditioning.* Retrieved from http://www.simplypsychology.org/operant-conditioning.html

McLeod, S. A. (2012). Carl Rogers. Retrieved from http://www.simplypsychology.org/carl-rogers.html

Mehrabian, A. (1971). *Silent messages.* Belmont, CA: Wadsworth.

Merriam, S., & Associates. (2007). *Non-western perspectives on learning and knowing.* Miramar, FL: Kreiger Publishing Company.

National League for Nursing. (2012). *Annual survey of schools of nursing, Fall 2011.* Retrieved from www.nln.org/research/slides/index.htm

National Survey of Student Engagement. (2012). *Promoting student learning and institutional improvement: Lessons from the NSSE at 13.* Bloomington, IN: Indiana University Center for Postsecondary Research.

Nilson, L. (2010). *Teaching at its best* (3rd ed.). San Francisco, CA: Jossey-Bass.

Pashler, H., McDaniel, M., Rohrer, D., & Bjork, R. (2008). Learning styles: Concepts and evidence. *Psychological Science in the Public Interest, 9,* 106–119.

Petty, G. (2004). Constructivist teaching. Retrieved from http://www.geoffpetty.com/activelearning.html

Phillips, C. (2010). *Socrates café.* New York, NY: W.W. Norton.

Pavlov, I. (1927). *Conditioned reflexes.* London: Oxford University Press.

Robert Wood Johnson Foundation. (2012). Men slowly change the face of nursing education. Retrieved from http://www.rwjf.org/en/about-rwjf/newsroom/newsroom-content/2012/04/men-slowly-change-the-face-of-nursing-education.html

Rocca, K. (2010). Student participation in the college classroom: An extended multidisciplinary literature review. *Communication Education, 59,* 185–213. doi:10.1080/03634520903505936

Schunk, D. H. (2012). *Learning theories: An educational perspective.* Boston, MA: Pearson.

Schunk, D. H., & Zimmerman, B. J. (2012). *Motivation and self-regulated learning: Theory, research, and applications.* New York, NY: Routledge.

Schunk, D. H., Pintrich, P. R., & Meece, J. L. (2008). *Motivation in education: Theory, research, and applications* (3rd ed.). Upper Saddle River, NJ: Prentice Hall.

Skinner, B. F. (1953). *Science and human behavior.* New York, NY: Free Press.

Sousa, D. (2011). *How the brain learns* (4th ed.). Thousand Oaks, CA: Corwin Press.

Sternberg, R., Grigorenko, E., & Zhang, L. (2008). Styles of learning and thinking matter in instruction and assessment. *Perspectives on Psychological Science, 3,* 486–506.

Suinn, R. (2013). Teaching culturally diverse students. In M. Svinicki & W. McKeachie (Eds.), *McKeachie's teaching tips: Strategies, research, and theory for college and university teachers* (14th ed., pp. 150–171). Belmont, CA: Wadsworth.

Svinicki, M., & McKeachie, W. (2013). *McKeachie's teaching tips: Strategies, research, and theory for college and university teachers* (14th ed.). Belmont, CA: Wadsworth.

Thorndike, E. L., & Gates, A. I. (1929). *Elementary principles of education.* New York, NY: MacMillan.

Utley, R. (2011). *Theory and research for academic nurse educators.* Boston, MA: Jones and Bartlett.

Velez, J., & Cano, J. (2008). The relationship between teacher immediacy and student motivation. *Journal of Agriculture Education, 49*(3), 76–86.

Weimer, M. (2012). Ten ways to promote student engagement. *Faculty Focus.* Retrieved from http://www.facultyfocus.com/articles/effective-teaching-strategies/10-ways-to-promote-student-engagement/

Weinstein, C. E., Acee, T. W., & Jung, J. (2010). Learning strategies. In B. McGaw, P. L. Peterson, & E. Baker (Eds.), *International encyclopedia of education* (3rd ed., pp. 323–329). New York, NY: Elsevier.

Weinstein, C. E., Acee, T., Stano, N., Meyer, D., Husman, J., McKeachie, W., & King, C. (2013). Teaching students how to become more strategic and self-regulated learners. In M. Svinicki & W. McKeachie, (Eds.), *McKeachie's teaching tips: Strategies, research, and theory for college and university teachers* (14th ed., pp. 291–304). Belmont, CA: Wadsworth.

Wilson, M., & Gerber, L. (2008). How generational theory can improve teaching: Strategies for working with "Millennials." *Currents in Teaching and Learning, 1*(1). Retrieved from http://www.worcester.edu/currents/archives/volume_1_number_1/currentsv1n1wilsonp29.pdf

Winne, P. H., & Hadwin, A. F. (2012). The weave of motivation and self-regulated learning. In D. Schunk, & B. J. Zimmerman (Eds.), *Motivation and self-regulated learning: Theory, research, and applications* (pp. 297–314). New York, NY: Routledge.

Wlodkowski, R. (2008). *Enhancing adult motivation to learn* (3rd ed.). San Francisco, CA: Jossey-Bass.

Wlodkowski, R. (2010). Enhancing adult motivation to learn: A comprehensive guide for teaching all adults. *Journal of Adult Education, 39*(2), 40–43.

Zimmerman, B. J. (2008). Investigating self-regulation and motivation: Historical background, methodological developments, and future prospects. *American Educational Research Journal, 45*(1), 166–183.

Zimmerman, B. J. (2011). Motivational sources and outcomes of self-regulated learning and performance. In B. J. Zimmerman & D. H. Schunk (Eds.), *Handbook of self-regulation of learning and performance* (pp. 408–425). New York, NY: Taylor & Francis.

Zimmerman, B. J., & Schunk, D. H. (2011). *Handbook of self-regulation of learning and performance.* New York, NY: Taylor & Francis.

Zimmerman, B. J., & Schunk, D. H. (2012). Motivation: An essential dimension of self-regulated learning. In D. H. Schunk & B. J. Zimmerman (Eds.), *Motivation and self-regulated learning: Theory, research, and applications* (pp. 1–30). New York, NY: Routledge.

Zusho, A., & Edwards, K. (2011). Self-regulation and achievement goals in the college classroom. In H. Bembenutty (Ed.), Self-regulated learning. *New Directions for teaching and learning, 126*(summer), 21–31. doi:10.1002/tl.441

3

Teaching Methods

DEBRA HAGLER AND BRENDA MORRIS

The most important question to ask about any teaching method is whether it is a good fit for the specific learning objectives, learners, teachers, and available resources. If the goal is to support students in mastering key course concepts and developing learning-related attitudes, values, beliefs, and skills (Slavich & Zimbardo, 2012), then the same teaching method will not work equally well for all situations. Nurse educators who would be appalled at the idea of treating each patient with identical interventions regardless of patients' individual needs might not be as concerned about using identical teaching methods for all learners and instructional purposes. Yet, choosing teaching methods congruent with specific learner needs and desired educational outcomes is critical to effective instruction.

This chapter describes a variety of teaching methods and offers guidance in selecting methods to fit the intended outcomes, learner characteristics, and available resources. Teaching methods are considered in relation to supporting learner development in the cognitive, affective, and psychomotor learning domains. Strategies are described for incorporating active learning and for promoting critical thinking. Expanded information on the use of educational technology is presented in Chapter 4 and on teaching through simulation in Chapter 5. Teaching methods for specific settings are described in later chapters as well: online teaching in Chapter 6, teaching in the learning laboratory in Chapter 7, and clinical teaching in Chapter 8.

SELECTING TEACHING METHODS

The educator selecting a teaching method should consider the fit of that method with the learning objectives, learner and teacher characteristics, and available resources. Of these factors, the single most critical aspect in choosing a teaching method is judging the fit of that method with the intended learning outcomes or objectives.

DOMAINS OF LEARNING

Learning can be described as development in one or more of three different domains: cognitive, affective, and psychomotor. Cognitive development, which involves thinking, cannot be directly observed but is seen through the behaviors or products of thinking. Affective development, which involves values and beliefs, cannot be directly observed either, and it is seen through attitudes, behaviors, and choices that express values.

Psychomotor development, which involves skilled movement, is directly observable in physical action. Program outcomes, course objectives (also referred to as outcomes), and module or daily objectives are written to reflect expected development across the three domains of learning. Nurses in practice rely on all three domains to provide care, so nurse educators need to design instruction, teach, and assess for student development in all three domains (Oermann & Gaberson, 2014).

Patients can view the physical care that nurses provide (psychomotor knowledge) and recognize that nurses have high ethical standards (Newport, 2012), which reflect nursing values and beliefs (affective knowledge). Patients, however, may not be aware of the intense thinking and planning that nurses engage in to promote health and prevent harm (cognitive knowledge). Despite the hidden nature of the thinking process in our observable work, the cognitive domain is often the easiest domain to address in writing objectives and in choosing teaching methods. In some teaching/learning situations, the affective and psychomotor aspects of learning are ignored or expected to develop without much attention, but educators who plan only for cognitive development should not be surprised when learners' beliefs and physical skills do not change with accumulation of information alone. Development in affective values and physical skills is often needed in concert with cognition for enacting complex new learning (Huckabay, 2009).

Some teaching strategies support learning in all three domains, whereas other strategies are more specific to learning in only one or two of the domains. Strategies chosen for a single class meeting do not need to represent each of the domains, but all domains should be included regularly for integrative experiences. It is important to note the hierarchical nature of each domain and to align the levels of learning objectives, teaching strategies, and evaluation methods. Descriptions of the levels within each learning domain and examples of activities that might be used to for teaching in that domain are in Tables 3.1, 3.2, and 3.3.

TABLE 3.1 Activities to Support Learning in the Cognitive Domain

Level	Definition	Examples of Teaching Strategies/Learning Activities
Remember	Recall previous information.	Practice definitions with flash cards, match items.
Understand	Comprehend the meaning.	Complete a crossword puzzle, represent images with words or words with images.
Apply	Use a concept in a new situation, carry out a procedure.	Interpret an equianalgesic chart to compare doses of two different narcotics.
Analyze	Distinguish between facts and inferences.	Discuss what is known versus what can be inferred about a patient's health situation.
Evaluate	Make judgments about the value of ideas or materials.	Compare a patient's activity plan with the collaborative goals set by the patient and health team.
Create	Build a structure or pattern from diverse elements.	Develop self-care learning materials for a patient or group of patients.

From Anderson et al. (2001).

TABLE 3.2 Activities to Support Learning in the Affective Domain

Level	Definition	Examples of Teaching Strategies/Learning Activities
Receive	Open to experience, willing to hear.	Listen to a lecture or story, watch a film.
Respond	React and participate actively.	Participate in discussions, ask questions, suggest interpretations.
Value	Attach values and express personal opinions.	Write a plan for personal health improvement.
Organize or conceptualize values	Reconcile internal conflicts; develop value system.	Write a philosophy of nursing that includes examples of nursing behaviors that reflect the philosophy.
Internalize or characterize values	Adopt belief system and philosophy.	Carry out a plan for personal health improvement.

From Krathwohl, Bloom, and Masia (1964).

TABLE 3.3 Activities to Support Learning in the Psychomotor Domain

Level	Definition	Examples of Teaching Strategies/Learning Activities
Imitation	Copy action of another; observe and replicate.	Watch a demonstration of how to safely log-roll a patient and repeat the action.
Manipulation	Reproduce activity from instruction or memory.	Practice positioning a patient with verbal coaching or written instructions for reference.
Precision	Execute skill reliably, independent of help.	Demonstrate coordination in using a walker.
Articulation	Adapt and integrate expertise to satisfy a nonstandard objective	Transfer patients from beds to chairs in a variety of situations.
Naturalization	Automated, unconscious mastery of activity and related skills at strategic level.	Practice taking blood pressures until able to accurately hear the pulse, watch the dial, and manipulate the equipment simultaneously.

From Dave (1970).

Supervising students practicing tracheal suctioning on task trainer manikins in the learning laboratory might support psychomotor skill development, but the activity lacks the context of care for a valued individual. Listening to an audio-recorded interview with a patient who has a debilitating disease with ineffective airway clearance might work well for supporting the affective objectives of valuing the patient perspective and cognitive objectives related to disease management, but not for psychomotor skill development. However, providing integrated care for an authentic patient in the clinical environment, a standardized patient in the clinical laboratory, or a simulated patient in the simulation laboratory can support development across all three domains. Nestel, Groom, Eikeland-Husebo, and O'Donnell (2011), in a systematic review of 47 educational simulation studies published from 2000–2010, found that the majority reported immediate improvements in learning after simulation-based interventions with positive outcomes involving skills, knowledge, and/or attitudes.

LEARNER CHARACTERISTICS

The characteristics of the intended learners, including their social and cognitive cultures, are important to consider in choosing teaching methods. Students who are not comfortable interacting with peers or learning in cooperation with peers need support to develop knowledge, skills, and attitudes for professional-level communication and collaboration. Disagreeing in a way that remains respectful and still furthers the discussion is a complex communication skill to develop, yet planning for that development is often ignored, based on an assumption that students begin higher education with such skills. Beginning clinical students often express levels of anxiety that require enormous skill, time, and effort to manage (Hutchinson & Goodin, 2013). Teachers can anticipate and plan for additional attention on helping students learn to manage their anxiety, rather than being surprised when the anxieties arising in learning settings overtake the scheduled learning topics.

When teaching strategies do not fit well with the characteristics of the learners, there is a greater need for resources. When learners have not developed the prerequisite knowledge and skills to support them in a later learning goal, the need for other resources, such as instructional time, increases. For example, if students admitted to an online program are familiar and comfortable with online technology, then orientation and learning related to the technology do not require as much instructional time or focused attention. However, when students admitted to an online program have little previous experience or no positive experiences with online learning, teachers will need to plan for extra time and effort to support the learners in developing skills as new technologies are introduced.

TEACHER CHARACTERISTICS

It would be unreasonable to expect that a teacher should be skilled in using every teaching method. The teacher's own comfort level is important to manage so that the focus of attention stays on learners and the learning process. However, stretching that comfort level to consider how assumptions about learning affect teaching choices can open the door to considering new teaching methods (Weimer, 2010). There is more than one way to teach any topic, so educators can choose from methods that fit both the learning objectives and the teaching expertise.

RESOURCES

Teaching method choices are sustainable when they are realistic for the reasonably available resources. Resources to consider in choosing teaching methods include time, space, support staff, technology, and materials.

Time is a most precious resource—for both teachers and learners. The teacher's time plan for using a particular teaching method should include the time in preparation, direct instruction, and providing formative feedback/coaching students. The students' time to be considered includes accessing the materials needed, preparatory assignments, instructional time, and any follow-up assignments. An experience that requires extensive instructional time should be planned only for the most important course and program goals.

Physical spaces and course enrollment can facilitate interaction or constrain teaching methods and activities. Large-class sections and lecture rooms make group interaction challenging, but not impossible. Even in lecture halls with unmovable desks, students can interact in pairs or clusters. Deslauriers, Schelew, and Wieman (2011) reported improved student learning outcomes from focusing on active learning strategies rather than on lectures, despite a large enrollment.

Availability and access to *support staff* can make the difference in the outcomes of some learning activities. Librarians can be amazing resource persons for students and faculty struggling to search for clinical evidence. Writing center staff can be helpful for students learning to write in the discipline of nursing and for faculty developing writing assignments. Technology experts can help assure that classroom plans for new software use or online resources go smoothly. In settings without support staff, the teacher should plan learning activities with the understanding that troubleshooting library database searches, coaching students to use software, or managing other technical challenges will add to the teacher's responsibilities.

Technology is a resource and a means to an end. When students are learning to manipulate a stethoscope, it is reasonable to focus both on developing auscultation skills and on the stethoscope as a tool, because nurses can expect to use stethoscopes throughout their careers for obtaining assessment data that will support clinical decisions. At times, however, technology that is not the direct focus of a learning objective becomes the focus of a misguided instructional effort. For example, leadership students learning the important skill of realistically budgeting for a clinical project might be directed to use a specific format or software for an assignment. If the format or software that learners are directed to use will require live instruction or tutorials and extensive practice, the teacher must consider whether learning to use the tool is a reasonable investment of student time. A larger investment in time and effort might be appropriate when learners will use the software program or other technology in the future workplace; however, that high level of investment is generally not worthwhile for a single assignment.

Elaborate *materials* and plans might not be a better fit than simple and inexpensive materials and methods for supporting a particular objective. For example, when students are practicing their first urinary catheter insertions, catheterizing a high-fidelity human patient simulator may not improve learning over working with a simple and far less costly static pelvic model. However, when the students are integrating assessments and interventions in more complex situations, being able to hear the simulated patient speak and express discomfort may add a level of realism that engages the student and improves the overall learning experience (Rystedt & Sjöblom, 2012).

PLANNING FOR ACTIVE LEARNING

Higher education has often been linked with a type of learning where students passively listen to their professors' wise thoughts, but a shift to promoting more active learning requires student engagement far beyond attendance. A focus on learner engagement and active learning is aligned with a general trend away from teacher-centered strategies and toward strategies focused on what students learn (Ambrose, Bridges, DiPietro, Lovett, & Norman, 2010).

Safe nursing practice relies heavily on application of the sciences. According to the President's Council of Advisors on Science and Technology (2012), approaches that engage students in active learning (as compared to lecture) lead to improved information retention, critical thinking development, and student persistence in STEM fields (science, technology, engineering, mathematics). Nursing students who are learning to base their practice on evidence from the sciences can benefit from active learning strategies as well.

Lecture, a frequently used teaching method in higher education, may call to mind an image of a teacher on the auditorium stage talking at an audience of students while the students doze off to sleep. Nurse educators individually may assert that they do not rely on lecture. However, Shindell (2011) surveyed nurse educators who had recently taught one or more prelicensure didactic courses in accredited prelicensure U.S. nursing programs. In that study, 75% of the 375 responding educators reported lecturing for at least half of their average class sessions. Lecture can be insidious in settings outside the classroom as well: when the post-clinical conference, the clinical laboratory session, or the simulation debriefing time involves the teacher doing most of the talking, those sessions have been subtly converted to extra lectures. The students have slipped from their intended roles as active participants back to being more passive recipients.

Lecture is a common teaching method in the large enrollment science classes that nursing students may take as prerequisites to nursing program courses, as well as large enrollment courses in nursing programs. Faced with teaching a science-based course to an enrollment of several hundred students, lecturing to the entire group might seem like the teacher's only reasonably efficient option, but the evidence indicates otherwise. In a widely reported study comparing two teaching methods, students in large physics course sections demonstrated more learning progress with the use of active and deliberate classroom practice as taught by inexperienced teachers than with traditional lecture taught by a highly experienced teacher. Active learning strategies about the physics concepts improved student attendance, increased engagement, and led to more than twice the learning as was demonstrated in the lecture sections (Deslauriers et al., 2011).

When teaching consists only of delivering a lecture, educators seem to expect that students can transform the lecturer's words directly into the students' authentic nursing actions. However, telling a student to remember and employ a list of airway clearance measures for their future patients is very different from asking the student to determine what types of airway clearance measures might be suitable for a specific elderly patient with an abdominal incision who is unable to sit up or walk. Applying principles and concepts to new situations requires active practice and coaching.

ACTION AND REFLECTION

Two processes are important for active learning: action and reflection. Taking part in meaningful activity followed by reflecting on the learning processes and outcomes transforms the learner from a passive recipient of someone else's thoughts to an active constructor of knowledge and meaning. This does not mean that all passive strategies should be abandoned. Interposing active and passive strategies together can create a rich opportunity for students to actively participate in learning and practice doing what they are expected to learn. For instance, a class session on substance abuse might be changed from continuous lecture to a series of activities: students completing a classroom survey of attitudes, pairing for brief discussion, participating in a large group discussion, viewing a related film clip, analyzing a short case study in a small group, synthesizing recommendations from the case analysis, and summarizing key learning points.

The passive activities of reading textbook chapters or watching a film can be shifted to more active learning by pairing those activities with specific reflection activities and expectations. Simple instructions can help the student become an active participant. "While you read this passage (or watch this film clip) about a recent news event, identify at least three specific opportunities for health promotion at the individual, family, and community level. Bring your list for discussion to the next class session." Rather than the teacher identifying extensive lists of examples for new concepts, asking the learners to identify and share additional examples of the concept in the environment tests their understanding of the concept and helps them find individual meanings for a concept.

DEVELOPING HIGHER LEVEL THINKING

Educators highly value critical thinking and aim to foster the development of critical thinking abilities among their graduates. Elder and Paul (2010) define critical thinking as "the process of analyzing and assessing thinking with a view to improving it" (p. 38). Terms that have similar meanings to critical thinking and are occasionally used interchangeably include higher order or higher level thinking, metacognition, critical reflection, and reflective thinking.

There are two aspects of critical thinking: ability and disposition. *Critical thinking ability* involves using higher level thinking skills such as conceptualizing, applying, analyzing, interpreting, inferring, explaining, evaluating, and synthesizing. *Critical thinking disposition* defines the characteristics of the ideal critical thinker: being habitually inquisitive, open-minded, mindful of alternatives, well-informed, fair-minded, and honest in facing personal biases (Ennis, 2010; Facione, 1990). Critical thinking incorporates the elements of thought and applies the universal intellectual standards.

The ability to think critically is discipline neutral; however, the context in which critical thinking is applied may be discipline specific. For example, how a nursing graduate applies critical thinking to nursing practice is very different from how an engineering graduate applies critical thinking to engineering practice. Both of these graduates may use similar higher-order thinking skills; however, the context in which these thinking skills are applied will be different.

TEACHING METHODS TO PROMOTE CRITICAL THINKING

There are many teaching methods that promote the development of critical thinking, including case studies, concept mapping, collaborative learning, problem-based learning (PBL), service learning, and gaming. Teachers can structure learning activities to develop critical thinking by focusing attention on reflection, providing reasons, and developing alternatives.

Teachers may support learners to reflect on a situation or experience by posing questions or structuring a written assignment to include reflection. Posing questions such as "How do you know?" and "What are the reasons?" help learners identify the reasons for their views and remind them to seek reasons for others' views (Ennis, 2010). To encourage learners to develop alternative hypotheses and evaluate alternate points of view, the teacher can prompt the learner to explain from a different perspective. Including targeted questions such as those in Table 3.4 help learners apply the Universal Intellectual Standards to their thinking (Elder & Paul, 2010).

TABLE 3.4 Questions Based on Universal Intellectual Standards Essential to Sound Clinical Reasoning

Standard	Questions
Clarity	Could you elaborate further on that point? Could you express that point in another way? Could you give me an illustration? Could you give me an example?
Accuracy	Is that really true? How could we check that out? How could we find out if that is true? What evidence is there to support the validity of your clinical thinking?
Precision	Could you give me more details? Could you be more specific?
Relevance	How is that connected to the question? How does that bear on the issue?
Depth	How does your answer address the complexities in the question? How are you taking into account the problems in the question? Are you dealing with the most significant factors?
Breadth	Do we need to consider another point of view? Is there another way to look at this question? What would this look like from the point of view of a conflicting theory, hypothesis, or conceptual scheme?
Logic	Does this really make sense? Is this consistent with what we know about the issue or problem?
Significance	Is this the most important problem to consider? Is this the central idea to focus on? Which of these facts are most important?
Fairness	Do I have a vested interest in this issue? Am I representing the viewpoints of others in a way that is fair and balanced?

From Hawkins, Elder, and Paul (2010), pp. 11–12. Reprinted by permission, 2013.

TEACHING METHODS

In the following section, a variety of teaching methods are described in categories such as independent learning methods, small-group methods, and large-class methods. However, each of the methods can be used in more than one way. For instance, reading is described as an independent learning activity, but there may be times that reading aloud in the classroom suits the instructional purpose. Discussion can take place in pairs, small groups of three to four, or with the entire class.

INDEPENDENT LEARNING METHODS

Reading

Assigning passages for students to read in a textbook or scholarly journal is a simple instructional plan, but many students find that reading is a difficult way to learn. Learning through reading requires understanding, then interpreting and synthesizing the text into useful application.

Students often report starting at the beginning of the assigned reading for the week, reading some of the assignment every day, but never finishing a week's reading before the next week's assigned chapters are due. By default, the chapters at the end of each week's list are the least likely to have been read. Two simple instructional strategies can improve the reading to learn experience: limiting the assignment to the most pertinent readings, and identifying the recommended sections by priority order rather than sequential order. Rather than assigning 10 chapters totaling 800 pages each week, assigning only the most important passages from each chapter or the most important chapters improves the possibility that students might be able to finish a week's reading assignment. Prioritizing the passages among the assigned readings that are required versus those recommended for enrichment or review helps students make informed choices.

Teachers also help students improve reading comprehension by suggesting specific comprehension strategies along with reading assignments. Levels of support for comprehension increase as the teacher introduces reading strategies, provides the rationale for a particular strategy, and even models the strategy (Zhang, 2011). Three broad categories of reading strategies include problem-solving strategies, support strategies, and global strategies (Mokhtari & Reichard, 2002). Problem-solving strategies deal with cognitive and metacognitive approaches such as reading slowly and carefully or paying close attention. Support strategies include approaches such as taking notes while reading or paraphrasing/summarizing text. Global strategies invoke the meaning and purpose of the reading, and the use of context.

Strategies that teachers can recommend or model for improving reading comprehension are listed in Table 3.5. Many of the strategies can be incorporated in both classroom and online activities.

TABLE 3.5 Teaching Strategies for Improving Reading Comprehension

Type of Strategy	Rationale	Activities to Recommend and Model
Activate prior knowledge	Connecting learners' existing information and experiences to a new topic improves understanding and memory.	Preview headings or key concepts, make predictions.
Use graphic organizers	Using visual representations helps students identify, organize, and remember important ideas.	Create timelines, framed outlines, concept maps, story maps, and Venn diagrams.
Teach comprehension monitoring strategies	Students keeping track of their understanding as they read and implementing "fix-up" strategies when identifying breakdown.	Keeping track: Note confusing or difficult words and concepts, create images, stop after each paragraph to summarize, and generate questions. When understanding breaks down: re-read, re-state, use context to figure out unknown words or ideas.

(continued)

TABLE 3.5 Teaching Strategies for Improving Reading Comprehension (*continued*)

Type of Strategy	Rationale	Activities to Recommend and Model
Teach summarization skills	Consolidating large amounts of information (several paragraphs or passages) into key ideas.	Identify topic sentences, identify words or concepts that represent a list of related terms, practice summarizing, and use graphic organizers to summarize.
Teach students to ask and answer questions	Asking questions before, during, and after reading supports engagement and understanding.	Ask explicit and inferential questions, identify whether the answers to teacher's questions are likely to be found in text or require an inference.
Multi-component comprehension strategy Instruction	Combining several comprehension strategies into an organizational system for reading.	Teach students to independently use strategies. Support students in generalizing strategy use across contexts and courses. Actively engage students in using comprehension strategies through cooperative learning, group discussions, and other interactions.

From Boardman (2008).

Writing

Clear writing is important across nursing roles and settings. "Nurses document patient care, communicate via writing with each other and colleagues in other disciplines, create educational materials for patients and staff, develop organizational policies and procedures, and compose material for publication" (Troxler, Vann, & Oermann, 2011, p. 280). Writing effectively is a means for health care career progression: crystallizing complex and sometimes opposing ideas into a coherent written message is a critical leadership skill. Gimenez (2012) suggested that future development of the nursing discipline depends on educators explicitly teaching students to participate in constructing nursing knowledge through writing. Exhibit 3.1 identifies core competencies that can be developed through writing.

However, communicating effectively in writing is not easy. The basic writing skills that students attain in secondary schools do not extend to the types of writing needed for professionals. Examples of common writing assignments used in higher education to prepare nurses for professional writing are provided in Exhibit 3.2.

Students are admitted to nursing programs with a wide range of writing skills. Nursing faculty members can expect to teach students how to write using vocabulary and formatting requirements specific to health professions as well as to support students in remediating basic writing skills. Many schools have student support services available for writing development and remediation, but those services do not take the place of nursing faculty emphasizing written communication consistently throughout the curriculum.

EXHIBIT 3.1 Core Competencies of Advanced Writing

• Organization	• Process
• Argument, evidence, and logic	• Accuracy
• Audience and voice	• Scholarly identity
• Content	• Sources
• Mechanics, grammar	• Expression
• Conceptualization and developing ideas	• Critique

From Ondrusek (2012). Reprinted with permission, 2013.

EXHIBIT 3.2 Types of Writing Assignments

• Appraisal	• Narrative
• Book report	• Pamphlet
• Blog	• Patient instructions
• Care plan	• Poetry
• Case analysis	• Policy/Procedure
• Critique	• Process reflection
• Evidence synthesis	• Project proposal
• Film report	• Research paper
• Journal	• Summary
• Letter	• Technical description
• Memo	• Wiki

There are a number of strategies for helping students develop effective writing skills, including the use of assignment rubrics, successive drafts, and feedback from peers and instructors. Table 3.6 indicates teaching strategies that support students' writing skills development.

Reflection

Benner, Sutphen, Leonard, and Day (2009) describe the process of helping students learn to identify what is important in a given situation as *teaching for salience*. One of the key strategies they describe as an exemplar of good teaching is that of helping learners reflect on practice. Coaching for reflection requires active engagement of the teacher, whereas reflecting requires active engagement of the learner. Exhibit 3.3 provides a list of questions that could frame reflection in a dialogue or in a writing activity such as journaling or blogging.

Contract Learning

There are several variations to contract learning, depending on the format of the course, the level of learners, and the purpose. These include a team learning contract, a contract learning approach, or an individual learning contract with a student.

Team Learning Contract. Teachers may use a team learning contract to specify performance behaviors for members completing a group assignment. A team learning contract is helpful because the learners define what behaviors and outcomes are

TABLE 3.6 Strategies for Improving Writing and Structuring Writing Assignments

Strategy	Teacher's Action	Rationale
Detailed rubrics	Provide specific criteria for content and quality.	Communicate expectations.
Exemplar papers	Share excellent papers written by previous students (with their permission) as examples.	Clarify intended level and scope of assignment.
Drafts with feedback	Provide feedback on successive versions of the work.	Expect revision of the initial draft.
Sequential section writing	Provide feedback and guidance on one section or aspect of a larger project before the next section is written.	Redirect efforts early.
Peer coaching	Facilitate student peers providing feedback to one another and revising their own work before they submit for teacher feedback.	Learn from how others conceptualize. Learn to give and receive effective feedback about writing.

From Sallee, Hallett, and Tierney (2011); Troxler et al. (2011); Peinhardt and Hagler (2013).

EXHIBIT 3.3 Questions to Frame Reflection

- What is new to you about this material?
- What did you already know?
- Does any point contradict what you already knew or believed?
- What patterns of reasoning (or data) does the speaker/author offer as evidence?
- How convincing do you find the speakers'/authors' reasoning or data?
- Is there any line of reasoning that you do not follow?
- Is this reasoning familiar to you from other courses?
- What don't you understand?
- What questions remain in your mind?

From Nilson (2010), p. 169. Reprinted with permission, 2013.

acceptable to the team, and the team is accountable for enforcing the contract standards among members (Nilson, 2010). This type of approach is useful with adult learners who want to set performance parameters and team behavior expectations.

Contract Learning. Educators may use a contract learning approach to managing a course. Using this approach, the teacher provides the learner with a menu of options available to demonstrate course learning outcomes, and establishes the minimum standards for satisfactory performance. The learner contracts with the teacher for the number and types of learning assignments that will be completed to achieve the desired level of performance. This approach allows the motivated, self-directed learner the ability to contract with the teacher to complete a series of learning assignments that demonstrate a high level of course performance (Nilson, 2010). One drawback to this approach is that it may be challenging for learners who are less motivated, not self-directed, or unable to articulate learning needs.

Individual Learning Contract. A learning contract specifies what the learner must accomplish to meet the course outcomes. The learning contract will specify individual student learning objectives, learning assignments, evaluation methods, and deadlines (Nilson, 2010). Depending on the structure of the course and the purpose of the learning contract, the teacher may initiate the learning contract, or the learner may initiate it. It is common for teachers to initiate the learning contract as a tool to clarify requirements with a student who is not meeting course expectations. In contrast, a student-initiated learning contract allows the self-directed student to individualize a learning experience.

Learning contracts are frequently used to guide directed or independent study courses, graduate courses, and fieldwork. Learning contracts may also be used with undergraduate students, or to help students who need to work at their own pace. The principles of andragogy support the use of learning contracts to help facilitate adult learning. In nursing education, it is common to use learning contracts to establish learning outcomes, assignments, and deadlines for clinical practice or practicum courses. The teacher provides the overall structure and expectations for establishing the learning contract. Both the teacher and learner mutually agree on the requirements of the learning contract. A well-written learning contract includes the following items: measurable learning objectives; learning activities and resources required to meet the objectives; deliverables or evidence to demonstrate that the outcomes have been met; and the specific criteria for evaluation.

Concept Mapping

Concept mapping is commonly used as an instructional method to facilitate the development of critical thinking. Concept mapping encourages active learning by helping students connect related concepts, understand interrelationships between concepts, and construct a visual representation of how concepts relate to one another (Chabeli, 2010; Henige, 2010). Concept mapping may be more effective at promoting knowledge retention and transfer than passive teaching methods such as reading text or attending lectures (Henige, 2010). Concept mapping is an appropriate teaching strategy when the faculty member is teaching cognitive information and wants to facilitate active learner participation.

Students construct a concept map to provide a visual representation of a concept. This approach allows students to "meaningfully connect, link and integrate new ideas, thoughts, concepts and statements to their existing body of knowledge" (Chabeli, 2010, p. 71). Concept mapping allows students to describe the bigger picture of the phenomenon by linking, cross-linking, and describing the relationships (Chabeli, 2010; Henige, 2010). The concept map helps the faculty member to assess a student's understanding of the concept and the connections among concepts.

Concept maps may be unstructured or highly structured. A commonly used structure for concept mapping involves placing the major concept in the center of the map and locating subconcepts around the major concept.

In nursing education, concept mapping is used to help students organize assessment data, integrate interventions and the nursing process, and understand the interrelationships among data. One advantage of concept mapping is that it allows students to build on prior knowledge and assimilate new information in a way that is meaningful to the student. Other advantages include facilitation of active engagement with content, the development of deductive and inductive reasoning, and the ability to cluster information. Concept mapping is effective for visual learners.

Variations of concept mapping include mind mapping and argument mapping. Mind maps have a high level of abstraction and use lines and associative words to link pictures, words, and diagrams to form a map of the associations between ideas. Argument maps have a low level of abstraction and use boxes, lines, and linking words to show the inferences between claims and supporting evidence (Davies, 2011). These different forms of knowledge mapping help foster meaningful learning, allow learners to scaffold or build upon previous learning, and facilitate critical thinking.

Self-Paced Modules/Reusable Learning Objects

A reusable learning object (RLO) is a small, self-contained educational unit that may include objectives, content, interactive learning activities, animations, narrated text, visual images, self-assessments, and feedback tools (Windle, McCormick, Dandrea, & Wharrad, 2011). RLOs may be used to introduce new content, reinforce or clarify existing content, or provide demonstrations (Nilson, 2010). They may be used independently or combined with other RLOs to teach larger content areas. Some teachers use RLOs when they "flip" the classroom by having the learners review the RLO prior to coming to class and using class time for more active learning activities.

When developing and designing an RLO, it is important for the teacher to keep the RLO focused on a small area of content, clearly define the scope of the RLO, and incorporate strategies that facilitate ease of navigation and interactivity. Some teachers use a storyboard approach to help facilitate the development of RLOs. Most RLOs are between 2 and 15 minutes in length.

The benefits of RLOs include the ability of the student to engage in self-paced learning, actively engage with content, review content, and perform self-assessment to identify learning needs. Learners highly value the flexible anytime and anywhere access that RLOs afford and appreciate the opportunity to review challenging content while advancing at their own pace. RLOs can be more effective than traditional lecture. Windle et al. (2011) found that learners in an RLO cohort answered more questions correctly than learners in the traditional lecture format.

SMALL-GROUP METHODS

Discussion

A good discussion is engaging, explores diverse ideas, and helps participants clarify their own thinking in the face of colleagues' alternative ideas. However, poorly planned classroom discussions can take up a large amount of time with little learning impact. Even after a well-focused discussion, students may not understand what points in the discussion are important to remember or apply in future work. Periodic restatements and summaries by group members can help everyone stay on track and remember key points.

A clear learning objective and agreed-upon ground rules help frame a discussion. Will students raise their hands, speak out at will, or indicate in some other way that they would like to have the floor? Is participation from all required or optional? How will the group manage those who dominate the discussion, avoid participation, move off topic, or show disrespectful behavior to other group members? The process of setting group discussion norms collaboratively creates a good starting point for a respectful and scholarly discussion. Examples of teacher responses that enhance discussion are in Table 3.7.

TABLE 3.7 Teacher Responses That Facilitate Discussion

If student contribution is...	Possible Teacher's Response to Facilitate Discussion
accurate	Provide some reinforcement such as a nod or brief affirming statement.
correct but only one of many	Ask another student to extend or add to the response; avoid early closure.
incomplete	Follow up with a question that directs the student to include more information.
unclear	Try to rephrase it; then ask if this is what the student means.
seemingly wrong	Follow up with one or more gentle Socratic questions designed to lead the student to discover the error. Invite the student to explain, clarify, or elaborate.

Adapted from Nilson (2010). Reprinted with permission, 2013.

Experiential Learning

Activities that engage the senses help learners understand and recall concepts. Trying to breathe through a straw for several minutes evokes both physical sensations to remember and a beginning sense of understanding how arduous and frightening it can be to feel short of breath. Taking part in a group exercise such as building a bridge with dry spaghetti or assembling a puzzle can open frank discussion about the dynamics of working in groups to complete tasks. Sorting a collection of items in three different ways helps promote understanding of competing classification systems or nomenclatures. Although doing kinesthetic activities in class takes time, the additional understanding that learners develop through the activity and facilitated reflection is valuable for lasting learning (Yoder-Wise & Kowalski, 2012).

Case Study

A case study is "a story with an educational message" (Herreid, 2011, p. 31). Case studies may be included in a lecture, discussion, or small-group learning activity in classroom or online environments. Case studies actively engage learners by providing opportunities to apply concepts or content to real or simulated scenarios (Nilson, 2010). In large classes, educators can use an audience response system to engage learners and increase interaction around case decisions.

Case studies may present a one-time snapshot of the situation or a continuous, unfolding story over time. Some case studies use a sequential-interactive approach where the learners move through the case study by making decisions or narrowing down solutions and requesting additional information from the teacher to ultimately solve the case (Nilson, 2010). Whatever approach is used for the case study, it is important for the teacher to debrief the learners by discussing the problems and solutions identified through the case study with the learners.

In nursing education, case studies can provide practice opportunities in assessing situations and making decisions. Case studies vary in length from short bullet-style cases (two to three sentences), through minicases or vignettes (two to three paragraphs), to lengthy multipage cases (Nilson, 2010). Teachers may purchase or create the case studies; frequently, nurse educators develop their own case studies based on prior clinical practice experiences. When creating a case study, the teacher develops objectives and questions that correspond with the case study to engage the learner and foster the development of higher level thinking abilities (analysis, synthesis, evaluation).

Cooperative Learning

Cooperative learning is a "form of highly structured group work that focuses on problem solving" (Millis, 2009, p. 17). Cooperative learning increases retention, engages learners, facilitates critical thinking, and promotes deeper learning. Teachers facilitate students' positive interdependence, individual accountability, and group processing by assigning tasks that require cooperation and cannot be completed alone (Millis, 2010). Educators build individual accountability into cooperative learning activities by having learners complete self, peer, and group evaluation of contributions to the group's project and functioning. Learners who participate in cooperative learning activities learn group processing skills such as managing group dynamics, ensuring participation by all group members, treating group member's contributions with respect, and arriving at group consensus. Teachers can incorporate heterogeneity into cooperative learning by forming groups with diversity in characteristics such as individual ability, diverse perspectives, gender, academic major, or age. Group heterogeneity provides the opportunity to work with and learn from others who are different.

The teacher's role in cooperative learning is to provide a structure that facilitates problem solving, assists learners in managing group process, and helps learners to synthesize and apply their learning. It is important for the teacher to clearly articulate the purpose of the cooperative learning activity, help the learners understand the value of the learning activity, provide clear instructions, and facilitate closure on completion of the learning activity. When creating groups for cooperative learning, the teacher should strive to keep the groups small in size, usually between two and four students; base group membership on principles of group heterogeneity; and allow the groups to worktogether long enough to form positive relationships (Millis, 2002). Teaching methods that promote cooperative learning can be used in traditional classroom or online learning environments, including think-write-pair-share, group investigations, three-step interviews, wikis, blogs, threaded discussions, and the use of clickers for interactive academic gaming.

Problem-Based Learning (PBL)

PBL is a student-centered active learning method that guides students to solve context-dependent, real-world problems through collaborative group work (Oja, 2011). Benefits of PBL include development of critical thinking skills, collaborative work competence, and effective team communication (Chunta & Katrancha, 2010; Oja, 2011). PBL allows students to be actively engaged in their learning, acquire new information in the context in which they will be using it, and create a link between theory and practice. Some educational programs deliver the entire curriculum using a PBL approach, whereas other programs use PBL techniques to deliver selected learning experiences. PBL has been used as a teaching-learning method in traditional theory-based, online, and clinical practice courses as well as to facilitate nursing staff development (Chunta & Katrancha, 2010).

The many different approaches to PBL share common attributes, including that (a) problems are used as the central focus to initiate or motivate learning, (b) students collaborate in small groups and work over a period of time to solve problems, (c) a faculty member serves as facilitator of learning and coach for managing group processes, (d) students initiate and direct learning, and (e) the curriculum includes limited or no lectures and provides time for self-study (Oja, 2011; Schmidt, Rotgans, & Yew, 2011).

There are four basic stages in implementing a PBL method. The first stage is problem analysis, where introductory information is given to the students, and the group identifies what is known and unknown about the situation. The second stage is brainstorming, where the group identifies resources to meet learning needs. During this stage, the group may also pose questions to the facilitator or their peers to clarify the situation. The third stage is self-directed learning, where each group member researches and gathers information to share. The final stage is solution testing, where group members share resources and information. During this stage, the group begins to test solutions by applying new knowledge to solve the situation. This process is ongoing until the group reaches a consensus that the problem or situation is resolved (Chunta & Katrancha, 2010).

PBL requires the teacher to actively facilitate group learning rather than deliver content. Because PBL relies on students building upon prior content knowledge, PBL may not be the most effective teaching method for entirely new content. It can take students time to adapt to active teaching methods, such as PBL, if they have been previously socialized to more passive teaching methods. To help students transition, the teacher can introduce PBL gradually and explain how the roles of educator and student are different in PBL.

Simulation, Standardized Patients, Role Play, and Drama

"Simulation is a technique, not a technology, to replace or amplify real experiences with guided experiences, often immersive in nature, that evoke or replicate substantial aspects of the real world in a fully interactive fashion" (Gaba, 2007, p. 126). The range of fidelity, or faithfulness, to reality in simulation is wide. At the low-fidelity end, learners practice injecting a medication into a practice pad or even a piece of fruit to feel the sense of puncturing through a barrier, while at the high end of simulation fidelity, learners provide care to standardized patients enacting health conditions or manikins programmed with realistic physiologic responses.

Simulation can support learning in the cognitive, affective, and psychomotor domains. Gropelli (2010) provided an example of using simulation to teach nursing ethics. Participating in a scripted drama or theatrical presentation is a specific type of role play that has been used to help nursing students learn about end-of-life care. Roles or drama are most effective for learning experiences when followed by thoughtful debriefing and reflection (Welsh & Lowry, 2011). Teaching with clinical simulation is described in detail in Chapter 5.

Teaching Others and Presentations

There is nothing like developing a presentation to encourage immersion in a topic. Through preparing and giving presentations, students have the opportunity to learn the same way that many teachers have learned unfamiliar content themselves. Organizing a presentation forces thinking about what information is needed, what the audience already knows, and how to explain a complex topic. Presentations focus on information in a chosen or assigned content area but have the additional advantage of providing real practice in the authentic workplace skill of teaching or explaining a concept to others.

Although the student presenter has an active role in learning through the preparation and delivery of a presentation, the other students observing the presentation stay in the positions of passive learners unless their roles are restructured. Assigning the audience members to some of the roles traditionally held by the teacher, such as moderator, timekeeper, provider of positive feedback, and provider of suggestions for further improvement changes the experience of the audience members to active participants in the learning. Engaging each of the students in some role helps adjust the experience to be more collegial and avoid a presenter/audience distinction.

Recording their presentations provides students the opportunity to see how they look and sound as presenters, and it allows for repeated or asynchronous viewing. Class members can provide feedback live or through online interactive video software programs (Smith & Sodano, 2011).

Service Learning

Service learning, a form of experiential education, extends opportunity beyond the classroom by allowing students to solve problems and apply generalized or abstract knowledge to the context of a real-world problem (Seifer & Connors, 2007; Taggart & Crisp, 2011). The evidence suggests that student participation in service learning increases engagement in learning, promotes a positive attitude toward civic involvement, and improves academic outcomes such as persistence, retention, and course completion (Taggart & Crisp, 2011). Service learning is distinguished from volunteer work by the primary goal of learning through providing service.

To effectively implement service learning, the teacher facilitates discovery learning and critical reflection to ensure that new knowledge, concepts, and skills are meaningfully linked to the learner's personal experiences (Seifer & Connors, 2007). Characteristics of effective service-learning experiences include joint planning between the academic institution and community partner, reciprocity between partners, clearly defined roles and responsibilities, effective communication among all parties, and a comprehensive student orientation to the service-learning project.

LARGE-CLASS METHODS

Lecture

A well-organized and enthusiastic lecture can be an inspiring event, while a lecture in which the presenter reads the slides aloud can lead to learners daydreaming. Exhibit 3.4 describes advantages of lecture as a teaching method.

EXHIBIT 3.4 Advantages of Lecturing

- Inspiring teachers can stimulate student interest.
- Textbooks can be supplemented with the most current information.
- Lecturing may give the teacher a sense of controlling the classroom.
- All students are exposed to the same information.

From Millis (2012).

Teachers organizing and preparing lectures may learn about the intended content through their own active engagement in the process; however, the students attending a lecture often remain passive. Teachers who are afraid they might not know the answers to student questions might be relieved to read from slides or notes without much interaction, while learners who are uncomfortable with communication might be relieved to listen to a lecture and avoid interacting with peers or teachers. However, unless students are engaged, they are unlikely to remain attentive and retain information from the lecture.

The key to keeping students engaged is to divide a longer lecture into several mini-lectures and stop talking every few minutes while students participate in active thinking tasks. Tasks that help students understand what they are hearing might be generating examples of the concept under discussion, taking part in a kinesthetic activity related to the concept, or applying the concept to solve a problem. Even in a large lecture hall with fixed seating, students can do a think-write-pair-share, draw an illustration, or respond using a student-response system to assess their understanding of the content (Gill, 2011). Exhibit 3.5 describes teacher actions that improve the effectiveness of lectures.

EXHIBIT 3.5 Suggestions for an Effective Lecture

- Determine intended learning outcomes
- Budget extra time for questions and interaction
- Subdivide content in 15-minute chunks
- Intersperse lecture with learning activities
- Use attention grabbers to begin
- Incorporate visuals, examples, and restatements
- Engage students in recapping key points

From Nilson (2010).

Questioning

Questions are a powerful tool for understanding what learners are thinking and helping learners organize and expand their thinking. However, a teacher's question can strike fear into the heart of a learner who is overly worried about what answer the teacher expects.

Brookfield (2012) describes supporting development of critical thinking through asking learners first about the general ideas or concepts being presented, then later asking more direct questions about the learner's own ideas. He suggests a process of asking learners questions related to identifying their assumptions, checking their assumptions, seeing multiple viewpoints, and taking informed actions.

One strategy to improve teaching skill in questioning is to identify pertinent questions related to Paul's Elements of Thought and ask the individual or group to respond to them. Table 3.8 provides examples of questions teachers might ask to facilitate deeper and more expansive thought on a clinical situation or other topic.

Not all queries are posed in the form of a question. A request that begins with "please share…" or "tell me more…" implies a question, yet may sound less threatening than a direct question. A specific type of questioning is Socratic questioning, in which the teacher leads the student or group to uncover their knowledge and make connections among concepts through a series of exploratory questions.

Demonstration/Return Demonstration

Demonstration, a teaching method frequently used in clinical practice and laboratory settings, may be incorporated into classroom sessions through display of experiments or problem-solving techniques (Nilson, 2010). Demonstration facilitates learning for students who learn through assimilation or convergence, or who consider themselves visual learners. A return demonstration by the learner supports a kinesthetic preference in learning. Demonstration is discussed more fully in Chapter 7.

Educational Games

Educational games are effective in reinforcing knowledge, building a sense of community, and creating a relaxed atmosphere that facilitates comprehension of content (Blakely, Skirton, Cooper, Allum, & Nelmes, 2009). Many students perceive games

TABLE 3.8 Using a Checklist for Clinical Reasoning to Generate Questions

Element of Reasoning	Example Questions
All clinical reasoning has a PURPOSE.	Can you state your purpose clearly? What is the objective of your clinical reasoning? Does your reasoning focus throughout on your clinical goal? Is your clinical goal realistic?
All clinical reasoning is an attempt to figure something out, to settle some QUESTION, to solve some PROBLEM.	What clinical question are you trying to answer? Are there other ways to think about the question? Can you divide the question into subquestions? Is this a question that has more than one right answer, or can there be more than one reasonable answer? Does this question require clinical judgment rather than facts alone?
All clinical reasoning is based on ASSUMPTIONS.	What assumptions are you making? Are they justified? How are your assumptions shaping your point of view? Which of your assumptions might reasonably be questioned?
All clinical reasoning is done from some POINT OF VIEW.	What is your point of view? What insights is it based on? What are its weaknesses? What other points of view should be considered in reasoning through this problem? What are the strengths and weaknesses of these viewpoints? Are you fairmindedly considering the insights behind these viewpoints?
All clinical reasoning is based on DATA, INFORMATION, and EVIDENCE.	To what extent is your reasoning supported by relevant data? Do the data suggest explanations that differ from those you have given? How clear, accurate, and relevant are the data to the clinical question at issue? Have you gathered data sufficient to reach a valid conclusion?
All clinical reasoning is expressed through, and shaped by, CONCEPTS and THEORIES.	What key concepts and theories are guiding your clinical reasoning? What alternative explanations might be possible, given these concepts and theories? Are you clear and precise in using clinical concepts and theories in your reasoning? Are you distorting ideas to fit your agenda?
All clinical reasoning contains INFERENCES or INTERPRETATIONS by which we draw CONCLUSIONS and give meaning to data.	To what extent do the data support your clinical conclusions? Are your inferences consistent with each other? Are there other reasonable inferences that should be considered?
All clinical reasoning leads somewhere, that is, has IMPLICATIONS and CONSEQUENCES.	What implications and consequences follow from your reasoning? If we accept your line of reasoning, what implications or consequences are likely? What other implications or consequences are possible or probable?

From Hawkins et al. (2010), pp. 5–7. Reprinted by permission, 2013.

as positive and motivational; however, some learners experience anxiety, embarrassment, and intimidation with the peer competition aspect of gaming (Blakely et al., 2009).

Educational games can be high or low technology and are classified by genre such as adventure, music, puzzle, racing, role play, simulation, sports, and strategy. Learners playing high-tech simulation or strategy games may use virtual reality or interactive video gaming to experience real-life situations or events that facilitate learning and decision making. Teachers are using three-dimensional virtual reality (such as Second Life®) to provide experiential virtual environments where learners are immersed in real-time interactions (Skiba, 2009). Low-tech games such as question-and-answer board games, team quizzes, card games, and tossing the ball to answer the question on-the-spot are effective in reinforcing learning.

The teacher should match the fit between the goal for the education session (i.e., delivering new content or reinforcing information) and the readiness of the learners to participate in the game. To effectively use gaming, teachers should be confident in their ability to lead the gaming session and be able to adjust it, dependent on the learners' responses. Logistical factors such as the amount of time, class size, and the teaching environment might be constraints to implementing gaming.

Film

Cinemeducation is the use of movies or film clips to teach concepts, facilitate discussion, and foster critical thinking (Wilson, Blake, Taylor, & Hannings, 2013). Movies create a controlled learning environment to facilitate learning and an opportunity to experience some situations firsthand (Wilson et al., 2013). One drawback of using movies is that sometimes learners make unsupported inferences about what they observe and they may not have the opportunity to ask questions as they would in a live practice situation. The teacher can ask specific questions to guide learners in identifying inferences from the movie and considering additional information they would obtain if they could interact with the characters.

The teacher should preview the film and ensure that it supports the desired concept, then provide learners with objectives to guide the experience and reflective questions to stimulate critical thinking. The students might submit responses to the teacher for evaluation or discuss responses with peers. Another approach is to have them write about specific concepts seen in the movie. Wilson et al. (2013) used this type of approach to teach family assessment; after viewing a full-length film that depicted a problem affecting a family or public health, learners completed a formal family assessment based on data presented in the film.

Debate

Debate helps learners develop communication skills, structure logical arguments, and engage in rebuttals. Teachers can use debate with small or large groups of learners. A common format for debate involves assigning groups of learners opposing positions on a controversial topic. The teacher provides the structure, facilitates learners' argument development, poses logical questions, manages group dynamics and interpersonal communications, and facilitates learners' reflection. Nurse educators frequently use debate to facilitate thinking about ethical issues. Debate encourages learners to develop logical arguments and impromptu fact-based responses about controversial issues.

Narrative Pedagogy/Storytelling

The use of stories for teaching and learning is naturally engaging and highly flexible. Storytelling formats can range from a simple face-to-face verbal or audio recording recounting an experience to a polished multimedia production. "Narrative requires

EXHIBIT 3.6 Typical Features of Narratives/Stories

- Specific rather than generic events
- Specific time and place settings
- People are involved in the events
- Include moment-by-moment thoughts, feelings, and sensory perceptions
- Include a setting, theme, plot, and resolution
- Audience members feel as if they have entered a different world

From Sanford and Emmott (2012).

readers to produce rich and complex mental representations. It offers one of the major means through which the experiences of other people, different cultures, and distant times may be conveyed, and it expands our virtual experience of the world. Typically, narratives manipulate not only our knowledge of things, but also our impressions of how people feel, judge, and react in a multitude of situations" (Sanford & Emmott, 2012, p. xi).

The same experience can be told as a story from different perspectives and with different themes in mind. For example, stories told on a nursing unit to newly hired staff may have the purpose of a cautionary tale, an orientation to the unit culture, establishment of a hierarchy, or providing other information. Exhibit 3.6 describes features common to narratives and stories used to teach.

Although storytelling is common to many purposes, educators have systematically investigated the use of narrative in nursing. "Narrative pedagogy is a research-based interpretive phenomenological pedagogy that gathers teachers and students into converging conversations wherein new possibilities for practice and education can be envisioned" (Ironside, 2006, p. 479).

The wide availability of digital media has provided many options for narratives, including videos and podcasts. A simple recording of a story in the patient's own voice could provide the prompt for an engaging class discussion or other assignment. Teachers need to obtain written permission from the storyteller before recording and sharing narratives.

SUMMARY

The educator selecting a teaching method should consider the fit of that method with the learning objectives, learner and teacher characteristics, and available resources. Of these factors, the single most critical aspect in choosing a teaching method is judging the fit of that method with the intended learning outcomes or objectives.

Learning can be described as development in one or more of three different domains: cognitive, affective, and psychomotor. Some teaching strategies support learning in all three domains, whereas other strategies are more specific to learning in only one or two of the domains.

The characteristics of the intended learners, including their social and cognitive cultures, are important to consider in choosing teaching methods. A teacher does not have to be skilled in using every method. It is important for the teacher to be comfortable with the methods chosen so that the focus of attention stays on learners and the learning process. Choices of teaching method are sustainable when they are realistic for the reasonably available resources. Resources to consider in choosing teaching methods include time, space, support staff, technology, and materials.

A focus on learner engagement and active learning is aligned with a general trend away from teacher-centered strategies and toward strategies focused on what students learn. Two processes are important for active learning: action and reflection. Taking part in some meaningful activity followed by reflecting on the learning processes and outcomes transforms the learner from a passive recipient of someone else's thoughts to a constructor of knowledge and meaning. There are many teaching methods for active learning that promote the development of critical thinking. These include case studies, concept mapping, collaborative learning, PBL, service learning, and gaming.

Teaching methods were categorized in this chapter as independent learning, small-group, and large-class methods. However, each of the methods can be used in more than one way. Independent learning methods include reading; writing; reflection; contract learning (including a team learning contract, contract learning approach to a course, and an individual learning contract); concept mapping; and RLOs. Small-group methods presented in the chapter were discussion; experiential methods; case study; cooperative learning; PBL; simulation (including standardized patients, role play, and drama); presentations; and service learning. Large-class methods include lecture, questioning, demonstration, educational games, film (and other media), debate, and narrative pedagogy/storytelling. Each of these teaching methods was discussed in the chapter.

REFERENCES

Ambrose, S. A., Bridges, M.W., DiPietro, M., Lovett, M.C., & Norman, M.K. (2010). *How learning works: Seven research-based principles for smart teaching.* San Francisco, CA: Jossey-Bass.

Anderson, L.W., Krathwohl, D. R., Airasian, P., Cruikshank, K. A., Mayer, R. E., Pintrich, P. R., & Wittrock, M. (2001). *A taxonomy for learning, teaching, and assessing: A revision of Bloom's taxonomy of educational objectives.* New York, NY: Longman.

Benner, P., Sutphen, M., Leonard, V., & Day, L. (2009). *Educating nurses: A call for radical transformation.* San Francisco, CA: Jossey-Bass.

Blakely, G., Skirton, H., Cooper, S., Allum, P., & Nelmes, P. (2009). Educational gaming in the health sciences: Systematic review. *Journal of Advanced Nursing, 65,* 259–269. doi: 10.1111/j.1365–2648.2008.04843.x

Blakely, G., Skirton, H., Cooper, S., Allum, P., & Nelmes, P. (2010). Use of educational games in the health professions: A mixed methods study of educators' perspective in the UK. *Nursing and Health Sciences, 12,* 27–32. doi: 10.1111/j.1442–2018.2009.00479.x

Boardman, A. G., Roberts, G., Vaughn, S., Wexler, J., Murray, C. S., & Kosanovich, M. (2008). *Effective instruction for adolescent struggling readers: A practice brief.* Portsmouth, NH: RMC Research Corporation, Center on Instruction.

Brookfield, S. (2012). *Teaching for critical thinking: Tools and techniques to help students question their assumptions.* San Francisco, CA: Jossey-Bass.

Chabeli, M., (2010). Concept mapping as a teaching method to facilitate critical thinking in nursing education: A review of the literature. *Health SA Geshondheid, 15*(1), 1–7. doi: 10.4102/hsag.v15i1.432

Chunta, K., & Katrancha, E. (2010). Using problem-based learning in staff development: Strategies for teaching registered nurses and new graduate nurses. *Journal of Continuing Education in Nursing, 41,* 557–564. doi: 10.3928/00220124–20100701–06

Dave, R.H. (1970). Developing and writing educational objectives (psychomotor levels). In R. J. Armstrong (Ed.), *Developing and writing behavioral objectives.* Tucson, AZ: Educational Innovators Press.

Davies, M. (2011). Concept mapping, mind mapping and argument mapping: What the differences and do they matter? *Higher Education, 62,* 279–301. doi:10.1007/s10734–010–9387–6

Deslauriers, L. Schelew, E., & Wieman, C. (2011) Improved learning in a large-enrollment physics class. *Science, 332,* 862. doi: 10.1126/science.1201783

Elder, L., & Paul, R. (2010). Critical thinking: Competency standards essential for the cultivation of intellectual skills, part 1. *Journal of Developmental Education, 34*(2), 38–39.

Ennis, R. (2010). *A super-streamlined conception of critical thinking*. Retrieved from www .criticalthinking.net

Facione, P. (1990). *The APA executive summary of the Delphi report. Critical thinking: A statement of expert consensus for purposes of educational assessment and instruction* (American Philosophical Association ERIC Doc. No.: ED 315 423). Retrieved from www.insightassessment.com/CT-Resources

Gaba, D. (2007). The future vision of simulation in healthcare. *Simulation in Healthcare, 2*(2), 126–135. doi: 10.1097/01.SIH.0000258411.38212.32

Gill, R. (2011). Effective strategies for engaging students in large-lecture, non-majors science courses. *Journal of College Science Teaching, 41*(2), 14–21.

Gimenez, J. (2012). Disciplinary epistemologies, generic attributes and undergraduate academic writing in nursing and midwifery. *Higher Education, 63*(4), 401–419. doi: 10.1007/s10734–011–9447–6

Gropelli, T. M. (2010). Using active simulation to enhance learning of nursing ethics. *Journal of Continuing Education in Nursing, 41*(3), 104–105. doi: 10.3928/00220124–20100224–09

Hawkins, D., Elder, L. & Paul, R. (2010). *Thinker's guide to clinical reasoning*. Dillon Beach, CA: Foundation for Critical Thinking.

Henige, K. (2010). Use of concept mapping in an undergraduate introductory exercise physiology course. *Advances in Physiology Education, 36*, 197–206. doi: 10.1152/advan.00001.2012

Herreid, C. F. (2011). Case study teaching. *New Directions for Teaching and Learning, 128 (Winter)*, 31–40. doi:10.1002/tl.466

Huckabay, L. (2009). The effect of creating a mental set on cognitive learning and affective behaviors of nursing students. *Nursing Forum, 4*, 222–234. doi: 10.1111/j.1744–6198.2009.00148.x

Hutchinson, T. L., & Goodin, H. J. (2013). Nursing student anxiety as a context for teaching/learning. *Journal of Holistic Nursing, 31*(1), 19–24. doi: 10.1177/0898010112462067

Ironside, P. M. (2006). Using narrative pedagogy: Learning and practicing interpretive thinking. *Journal of Advanced Nursing, 55*, 478–486. doi: 10.1111/j.1365–2648.2006.03938.x

Krathwohl, D. R., Bloom, B. S., & Masia, B. B. (1964). *Taxonomy of educational objectives: The classification of educational goals. Handbook II: Affective domain*. New York, NY: David McKay.

Millis, B. (2002). *IDEA paper # 38: Enhancing learning- and more! – Through cooperative learning*. Manhattan, KS: The IDEA Center. Retrieved from www.theideacenter.org/research-and-papers/idea-papers/idea-paper-no-38

Millis, B. (2009). Becoming an effective teacher using cooperative learning: A personal odyssey. *Peer Review, 11*(2), 17–21.

Millis, B. (2010). *New pedagogies and practices for teaching in higher education: Cooperative learning in higher education: Across the disciplines, across the academy*. Sterling, VA: Stylus Publishing.

Millis, B. (2012). *IDEA Paper #53: Active learning strategies in face-to-face courses*, Manhattan, KS: The IDEA Center, Available at www.theideacenter.org/sites/default/files/paperidea_53.pdf

Mokhtari, K., & Reichard, C. A. (2002). Assessing students' metacognitive awareness of reading strategies. *Journal of Educational Psychology, 94*, 249–259.

Nestel, D., Groom J., Eikeland-Husebo, S., & O'Donnell, J. M. (2011). Simulation for learning and teaching procedural skills: the state of the science. *Simulation in Healthcare, 6*(7):S10–S13. doi: 10.1097/SIH.0b013e318227ce96

Newport, F. (2012). Congress retains low honesty rating: Nurses have highest honesty rating; car salespeople, lowest. *Gallup Politics*. Retrieved from www.gallup.com/poll/159035/congress-retains-low-honesty-rating.aspx

Nilson, L. B. (2010). *Teaching at its best: A research-based resource for college instructors*. San Francisco, CA: Jossey-Bass.

Oermann, M. H., & Gaberson, K. B. (2014). *Evaluation and testing in nursing education* (4th ed.). New York, NY: Springer.

Oja, K. J. (2011). Using problem-based learning in the clinical setting to improve nursing students' critical thinking: An evidence review. *Journal of Nursing Education, 50*, 145–151. doi: 10.3928/01484834–20101230–10

Ondrusek, 2012, What the research reveals about graduate students' writing skills: A literature review. *Journal of Education for Library and Information Science, 53*, 176–188.

Peinhardt, R., & Hagler, D. (2013). Peer coaching to support writing development. *Journal of Nursing Education, 52*, 24–28. doi: 10.3928/01484834–20121121–02

President's Council of Advisors on Science and Technology. (2012). *Engage to excel: Producing one million additional college graduates with degrees in science, technology, engineering, and mathematics.* Retrieved from www.whitehouse.gov/sites/default/files/microsites/ostp/pcast-engage-to-excel-final_feb.pdf

Rystedt, H., & Sjöblom, B. (2012). Realism, authenticity, and learning in healthcare simulations: Rules of relevance and irrelevance as interactive achievements. *Instructional Science, 40*, 785–798. doi: 10.1007/s11251–012–9213-x

Sallee, M., Hallett, R., & Tierney, W. (2011). Teaching writing in graduate school. *College Teaching, 59*(2), 66–72. doi: 10.1080/87567555.2010.511315

Sanford, A. J., & Emmott, C. (2012). *Mind, brain and narrative.* Cambridge, UK: Cambridge University Press.

Schmidt, H., Rotgans, J., & Yew, E. (2011). The process of problem-based learning: What works and why. *Medical Education, 45*, 792–806. doi: 10.1111/j.1365–2923.2011.04035.x

Seifer, S., & Connors, K. (Eds.). (2007). *Community campus partnerships for health: Faculty toolkit for service-learning in higher education.* Retrieved from www.servicelearning.org/library/resource/7120

Shindell, D. L. (2011). *Factors which influence the use of active learning strategies by nursing faculty.* Ann Arbor, MI: ProQuest, UMI Dissertations Publishing.

Skiba, D. (2009). Nursing education 2.0: A second look at Second Life. *Nursing Education Perspectives, 30*, 129–131.

Slavich, G. M., & Zimbardo, P. G. (2012). Transformational teaching: Theoretical underpinnings, basic principles, and core methods. *Educational Psychology Review, 24*, 569–608. doi: 10.1007/s10648–012–9199–6

Smith, C., & Sodano, T. (2011). Integrating lecture capture as a teaching strategy to improve student presentation skills through self-assessment. *Active Learning in Higher Education, 12*(3), 151–162. doi: 10.1177/1469787411415082

Taggart, A., & Crisp, G. (2011). Service learning at community colleges: Synthesis, critique, and recommendations for future research. *Journal of College Reading and Learning, 42*(1), 24–44.

Troxler, H., Vann, J. C., & Oermann, M.H. (2011). How baccalaureate nursing programs teach writing. *Nursing Forum, 46*, 280–288. doi:10.1111/j.1744–6198.2011.00242.x

Weimer, M. (2010). *Inspired college teaching: A career-long resource for professional growth.* San Francisco, CA: Jossey-Bass.

Welsh, D., & Lowry, R. C. (2011). Nursing students and end-of-life care: A play. *Nursing Education Perspectives, 32*, 414–416.

Wilson, A., Blake, B., Taylor, G., & Hannings, G. (2013). Cinemeducation: Teaching family assessment skills using full-length movies. *Public Health Nursing, 30*, 239–245. doi: 10.111/phn.12025

Windle, R. J., McCormick, D., Dandrea, J., & Wharrad, H. (2011). The characteristics of reusable learning objects that enhance learning: A case-study in health-science education. *British Journal of Educational Technology, 42*, 811–823. doi: 10.1111/j.1467–8535.2010.01108.x

Yoder-Wise, P., & Kowalski, K. (2012). *Fast facts for the classroom nursing instructor: Classroom teaching in a nutshell.* New York, NY: Springer Publishing Company.

Zhang, Y. (2011). Supporting adult learners' use of reading strategies through effective literacy scaffolding. *International Forum of Teaching and Studies, 7*(2), 20–31.

4

Integrating Technology in Education

HELEN B. CONNORS AND KATHY TALLY

Technology permeates every aspect of our lives, including education. The rapid advances and constant pace of change in technology create challenges and opportunities for teaching and learning. Nationally and internationally, education leaders and policymakers are promoting efforts to transform education to improve student achievements and readiness for life-long learning and career options. Education leaders, policymakers, parents, teachers, and students all seem to agree that technology is an essential component of education. The more educators use technology, the more they recognize and value its strong positive effects on student learning and engagement and its connection to 21st-century skills. This means that educators must be prepared to adopt existing technologies and explore emerging technology tools; they must be collaborators in learning, constantly seeking new knowledge and skills along with their students as the technology evolves. Technology is helping teachers to expand beyond linear, text-based learning and to engage students who have a variety of learning styles. The role of technology in education has evolved from a contained "computer class" into a versatile learning tool set that changes how faculty demonstrate concepts, assign projects, assess progress, and increase access to education. Educators should not use technology because they can, but rather integrate appropriate technology in the curriculum based on quality standards and pedagogical approaches that support best practices and improve the student's ability to meet learning outcomes.

Successful integration of technology in the curriculum requires a paradigm shift and new set of necessary competencies as technology continues to evolve. Technology can mean different things to different people. This chapter focuses on technology integration that supports achievement of learning outcomes with attention to curriculum and classroom alignment that increases rigor, relevance, and relationships. Technology will continue to disrupt education, and the disruption will change as technology changes over time. The goal is to explore and embrace technology tools that support good teaching practices. Technology is the tool—pedagogy and quality promote its use in nursing education.

BACKGROUND

Technology is commonly thought of as gadgets, instruments, machines, and devices; however, in today's world, most educators refer to technology for the classroom as equipment, particularly electronic equipment. Educational technology, especially computers and computer-related peripherals, have expanded rapidly over the last few decades. The continued development and expansion of the Internet in the 1980s laid the foundation for networking capabilities. Then, with the availability of the web in the 1990s, followed by Web 2.0 tools in the early 2000s, digitalized communication and networking in education exploded taking on many forms and changing the face of education. In addition, the more recent emergence of mobile devices and ubiquitous technology gave new meaning to teaching and learning and challenged educators to look at new education paradigms. It also challenged faculty, administrators, and policymakers to question the quality, evaluate outcomes, and establish standards for technology-based education.

These emerging technologies are examples of disruptive innovations that have changed the education marketplace over the past decade, pushing the boundaries of higher education and providing new and disruptive pathways to offer higher education. The increasing number of pathways has not only created greater education market competition, but a strong emphasis on developing quality programs and the need for standards to evaluate and guide continuous improvement processes that reflect ongoing changes in technology-based education.

THE INTERNET AND THE WEB

The Internet and the web are frequently used interchangeably, although they are not one and the same. The Internet is the hardware—it is a collection of computer networks connected through either copper wires, fiber optic cables, or wireless connections. The web is considered the software—it is a collection of web pages connected through hyperlinks and universal resource locators (URLs) or addresses to specific locations so that information that is sent or retrieved is located and delivered to the requesting computer or end-user. The web depends on the Internet to make it work. The web is a complex and highly organized set of electronic pathways similar to highways and interstate systems used by people to travel from one point to another in search of information. A request for information travels across the Internet to reach resources that are located in different sites on the web. Once those resources are located, that information, which may include files or media, is sent to the requesting computer/user.

Educators using technology to teach need to have a basic understanding of how information travels along these pathways. This is particularly important as we explore more robust teaching technologies including virtual worlds, web-conferencing, and content delivery using different types of media such as podcasts (audio files) and vodcasts (video files). Text-based information transfers to the requesting computer/user at a much faster rate than larger files like audio and video, or rich media found in virtual worlds. All this information travels in packets; the larger the file, the greater number of packets required for travel from one location to another. Having the right Internet connection and hardware are essential for students to be successful in accessing the teaching technologies and content used in media rich online learning environments. It is recommended that the teacher include guidelines in the course syllabi and program description about the type of Internet connection that is needed. The statement in Exhibit 4.1 is an example of the information the teacher might include in the syllabus. It can be modified to reflect the specific teaching technologies.

EXHIBIT 4.1 Sample Statement on Internet Connection

General technology requirements include the use of a broadband Internet connection for all online or hybrid courses. The most reliable broadband connections are cable and DSL. Although satellite, which is often used in rural areas where cable or DSL are not available, and wireless cards purchased through mobile Internet providers are also broadband connections, these two broadband connections can be less reliable, producing intermittent connections and slower Internet speed. That can interfere with successful web-conferencing session, robust information transfer of course content, and connections during online assessments delivered via a learning management system.

Additionally, we recommend that you do not use a wireless connection when taking online assessments or participating in high-stakes web-conferencing events such as applied demonstrations. Instead, connect your computer directly to the router with an Ethernet (Internet connection) cable.

The web is considered one of several services provided by the Internet. Other services over the Internet include e-mail, chat, and file transfer services. All of these services are readily available to consumers for use by businesses, educational institutions, government, and individuals creating their own networks or platforms. The Internet is a huge network that is available to anyone and most anywhere around the world.

The original purpose of the web was to communicate and share information. The development of the web dramatically changed methods of communication and sharing information and ultimately changed the way people learn. Web-based learning means using the web as the teaching and learning strategy. It reduces time and space barriers to learning and coupled with an array of emerging integrated technologies, makes learning self-directed, active, accessible, and engaging.

The Internet has changed how we interact with time. We now can be learning all the time, whenever we want, and wherever we want. Because of that, there has been explosive growth in online education, with entire courses and selected parts of a course taught via the web. With this shift in education strategy, the role of the instructor transformed from that of giving knowledge to students to one of moderating and facilitating learning. Today, the web can be accessed from virtually anywhere through the Internet, allowing flexibility for teaching and learning any time and any place. Students and faculty can work collaboratively via the web to share ideas, knowledge, and skills. The degree of using the web in a course can range from the web supplementing classroom learning, a mix of traditional classroom activities and online activities, and courses and programs that are offered completely online, to massive open online courses (MOOCs) in which anyone with Internet access can engage in the course and choose their level of participation (Thompson, 2011).

In 2011, approximately 6.7 million college students, or approximately one-third of all college enrollees, were taking one or more courses online. This number increases substantially each year (Allen & Seaman, 2012). Creative uses of the web are helping to provide and enhance education while creating a disruptive force in higher education as open access to learning and emerging technologies challenge traditional education models until they change.

Over the past decade there has been excitement within the education community about Web 2.0 technologies. Web 2.0 is an umbrella term for a host of recent Internet applications such as social networking, wikis, folksonomies, virtual societies, blogging, multiplayer online gaming, and "mash-ups." These applications differ in form and function; however, all these applications share a common characteristic of supporting Internet-based interaction between and within groups, which is why the term "social software" is often used to describe Web 2.0 tools and services.

In addition to the Internet, many other technologies, such as simulation and virtual worlds, iPads and tablet devices, smartphones, gaming, and learner response systems, among others, are transforming education. These technologies are evolving quickly, and the pace seems to increase each year. Educators need to keep current with the emerging instructional technologies to ensure they are adopting the best tools to support active learning, use student and faculty time productively, improve learning outcomes, and prepare students for lifelong learning and successful careers. Technology implementations in schools and classrooms, no matter how big or small, will benefit from thoughtful strategic planning and evaluation.

TECHNOLOGY TOOLS: PRESENT AND FUTURE

LEARNING MANAGEMENT SYSTEMS

One of the most common tools used to support technology integration in education today is a learning management system (LMS). The International Forum of Educational Technology & Society (IFETS) defines an LMS as a collection of e-learning tools available through a shared administrative interface (Avgeriou, Papasalouros, Retalis, & Skordalakis, 2003). LMSs' interface technologies vary from simple to complex in how they are used and what tools support and deliver online content. LMSs have been adopted widely by educational institutions across the globe to meet specific needs and requirements of increasing education demands. Educators and instructional designers working together can effectively use LMS tools to develop and deliver online course components that maximize the technology inherent in most LMSs. The outcome can result in high-quality courses that reduce faculty workload and provide students with access to information and learning tools that facilitate the highest levels of learning in a completely online environment, blended courses (integrating face-to-face and online activities), or a web-component that reinforces content delivered in a face-to-face classroom (Avgeriou et al., 2003). A few examples of proprietary LMSs include Blackboard, Desire2Learn, and Canvas. Examples of open source systems available include Sakai and Moodle. New systems are being developed as demand continues to increase with the expansion of online course offerings and programs.

WEB 2.0 TOOLS

Web 2.0 is a second generation of the web that provides users the opportunity to interact and collaborate with each other, as opposed to websites that limit them to passive viewing of the content. Web 2.0 and similar emerging technologies are new tools and ways of creating, collaborating, editing, and sharing user-generated content online. Some basic examples of Web 2.0 tools are weblogs, wikis, video casting, social bookmarking, social networking, podcasts, and picture sharing tools. There are a growing abundance of Web 2.0 applications that are readily available, making technology easier to use and more accessible to faculty and students.

Many of these applications are free and can be integrated into a course to support all levels of Bloom's digital taxonomy. The digital taxonomy follows the learning process on a continuum of lower order thinking skills (LOTS) to higher order thinking skills (HOTS). It is not about the tools but is about integrating the tools to engage students and enhance the learning outcomes. Over the years, Bloom's taxonomy of educational objectives has been revised to address new behaviors and learning opportunities that have been enriched by technologies (Bloom, Englehart, Furst, Hill, & Krathwohl, 1956).

Examples of Bloom's digital taxonomy and potential technologies to support the desired learning outcomes are available at http://edorigami.wikispaces.com. Other excellent sites for sharing Web 2.0 applications that support Bloom's taxonomy are http://pinterest .com/esheninger/web-2-0-tools-for-educators and the Multimedia Education Resource for Learning and Online Teaching (MERLOT) www.merlot.org. These are dynamic websites that change frequently as educators add new applications and assessments.

WEB 3.0

Imagine what will happen as the web "gets smarter" and can assist in organizing, integrating, and evaluating the information it provides? This is currently referred to as the semantic web, or Web 3.0 (Markoff, 2006). Internet experts believe this next generation of the web will be similar to having a personal assistant—the more you use the web, the more your browser will learn about you and bring you specific information from a variety of sources that meets your needs. It will personalize learning and provide richer and more significant information based on your individual profile.

The semantic web will have profound implications for nursing education. When a user searches the web, it will bring the learner more than a list of websites to explore to find the most relevant information. Instead, it will provide a multimedia report integrating many sources including websites, scientific repositories, textbook chapters, blogs, speeches, videos, and others. The multimedia report will focus on knowledge areas that emerge from the individual's research (Ohler, 2008). Currently, much of faculty time is spent teaching students to identify legitimate information, organize and synthesize it, integrate it with other information from multiple sources, and ultimately produce new knowledge. This is the essence of critical thinking. With the technology doing much of this work for the learner, students can spend more time making sense of the synthesis, creating new knowledge, and applying the learning to real-world situations. Teachers will need new skills in the near future with a shift to Web 3.0.

CLOUD COMPUTING

Advances in hardware, software, and networking have generated opportunities for academic institutions to seek out alternative sources of information technology (IT) services such as cloud computing. Although there are many definitions of cloud computing, the National Institute of Standards and Technology (NIST) defines cloud computing as "a model for enabling ubiquitous, convenient, on-demand network access to a shared pool of configurable computing resources (e.g., networks, servers, storage, applications, and services) that can be rapidly provisioned and released with minimal management effort or service provider interaction" (Mell & Grance, 2011, p. 2). These evolving cloud-based services are purported to increase institutional flexibility and reduce operating cost, thus offering attractive alternatives to traditional information technology (IT) services on campus (Tamarkin & Rodrigo, 2011). Despite the promise of reducing operating costs, according to the Campus Computing Project (Green, 2012), there are small gains in the movement of critical campus operations to the cloud over the previous year's survey. The most gains have been with institutions moving e-mail, LMS, and customer relationship management operations to the cloud. Although there are performance benefits and cost savings to be realized in migrating to the cloud, the challenges faced by academic institutions are related to risk, trust, and control. The cloud computing space is an emerging paradigm with many promising opportunities; therefore, as this space advances, developing a campus-wide cloud strategy will continue to be important for most academic institutions (Grajek & Pirani, 2012; Green, 2012; Sultan, 2010).

MASSIVE OPEN ONLINE COURSES

With Internet access, Web 2.0 technologies, open-access (unrestricted access to scholarly publications), and cloud-based services, a new phenomenon in learning has occurred in higher education in the past few years. The original concept of a MOOC was a web course developed by experts in a specific field that people from all over the world could take for free and earn no course credit. Some MOOCs, however, have a fee and can be taken for credit. Most MOOCs typically have massive enrollments. With this kind of support for anywhere, anytime, and no-cost online learning, MOOCs have evolved at an unprecedented pace and moved to the center of a national discussion about the future of higher education. MOOCs have attracted millions of learners from all over the world to learn from top professors at elite universities. At this point, it is too early to determine the impact of MOOCs on higher education, but several projects are underway in the United States and internationally. For example, the University of Wisconsin system is piloting the use of MOOCs and other resources for creating several degree and certificate programs for adult and nontraditional students. For this competency-based curriculum, students use open resources, faculty provide individualized support through tutoring and coaching, and students earn credit by demonstrating knowledge they have acquired through regular assessments (UW Flexible Option, 2013).

SIMULATION, VIRTUAL WORLDS, AND GAMING

The use of simulators as teaching tools in health professions education has grown rapidly as a mechanism to improve the quality and safety of health care, much like airline simulators have improved the safety of air travel. As with other teaching tools, using simulation to improve patient safety requires full integration of its applications into the routine structure of the curriculum. The best outcomes occur when simulation is integrated across the curriculum rather than added on top of an already over-crowded curriculum.

Integrating simulation in the curriculum starts with a roadmap. This involves all faculty teaching across the curriculum and embeds simulation where it appropriately matches learning objectives, instead of viewing simulation exercises as independent learning experiences. The process of mapping simulation to the curriculum allows educators to develop unfolding cases where each successive simulation builds on preceding ones. As the curriculum progresses, the learner is expected to demonstrate increased knowledge and competencies. Mapping simulation to the curriculum creates efficiencies and develops an evidence-based simulation curriculum that engages both students and faculty across the academic program or programs.

For the most part, the word simulator in nursing and health professions education brings to mind the human patient simulator (HPS). This type of simulator is probably the most widely used; however, it is only one aspect of re-creating a realistic clinical environment for teaching patient care skills without harming patients. Today, emerging information and communication technologies, such as electronic health records (EHRs), telehealth technologies, and m-health, are changing health care delivery. Those changes need to be reflected in our education practices for graduates to be prepared with the health information technology (health IT) competencies needed for practice (Connors, 2006).

The clinical simulation environment provides an excellent opportunity to integrate health IT competencies with the curriculum. Merging EHR technology with laboratory simulation provides students with virtual clinical experiences that closely represent the increasingly automated practice environments (Warren, Meyer, Thompson, & Roche, 2010). Just like the HPS can be programmed to simulate patient care experiences, a simulated EHR can be used to simulate patient data and clinical decision-making scenarios to accompany the virtual case studies enacted through the HPS. In other words, the simulated patients have their own EHR-like environments, with access to clinical data to enable students to develop critical thinking skills and make data-driven decisions in a safe environment. An example of an Academic EHR integrated into the simulation curriculum is the Simulated E-hEalth Delivery System (SEEDS) at the University of Kansas (Connors, Warren, & Weaver, 2007; Warren & Connors, 2007; Warren, Manos, Meyer, & Roache, 2013). In 2000, through a partnership with a leading EHR software supplier, the company's well-established clinical information system was adapted to fit the education workflow of the academic environment and led to the creation of a virtual care delivery system supported with the EHR. The virtual care delivery system includes an acute care hospital, as well as outpatient environments such as school-based clinics, public health clinics, ambulatory care clinics, and home settings. The virtual care environments reflect all aspects of nursing and other health professions curriculum, and each simulated patient has his or her own EHR within the virtual environment.

The product adapted for use with the SEEDS program is called the Academic Education Solution (AES©) and is currently being used by a number of academic institutions in order to integrate informatics competencies in the curriculum. More recently, several other vendors developed Academic EHRs that are similar to the AES, thus providing schools with vendor choices to help simulate more closely the reality of practice in a technology-rich health care environment.

Virtual worlds such as Second Life©, Active Worlds, Wonderland, and World of Warcraft add another dimension to simulation. Virtual worlds are part of the Web 2.0 and future Web 3.0. For example, hundreds of colleges and universities across the globe are using Second Life to teach classes and as supplemental learning experiences (Skiba, 2009; Warren, Connors, & Trangenstein, 2011). In a virtual world, existing educational tools such as a PowerPoint presentation, images, and links to websites, course material, and 3-D objects can be aggregated into a dynamic learning hub. The uses of virtual worlds are varied and can be adapted to different needs. Gerald and Antonacci (2013) provide an example of a real-world approach to the use of this virtual learning space in their Second Life operating room simulation, which can be viewed in this article. Exhibit 4.2 displays some common applications for virtual worlds.

Game-based learning (GBL) is in the early stage of adoption in higher education. While there are many examples of simulation-based learning in nursing education in both real and virtual environments, there are few edugames used successfully in higher education. Edugames are beginning to expand, driven largely by growing consumer fascination with games and the abundance of mobile technology making gaming techniques readily available (Epper, Derryberry, & Jackson, 2012). In the health care sector, the University of Minnesota School of Nursing has partnered with the Minnesota Hospital Association and VitalSims to develop a series of interactive web-based games that engage nursing and other health profession students (Moore, 2012). These games, coupled with classroom and simulation laboratories, will be another valuable tool to better equip future nursing and health professionals. Some experts have projected wide-spread adoption of serious GBL in upcoming years (Johnson et al., 2013). Serious gaming in education is gaining additional support among researchers and educators

EXHIBIT 4.2 Common Applications for Virtual Worlds

Communication Scenarios. Virtual worlds (VWs) are being used to teach specific communication skills and working together as a team. For example, a health informatics class may meet virtually with different key individuals from a health facility to negotiate the terms and conditions for developing a database for the facility.

Collaboration. Second Life© gives students a common place to interact regardless of their physical location.

Staging an Exhibit. Students can present their final course project in a virtual auditorium or exhibit hall created in Second Life to display these projects to faculty and peers.

Virtual Campuses. Many colleges and universities are building a virtual presence to focus on learning resources, student centers, and marketing efforts.

Virtual Classrooms. Some nursing faculty are using the VW platform to deliver lectures embedded with PowerPoint, videos, links to websites and other virtual spaces, e-books and 3D models to create a dynamic learning hub.

Virtual Centers. Several research laboratories and centers such as the Ames Research Center, the Jet Propulsion Lab, and NASA have partnered to create a virtual presence in Second Life to provide a space to try out new ideas and host meetings and talks.

Conference Facilities. Second Life can be used to offer conferences, for example, to host seminars on health problems and treatments.

Technical Training. Nurse anesthesia faculty have developed a VW operating room simulation to assist first-year students with learning the basic induction procedure. This activity builds confidence and emphasizes important safety techniques.

Virtual Field Trip. These can provide experiences for learning to navigate VWs or as a final project. For example, a nursing student might visit the Virtual Ability Island to learn more about living with a disability or to address a problem area.

Simulated Experiences. With simulated experiences, occupational, physical therapy, and nursing students can develop skills in home assessment and recommending modifications in the home through a series of virtual home environments.

Research Studies. VWs are the subject of much academic research. In addition, researchers are exploring how VWs can help to practice and promote healthy behaviors such as activities involved in weight loss programs or managing posttraumatic stress disorders.

who recognize that GBL engages students and stimulates critical inquiry among them. Examples of universities exploring GBL are in Table 4.1.

MOBILE DEVICES

The pervasiveness of mobile devices such as smartphones, tablets, iPads, e-book readers, and other emerging mobile technologies used in everyday personal and work life is making its way into the classroom. Today, many students, faculty, and staff members arrive on campus with one or more mobile devices and expect to use these personal devices to access the network and its resources. They expect institutions to provide reliable wireless connectivity. This is known as the "Bring Your Own Device" (BYOD) or more recently as "Bring Your Own Everything" (BYOE) phenomena. This move to mobile computing on campus coincides with a push among educational publishers toward digital content, such as electronic textbooks, multimedia-rich applications, online videos, and other online tools for faculty and students. Schools of nursing programs and colleges and universities are struggling to meet these expectations and are finding that they need to rethink their IT strategies in order to enhance learning.

TABLE 4.1 University Research Centers Exploring Game-Based Learning

Research Center	Website
The Education Arcade at Massachusetts Institute of Technology	www.educationarcade.org
Games + Learning + Society at University of Wisconsin-Madison	www.gameslearningsociety.org
Center for Game Science at University of Washington	www.centerforgamescience.org/site
The Games for Learning Institute at New York University	www.g4li.org/about
Institute for Simulation & Training at University of Central Florida	www.ist.ucf.edu
Center for Transformational Media at Parsons The New School for Design	http://ctm.parsons.edu
Interactive Communications & Simulations at University of Michigan	http://ics.soe.umich.edu
GAMeS (Games, Animation, Modeling, and Simulation Lab) at Radford University	http://gameslab.radford.edu
3-D Game Lab at Boise State University	http://web1.boisestate.edu/extendedstudies/ educatorsdevelopment/workshops/ Professional-Education-3DGameLab.html
Serious Games Center at Purdue University	http://www.edci.purdue.edu/learning_design_ and_technology/Serious%20Games%20 Center.html

To successfully implement a campus-wide mobile computing initiative, there needs to be an institutional commitment to support these devices through the campus infrastructure as well as the pedagogical approaches in the classroom. Many institutions need to increase bandwidth, add access points and sufficient power, boost their network management capabilities, address security concerns, and hire or develop IT personnel who are familiar with a common variety of mobile device operating systems. The meaningful use of mobile devices and applications in the curriculum give users instant access to information and encourage student engagement, participation, and collaboration, while fostering a personal learning network. As nursing faculty members more fully integrate technology into the curriculum, improved learning outcomes may result. According to the Pew Research Center's Internet & American Life Project, mobility and wireless connectivity are creating new kinds of learners who are more self-directed in their acquisition and sharing of knowledge, more inclined to collaborate, and more reliant on feedback (Smith, 2010).

The rapid expansion of BYOD complements other trends in higher education, such as virtualization and technology-enriched classrooms. As with these other trends, faculty buy-in and support is critical to successful implementation. According to the 21st-Century Campus Report, the top challenge to increased classroom technology, as rated by faculty, administrators, and students, is the faculty's lack of technology knowledge and skill (2011 CDW-G 21st-Century Campus Report, 2011). Although 81% of the institutions surveyed provided technology-specific professional development, faculty members perceived that this approach did not meet their needs. Faculty suggested that the institutions offer discipline-specific faculty development and that tech-savvy faculty members lead the sessions. This same strategy could be used for preparing nurse educators.

LEARNING ANALYTICS

Learning analytics is the "measurement, collection, analysis and reporting of data about learners and their contexts, for purposes of understanding and optimizing learning and the environments in which it occurs" (1st International Conference on Learning Analytics and Knowledge, 2011). The Horizon Report indicated that learning analytics was associated with deciphering trends and patterns from educational large datasets, huge sets of student-related data, to further the advancement of a personalized, supportive system of higher education (Johnson et al., 2013). Traditionally, learning has been measured by student evaluation, analysis of grades, and attrition rates, as well as the faculty member's perception of the student. As more educational activities move online, an extraordinary amount of data about these learning activities is becoming captured and available.

Recent interest in how this unique information can be used to improve teaching and learning has emerged as the field of learning analytics. Initially, uses of student data were focused on at-risk students to improve outcomes. However, with advances in technology and its powerful tools, it is possible to use the data to personalize learning and provide student-specific coaching to result in more productive learning habits and improved outcomes. A report from the U.S. Department of Education Office of Educational Technology (2013) focuses on using these data to examine how people learn and create learning systems that support these best practices. As the field of learning analytics develops over the next few years, the goal is for the data and tools to provide a better understanding of learning outcomes and assessment in higher education, including nursing education.

RETHINKING THE EDUCATION PARADIGM

Technology enhances active learning, accommodates a variety of learning styles, and allows for communication, collaboration, and sharing among students. A technology-oriented strategy should support and facilitate learning, including critical thinking, problem solving, creativity, and innovation. The specific technology is chosen not because it is available and exciting, but because it is based on its fit with the learning pedagogy and goals of the nursing course or program. The pedagogy and goals provide the framework for nurse educators to decide on the best technology for their courses. When a school of nursing decides to offer technology-based courses or programs, a significant amount of attention should focus on the infrastructure, resources, and support. Lack of attention to any of these will result in foreseeable and preventable challenges (Hartman, 2008).

INFRASTRUCTURE

Investment in infrastructure is of utmost importance to ensuring success in transforming education in schools of nursing and colleges and universities. Schools are more reliant than ever before on an infrastructure that can support their evolving technological demands. This infrastructure must be secure, available 24/7, able to meet a wide range of applications, and adaptable to new technologies. At the same time, it must be transparent to the end users and expected to operate continuously. To accomplish these goals, campuses must develop and implement enterprise-wide strategic and operational technology plans that align with the institution's mission and goals. These plans should not be static, as almost every day new technologies are competing for infrastructure resources. The key to success is institutional and nursing program leadership commit-ted to supporting IT and using technology to improve institutional performance while maintaining efficiencies.

Alignment With Institution and School of Nursing Mission and Goals

Over the past three decades, colleges and universities have made substantial invest-ments in technological infrastructure such as course management systems, wireless networks, multimedia classrooms, and a wide array of technology tools to transform teaching and learning. There are many technologies available and ways to implement them, making it difficult for faculty members, including nurse educators, to keep pace and know whether the use of the technology is having an impact on learning outcomes (Hartman, 2008). Questions about technology integration persist, even after more than half a century of research documenting the use of technologies from television to mobile devices and the benefits of technologies for learning.

Reviews of the literature reveal that the emphasis of teaching and learning with technology has been on the technology itself. However, the technology alone does not transform education. In fact, there is a large body of research demonstrating no sig-nificant difference when the focus of the research is on the technology and not on the teaching practices (Means, Toyama, Murphy, Bakia, & Jones, 2010; Western Interstate Commission for Higher Education, 2010). As Graves (2005) suggested, all too often teachers "bolt on" the technology rather than redesign the teaching and learning pro-cess supported and enhanced by it. Because there are so many technologies for teachers to choose and ways to use them, and many faculty members with diverse pedagogi-cal approaches, most institutions have been unable to determine on an enterprise level whether the introduction of technologies is having a positive impact on student learn-ing outcomes (Hartman, 2008). The same is true at the level of the school of nursing or nursing department.

What is needed is an institutional approach to teaching and learning with tech-nology to determine efficiency, effectiveness, sustainability, and quality. A systematic approach may not be appropriate for all technology, but this approach is ideal for those technologies that have a broad applicability across the institution. A more individual-ized approach may be appropriate for specific technologies and for use in a specialized area of study such as nursing. However, to truly transform education with technol-ogy, technology integration needs to be part of the mission and goals of the institution, not used arbitrarily by a few educators across the institution. Unless the culture and structure of a school is compatible with and supportive of specific uses of technology, technology integration is not likely to succeed. When technology-enhanced education is part of the mission and goals of the institution, it is evident in all aspects of the pro-gram and should create an innovative culture that is necessary for truly transforming education.

Innovation is frequently defined as the introduction of something new that leads to a positive change: a new idea, method, or device. It is frequently viewed as necessary for quality improvement (Melnyk & Davidson, 2009). An innovative culture establishes innovation as a central theme in the organization's vision and purpose. With innovation as an integral part of the framework, the organization will not only embrace creative thinking, teaching, and learning that is outside the traditional processes, but it will also encourage and support such creativity through established practices such as hiring, coaching, mentoring, and rewarding faculty and staff. A culture of innovation provides a framework to assist institutions and nursing programs to turn disruptive innovation into productive innovation.

Pedagogy

Pedagogy is the study of the art and science of teaching and includes multiple theories of behavior that are based on the learning process or the observation and scientific study of how people learn. Learning theories were presented in Chapter 2. Most nursing faculty members learned in a teacher-centered model of instruction, with emphasis on the presentation of knowledge or a skill set that teachers perceived students needed to learn. In this case, the focus is on the teacher, who has control of the learning process. In these settings teachers are active and students are passive.

Over the past several decades, however, there has been the emergence of new learning theories, such as social constructivism and other student-centered pedagogical practices, that support new paradigms for teaching and learning (Hartman, 2008). These new learning pedagogies recommend that to best prepare 21st-century learners for the increasingly complex and interconnected global society in which they live and work, teachers should implement practices that involve interactive, problem-based, and technology-enriched teaching and learning.

Constructivism is a theory of learning founded on the premise that learners are actively involved and create their own learning through interaction with others and with the environment. They construct their own understanding of the world through experiential learning and reflection on their past experiences to build new knowledge (Bruner, 1966). In Bruner's (1996) more recent work, he expanded his theoretical framework to include the social and cultural aspects of learning. Modern constructivists believe that learning is a social process and is more active and self-directed than either behaviorism or cognitive theory. Much of today's instructional technologies promote constructivism principles of learning by creating learning environments that challenge students to work collaboratively to become actively engaged, self-directed lifelong learners inside and outside of formal learning spaces.

A goal for nurse educators is to use learning theory and best practice teaching strategies to guide technology integration and derive quality outcomes. Although technology has expanded the educational paradigm, good teaching has not changed. What has changed is the availability of technology tools to support teaching. Just as curriculum and pedagogy must be assessed and rethought, so must teaching and learning strategies. For example, Chickering and Gamson's (1987) Seven Principles for Good Practice in Undergraduate Education continue to be applicable in today's digital-enabled classrooms and web-based learning environments. Chickering and Ehrmann (1996) provide further evidence that technology integration encourages and supports each of the seven principles. Exhibit 4.3 displays the Seven Principles as applied to teaching and learning with technology.

Classroom Redesign

As technology and learning theories change, so does the design of the classroom. Across the country many educational institutions and schools of nursing are renovating existing learning space or constructing new learning environments. A key impetus in classroom space renovation or new construction is the need to accommodate new technologies and teaching strategies (Lippencott, 2009). Technology-enhanced education calls for a redesign of the traditional learning space and new pedagogical approaches to learning. The recent widespread adoption of technology and technology tools, along with the availability of wireless access, has challenged nurse educators to change pedagogical approaches to learning, which in turn has brought about a rethinking of classroom space.

EXHIBIT 4.3 Seven Principles for Good Practice in Education Applied to Teaching With Technology

1. Contacts between student and faculty (before, during, and after class)

2. Develops reciprocity and cooperation among students (team-based learning in web-enabled collaboration rooms via web conferencing, Skype, Facetime, and Social Media outlets)

3. Uses active learning techniques (simulation, VWs, student applied demonstrations, standardized patient interviews, all conducted in a virtual environment)

4. Gives prompt feedback (using LMSs for formative evaluations via quizzes that provide immediate feedback and multiple learning opportunities)

5. Emphasizes time on task (knowledge and comprehension task that are done as preparatory work to allow time on task to be directed to higher order learning, such as application and creation)

6. Communicates high expectations (knowledge acquisition occurs first in self-directed learning with high expectations for student–student and faculty–student interactions that are rich and engaging)

7. Respects diverse talent and ways of learning (teaching technology tools provide multiple modalities for the learner and allow rehearsal and repetition of content for all learning paces and learning styles)

From Chickering and Gamson (1987, 1996).

New learning spaces such as the active learning classroom are designed to facilitate a more active, student-centered pedagogy and take advantage of the room's potential. Typically, students bring their own computers to class and use the building's wireless capability to collaborate with peers in small groups to build new ideas and applications. The faculty member becomes a facilitator of learning, answering questions and making suggestions. Active learning classrooms are designed to facilitate hands-on activities and problems that require students to interact with each other to reach a solution. Students can display their work on large LCD screens mounted around the room to promote small- and large-group discussion. A clear goal in the redesign of learning spaces is to promote a change in pedagogy; therefore, the nurse educator's interest and motivation for making change in the curriculum and pedagogy through the use of technology must be taken into consideration during the redesign phase, or the active learning classroom may not be successful (Lippencott, 2009). Figure 4.1 is a photograph of an active learning classroom.

Although the literature on learning space suggests that design features have an impact on learning outcomes, there is little evidence-based research to support this assertion. Whiteside, Brooks, and Walker (2010) found that students attending classes in active learning classrooms had a significant positive effect on learning outcomes as measured by grades. The active learning classroom also had a positive influence on teaching and learning activities employed by faculty members and students in terms of lecture, discussion, coaching, and group activities. Further research is needed to explore the connections among learning spaces, pedagogical approaches, and student learning outcomes. As active learning classroom environments become more common in nursing education, it will be possible to conduct longitudinal studies of the impact of taking multiple courses in new learning spaces on broad strategic outcomes such as student enrollment and retention and failure rates.

FIGURE 4.1 Active learning classroom.

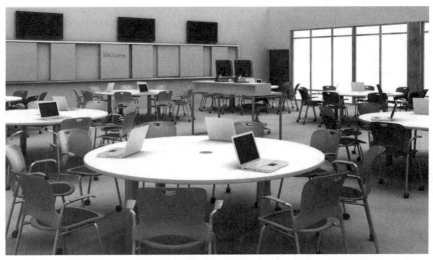

Image provided courtesy of Herman Miller, Inc. Reprinted by permission of Herman Miller, Inc. (2013).

Flipping the Classroom

A recent teaching revolution referred to as flipping the classroom is a good example of how technology and redesigned learning space can be used to structure learning. Flipping the classroom is a pedagogical approach that uses technology integration to provide students with knowledge- and comprehension-based learning activities that are provided via the web prior to coming to class in either a face-to-face, blended, or virtual learning environment. Flipping the classroom refers to swapping lecture time for active or applied learning in the classroom. This technique allows for more focused learning to take place in the classroom and engages students in a more active learning process (Kachka, 2012). It makes sense, because why should nursing faculty members use valuable class time for content delivery when there are other more efficient ways of doing that outside of class? Why should nursing students engage with the material alone and without the benefit of the faculty member's expertise? It would be better to do that during class time.

In a flipped classroom, students are accountable for prelearning activities that prepare them to discuss, apply, and assimilate what they have learned outside of class when they meet in a synchronous learning environment, either the traditional classroom or in a virtual classroom via the web. It is in the classroom environment (traditional or virtual) where they share and collaborate with their peers, and work in teams to expand their knowledge and incorporate their ideas with others. The teacher guides and facilitates higher learning, remediating, and scaffolding (providing instructional support to promote learning when first introduced to a new concept). Flipping the classroom requires flipping the minds of students and faculty. The concept of flipping the classroom is not new; it is the way the concept is applied and the use of assistive technology that is gaining attention. Flipping uses technology to replace passive learning such as lecture for a more active teacher–learner, student-centered interaction in the classroom. Flipping the classroom, however, does not guarantee student success. The nurse educator needs to embrace the concept and use effective teaching strategies that guide learning. Some examples of a flipped classroom model are included in Exhibit 4.4.

EXHIBIT 4.4 Examples of Flipping the Classroom

1. Students assume the teaching role via applied demonstrations of knowledge and assignments and present during the face-to-face or synchronous online web-conferencing sessions. The faculty member becomes the facilitator; the student becomes the educator.

2. Team-based learning approaches that help ensure students come to class prepared for learning include the use of individual quizzes by providing immediate feedback via an LMS assessment. In class, students are placed in teams, and they retake the quiz as a group, using discussion and collaboration to arrive at the correct answers.

3. Case studies that are embedded in the academic EHR can be reviewed by students prior to class and then presented in class. Students can be placed in teams to navigate the EHR and problem solve the case.

4. Educational games (e.g., Jeopardy, Who Wants to Be a Millionaire, Family Feud, etc.) can be used to review content to create a collaborative and competitive learning atmosphere. Examples can be found at http://jc-schools.net/tutorials/ppt-games

5. Chat rooms can be used in large classrooms to solicit feedback after mini-lectures or group discussion, allowing all students to have a voice.

6. Role-playing scenarios, with preassigned roles, can be performed during class.

7. Individual students or teams can be assigned topics to research in preparation for in-class debates on health care, health care reform, patient safety, or other topics.

DEVELOPING FACULTY COMPETENCIES AND MENTORING

Nursing faculty have been cited as a barrier to IT integration in nursing education programs because they lack knowledge and skills about new technologies and their potential (Institute of Medicine, 2010). Many faculty members are overwhelmed by the various technologies and challenged by the need to keep up with the ever changing course management systems, Web 2.0 technologies, and various software applications for classroom and clinical teaching. Although 81% of colleges and universities are providing technology-specific professional development, faculty members report that the approaches used most frequently, such as group meetings, seminars, online tutorials, one-to-one meetings, and peer mentoring, are not meeting their needs (2011 CDW-G 21st-Century Campus Report, 2011). Faculty suggested that professional development sessions would be more effective if the individuals who actually used the technology in the classroom led the training and if the sessions were targeted to the unique needs of specific academics. Most faculty members need to work with others to implement new pedagogical approaches and learn how to use technology.

The aim of faculty development should not focus on teaching nurse educators how to use the technology; rather the aim should be to understand what learning outcomes the teacher is attempting to achieve and suggest innovative technology and strategies to effectively reach those outcomes (Lippencott, 2009). For example, the University of Kansas School of Nursing joined with the schools of nursing at the University of Colorado, Indiana University-Purdue University Indianapolis, and Johns Hopkins University and the National League for Nursing to develop and implement the Health Information Technology Scholars (HITS) Program. This was one of the nine funded faculty development collaboratives supported by the Health Resource and Service Administration Bureau of Health Professionals, Integrating Technology into Nursing Education and Practice. The overall aim of the HITS program was to educate a cadre of well-informed nursing faculty to focus on real-world applications of technologies in their education practices. The 1-year program consists of online modules with discussion, webinars, a 3-day face-to-face workshop, and mentoring. Faculty applied for the program with a project that they intended to implement at their respective institutions. The faculty scholars engaged in active learning strategies by discussing their projects with their group and receiving feedback from the peer group as well as their mentor.

The success of this faculty development program can be attributed to targeting the learning to nurse educators' specific needs related to their technology project and goals, thus ensuring intrinsic motivation and personal relevance of the learning; using faculty experts and instructional designers to model pedagogies associated with new technologies; providing sustained mentorship and peer support through the group mentoring process; and fostering collaboration among faculty and institutions, which for many continued well after the faculty development program ended.

QUALITY FIRST, THEN TECHNOLOGY

Any nursing program, school of nursing, or institution that incorporates technology-based education should consider standards of quality equivalent to those for traditional educational approaches. Several comprehensive approaches to evaluating quality have been established. These various approaches use differing terminology to present evaluation criteria, including use of benchmarks, pillars, indicators, dimensions, best practices, and paradigms. Quality frameworks that exist for online, hybrid or blended, and face-to-face approaches to education include: (1) the International Association for K–12 Online Learning (iNACOL) standards, (2) the Sloan Consortium (Sloan-C) Framework, and (3) Quality Matters (QM). Although originally designed to assess online programs for quality indicators, for the most part the standards can be applied to courses and curricula that integrate technology. The three frameworks focus on indicators based on best practice standards on teaching and learning, sound instructional design principles, and research findings, and include tools to evaluate, create, and improve student learning environments through a continuous improvement process model.

International Association for K–12 Online Learning

In 2006, the North American Council for Online Learning conducted a review of course standards and adopted the Southern Regional Education Board (SREB) Standards for Quality Online Courses (SREB, 2006). The International Association for K–12 Online Learning (iNACOL) has continued the development of these standards. The standards for quality online courses are categorized into five areas:

1. Content
2. Instructional Design
3. Student Assessment
4. Technology
5. Course Evaluation and Management (iNACOL, 2011)

A scoring guide is available to rate the effectiveness of each standard using a 0 to 4 scale, with 0 indicating absent and 4 indicating very satisfactory.

The Sloan-C Quality Framework

The Sloan-C Quality Framework provides a general approach to evaluating quality in technology-based education (The Sloan Consortium, 2013). The framework identifies five pillars of quality:

Pillar I: Learning Effectiveness
Pillar II: Scale (Cost Effectiveness and Commitment)
Pillar III: Access
Pillar IV: Faculty Satisfaction
Pillar V: Student Satisfaction

The strengths of this framework are that for each pillar, goals, process/practices, evaluation metrics, and progress indices are identified. Effective practices linked to the Sloan-C Quality Framework have been identified, facilitating implementation of the framework to assess quality (Moore, 2011).

Quality Matters Program

The QM Program provides a robust rubric used to evaluate online, hybrid or blended, and technology-integrated courses. The rubric has eight standards with 41 specific standards and is complete with annotations that explain the application of the standards and relationships among them (Quality Matters Program, 2011). Courses are submitted for review to a team of experienced faculty who are trained to use the rubric to evaluate them. There is a scoring system and set of online tools to facilitate the review. The goal of the review is to provide constructive, specific, measurable, sensitive, and balanced feedback that guides faculty/course developers to implement changes based on the standards to improve course design. The eight standards are:

1. Course Overview and Introduction
2. Learning Objectives (Competencies)
3. Assessment and Measurement
4. Instructional Materials
5. Learner Interaction and Engagement
6. Course Technology
7. Learner Support
8. Accessibility

A key component imbedded in the QM rubric is the focus on alignment. During a course review, evaluators examine the alignment across the standards.

CHALLENGES AND OPPORTUNITIES

Creating effective learning environments with technology poses ongoing challenges as the technology and infrastructure for its use continue to evolve. When thinking about the next level of teaching with technology, academic leaders of nursing programs and nurse educators should reflect on how their students currently use technology and how increased use of social media, mobile applications, and emerging technologies might influence the technology classroom of the future. Nursing faculty need to keep current with the rapidly changing technology trends to ensure that the preparation of today's graduates is always focused on educating them for the world in which they live and work. Assisting nursing and other faculty in higher education with the instructional integration of IT continues to be a top priority. Despite the widespread agreement on the importance of digital media literacy, training in developing skills and techniques is lacking in formal and informal preparation for faculty (Johnson et al., 2013). Table 4.2 displays the top 10 technology challenges for institutions.

TABLE 4.2 Top Institutional Priorities and Emerging Technologies

Campus Computing Survey[a] Percent Reporting "Very Important"	Top 10 IT Priorities[b]
1. Assisting faculty to integrate technology into instruction (74%)	Updating IT professionals' skills and roles
2. Providing adequate user support (70%)	Supporting trends toward BYOD
3. Hiring and retaining qualified IT staff (69%)	Developing a campus-wide cloud strategy
4. Providing online education via the web and implementing and supporting mobile computing (61%)	Improving operational efficiency through the use of IT resources
5. Upgrading/enhancing network and data security (54%)	Integrating IT into institutional decision making
6. Financing the replacement of aging IT (50%)	Using analytics to support institutional outcomes
7. Upgrading and enhancing IT network (42%)	Funding IT strategically
8. Migrating to cloud computing (33%)	Transforming the institution's business with IT
9. Upgrading and enhancing administrative IT systems (24%)	Supporting the research mission through large datasets and analytics
10. Upgrading and enhancing emergency communication (16%)	Establishing and integrating IT governance

Horizon Report 2013[c]: Emerging Technologies and Their Impact on Higher Education

Near term (12 months)	Massive open online courses (MOOCs)
	Tablet computing
Mid-term (2–3 years)	Games
	Learning analytics
Far term (4–5 years)	3-D printing
	Wearable technology

BYOD, Bring Your Own Device; IT, information technology.
[a]Green (2012); [b]Grajek and Pirani (2012); [c]Johnson et al. (2013).

SUMMARY

The rapid advances and constant pace of change in technology create challenges and opportunities for teaching in nursing. The more nurse educators use technology, the more they recognize its positive effects on student learning and engagement and its connection to 21st-century skills. Nurse educators need to be prepared to adopt existing technologies and explore emerging technology tools. Technology is helping teachers to expand beyond linear, text-based learning and engage students who have a variety of learning styles. The role of technology in nursing education has evolved from a contained "computer class" into versatile learning tools that change how faculty demonstrate concepts, guide students' learning, assess progress, and increase access to nursing education.

Nurse educators should not use technology because they can, but rather integrate appropriate technology in their courses based on quality standards and pedagogical approaches that support best practices and improve students' ability to learn. This chapter explored technology integration and technology tools such as LMS, Web 2.0, Web 3.0, virtual words and gaming, and others, to support student achievement of learning outcomes with attention to curriculum and classroom alignment that increases rigor, relevance, and relationships. Classroom redesign, including flipping the classroom, was also discussed in the chapter. When a nursing program and faculty decide to offer technology-based courses or programs, a significant amount of attention should focus on the infrastructure, resources, and support.

Technology will continue to disrupt nursing education, and the disruption will change as technology evolves over time. The goal is to explore and embrace technology tools that support good teaching practices in nursing.

REFERENCES

1st International Conference on Learning Analytics and Knowledge. (2011, February 27-March 1). Banff, Alberta. Retrieved from https://tekri.athabascau.ca/analytics

2011 CDW-G 21st-Century Campus Report. (2011). Retrieved from www.cdwnewsroom. com/2011-cdw-g-21st-century-campus-report

Allen, I. E., & Seaman, J. (2012). *Conflicted: Faculty and Online Education, 2012.* Inside Higher Ed, Babson Survey Research Group and Quahog Research Group, LLC. Retrieved from www. eric.ed.gov/PDFS/ED535214.pdf

Avgeriou, P., Papasalouros, A., Retalis, S., & Skordalakis, M. (2003). Towards a pattern language for learning management systems. *Educational Technology & Society, 6*(2), 11–24.

Bloom, B. S., Englehart, M. D., Furst, E. J., Hill, W. H., & Krathwohl, D. R. (1956). *Taxonomy of educational objectives: The classification of educational goals. Handbook I: Cognitive domain.* White Plains, NY: Longman.

Bruner, J. (1966). *Towards a theory of instruction.* Cambridge, MA: Harvard University Press.

Bruner, J. (1996). *The culture of education.* Cambridge, MA: Harvard University Press.

Chickering, A. W., & Ehrmann, S. (1996). Implementing the seven principles: Technology as lever. Retrieved from www.tltgroup.org/programs/seven.html

Chickering, A. W., & Gamson, Z. F. (1987). Seven principles for good practice in undergraduate education. *AAHE Bulletin, 39*(7), 3–6.

Connors, H. R. (2006). Transforming the nursing curriculum: Going paperless. In C. Weaver & C. Delaney (Eds.), *Nursing and informatics for the 21st century: An international look at the trends, cases, and the future* (pp. 183–194). Chicago, IL: Healthcare Information and Management Systems Society.

Connors, H. R., Warren, J. J., & Weaver, C. (2007). HIT plants SEEDS in healthcare education. *Nursing Administration Quarterly, 31*, 129–133. doi:10.1097/01.NAQ.0000264861.49217.f0

Epper, R. M., Derryberry, A., & Jackson, S. (2012, August 9). *Game-based Learning: Developing an Institutional Strategy* (Research Bulletin). Louisville, CO: EDUCAUSE Center for Applied Research. Retrieved from www.educause.edu/ecar

Gerald, S., & Antonacci, D. M. (2013). A virtual world learning spaces: Developing a Second Life operating room simulation. *EDUCAUSE Review Online*. Retrieved from www.educause.edu/ero/article/virtual-world-learning-spaces-developing-second-life-operating-room-simulation

Grajek, S., & Pirani, J. A. (2012). The top-ten IT issues, 2012. *EDUCAUSE Review, 47*(3). Retrieved from www.educause.edu/ero/article/top-ten-it-issues-2012

Graves, W. H. (2005). Improving institutional performance through IT-enabled innovation. *EDUCAUSE Review, 40*(6), 78–99.

Green, K. (2012). *Campus Computing 2012: Mixed Assessments for IT Effectiveness*. Retrieved from www.campuscomputing.net/item/campus-computing-2012-mixed-assessments-it-effectiveness

Hartman, J. L. (2008). Moving teaching and learning with technology. *EDUCAUSE Review, 43*(6), 24–25.

International Association for K-12 Online Learning (iNACOL). (2011). *National Standards for Quality Online Courses: Version 2*. Vienna, VA: iNACOL. Retrieved from www.inacol.org/cms/wp-content/uploads/2013/02/iNACOL_CourseStandards_2011.pdf

Institute of Medicine. (2010). *The future of nursing leading change, advancing health*. Washington, DC: National Academy of Sciences.

Johnson, L., Adams Becker, S., Cummins, M., Estrada, V., Freeman, A., & Ludgate, H. (2013). *NMC Horizon Report: 2013 Higher Education Edition*. Austin, TX: The New Media Consortium.

Kachka, P. (2012). Understanding the flipped classroom: Part 1. *Faculty Focus*. Retrieved from www.facultyfocus.com/articles/teaching-with-technology-articles/understanding-the-flipped-classroom-part-1

Lippencott, J. K. (2009). Learning spaces involving faculty to improve pedagogy. *EDUCAUSE Review, 44*(2), 17–24.

Markoff, J. (2006, November 12). Entrepreneurs see a web guided by common sense. *The New York Times*. Retrieved from www.nytimes.com/2006/11/12/business/12web.html?pagewanted=all&_r=0

Means, B., Toyama, Y., Murphy, R., Bakia, M., & Jones, K. (2010). *Evaluation of evidence-based practices in online learning: A meta-analysis and review of online learning studies*. Washington, DC: United States Department of Education Office of Planning, Evaluation, and Policy Development.

Mell, P., & Granace, T. (2011). *The NIST definition of cloud computing*. The National Institute of Standards and Technology, United States Department of Commerce. Special Publication 800–145. Gaithersburg, MD: National Institute of Standards and Technology.

Melnyk, B. M., & Davidson, S. (2009). Creating a culture of innovation in nursing education through shared vision, leadership, interdisciplinary partnerships, and positive deviance. *Nursing Administration Quarterly, 33*, 288–295. doi:10.1097/NAQ.0b013e3181b9dcf8

Moore, J. C. (2011). A synthesis of Sloan-C effective practices. *Journal of Asynchronous Learning Networks, 16*(1), 91–115. Retrieved from http://sloanconsortium.org/jaln/v16n1/synthesis-sloan-c-effective-practices-december-2011

Moore, R. (2012). The serious side of gaming. Retrieved from www1.umn.edu/news/features/2012/UR_CONTENT_408880.html

Ohler, J. (2008). The semantic web in education. *EDUCAUSE Quarterly, 31*(4), 7–9. Retrieved from www.educause.edu/ero/article/semantic-web-education

Quality Matters Program. (2011) Quality Matters™ Rubric Standards 2011–2013 Edition with Assigned Point Values. MarylandOnline, Inc.

Skiba, D. J. (2009). EMERGING technologies center nursing education 2.0: A second look at Second Life. *Nursing Education Perspectives, 30*, 129–131.

The Sloan Consortium. (2013). The 5 Pillars. Retrieved from http://sloanconsortium.org/5pillars

Smith, A. (2010). Mobile Access 2010. *Pew Internet & American Life Project*. Retrieved from http://pewinternet.org/Reports/2010/Reputation-Management.aspx

Southern Regional Education Board (SREB). (2006). *Standards for Quality Online Courses*. Atlanta, GA: SREB. Retrieved from http://publications.sreb.org/2006/06T05_Standards_quality_online_courses.pdf

Sultan, N. (2010). Cloud computing for education: A new dawn? *International Journal of Information Management, 30,* 109–116.

Tamarkin, M., & Rodrigo, S. (2011). Evolving technologies: A view to tomorrow. *EDUCAUSE Review,* 46(6), 63–80. Retrieved from www.educause.edu/ero/article/evolving-technologies-view-tomorrow

Thompson, K. (2011). 7 things you should know about MOOCs. *EDUCAUSE Learning Initiative.* Retrieved from www.educause.edu/library/resources/7-things-you-should-know-about-moocs

U.S. Department of Education Office of Educational Technology. (2013). *Expanding Evidence Approaches for Learning in a Digital World.* Retrieved from www.ed.gov/edblogs/technology/evidence-framework

UW Flexible Option. (2013). Board of Regents—University of Wisconsin System. Retrieved from http://flex.wisconsin.edu

Warren, J. J., & Connors, H. R. (2007). Health information technology can and will transform nursing education. *Nursing Outlook,* 55(1), 59–60. doi:10.1016/j.outlook.2006.11.003

Warren, J. J., Connors, H. R., & Trangenstein, P. A. (2011). A paradigm shift in simulation: Experiential learning in Second Life. In V. K. Saba & K. A. McCormick (Eds.), *Essentials of nursing informatics* (pp. 619–631). New York, NY: McGraw Hill.

Warren, J. J., Manos, E. L., Meyer, M., & Roche, A. (2013). Integrating an academic electronic health record into simulations. In S. Campbell & K. Daley (Eds.), *Simulation scenarios for nursing educators: Making it real* (2nd ed., pp. 519–528). New York, NY: Springer Publishing Company.

Warren, J. J., Meyer, M. N., Thompson, T., & Roche, A. (2010). Transforming nursing education: Integrating informatics and simulations. In C. Weaver, C. Delaney, P. Weber, & R. Carr (Eds.), *Nursing and informatics for the 21st century: An international look at practice, trends and EHR technologies* (2nd ed., pp. 145–161). Chicago, IL: Healthcare Information and Management Systems Society.

Western Interstate Commission for Higher Education. (2010). *NSD No significant difference.* Retrieved from www.nosignificantdifference.org

Whiteside, A., Brooks, D. C., & Walker, D. (2010). Making the case for space: Three years of empirical research on learning environments. *EDUCAUSE Quarterly.* Retrieved from www.educause.edu/ero/article/making-case-space-three-years-empirical-research-learning-environments

5

Clinical Simulations in Nursing Education: Overview, Essentials, and the Evidence

PAMELA R. JEFFRIES, KRISTINA THOMAS DREIFUERST, DIANE S. ASCHENBRENNER, KATIE ANNE ADAMSON, AND ANDREA PARSONS SCHRAM

Traditionally, simulations have been used to provide opportunities for students to practice patient care in a safe environment before going into the clinical setting. However, in the current environment of increasing patient acuity and limited clinical placements, simulation can serve a broader role as an adjunct or replacement for traditional clinical hours. Moreover, the Institute of Medicine (2011) recently cited simulation as a critical ingredient for producing an adequate number of competent nurses. As simulation pedagogy progresses, it also will play an increasingly important role in both formative and summative student and nurse evaluation.

This chapter provides an overview of types of clinical simulations in nursing, as well as how to integrate and implement them into a nursing curriculum. The importance of how to create realism and suspending disbelief in the simulations are also discussed. In addition, debriefing approaches, evaluation processes to use when developing and implementing clinical simulations, and evidence on the use of clinical simulations beyond the point of asking whether the pedagogy actually works, but also how to make it work best, are highlighted.

DIFFERENT TYPES OF SIMULATION

There are a several different types of simulations that vary in the degree of fidelity or the ability of the simulation environment to best replicate the actual clinical environment (Jeffries & Rogers, 2007). This fidelity, or realism, allows the learner to become engaged within the simulation on a physical, conceptual, emotional, and experiential level (Rudolph, Simon, & Raemer, 2007).

MANIKIN-BASED SIMULATION

Manikin-based simulation has been used for hundreds of years, including the bronze acupuncture teaching statues from the Song Dynasty in China and Mrs. Chase, the classic nursing manikin used for task training since 1922 (Herrmann, 2008; Owen, 2012). Manikins, as human patient simulators (HPSs), vary in the amount and degree of technology and fidelity built into the devices. Simulation fidelity is defined as the extent to which a simulated experience is real or believable to the participants (INASCL Board of Directors, 2011). It can be thought of in two dimensions: *engineering fidelity*, or how authentic the simulation looks and feels, and *psychological fidelity*, or how realistic the behaviors and actions required mimic what is anticipated or expected (Norman, Dore, & Grierson, 2012). Fidelity is important to consider when developing simulations for students because it reflects the level of engagement that will be expected of participants as they are involved in the experience (Feinstein & Cannon, 2002) and to what lengths the nurse educator and simulation personnel will go to create it.

Manikins that are life-sized, have realistic anatomical structures, and contain technology that dynamically mimics changes in human physiology are called high-fidelity HPSs, whereas other full-sized manikins that can mimic physiologic changes only partially or not as rapidly are called medium-fidelity manikins (Lapkin, Levett-Jones, Bellchambers, & Fernandez, 2012). Low-fidelity HPSs are task trainers that are static and typically represent one function of the human body, such as an arm model used to practice venipuncture. These are particularly useful for novice students learning basic skills and general principles of patient care (Kardong-Edgren, Anderson, & Michaels, 2007).

High-fidelity HPSs are best used when learners are expected to successfully care for a patient with multiple abnormal physiologic findings within the simulation scenario. These manikins allow for changes of physiologic parameters within the simulation, either by programming ahead of the simulation or by changing the parameters within the simulation. This allows faculty to evaluate the learner's ability to respond rapidly to changes in the patient's condition or to demonstrate the physiologic effects of any given treatment (medications or interventions). Multiple physiologic parameters, including pupil dilation/constriction, respiratory and cardiac functions (breath and heart sounds, pulses, blood pressure, pulse oxygenation), and abdominal signs (bowel sounds), can be programmed depending on the type of high-fidelity HPS. High-fidelity HPS also allow learners to practice and refine psychomotor skills, such as providing basic and advanced life support or assisting at childbirth. When the simulation scenario requires only a limited number of physiologic changes or complex task training, using a medium-fidelity HPS might be sufficient.

The decision about what level of fidelity to select is predicated on what is available, the objectives of the experience, and the intended learner outcomes. Fidelity can also involve a variety of dimensions, including (a) physical factors such as environment, equipment, and related tools; (b) psychological factors such as emotions, beliefs, and self-awareness of participants; (c) social factors such as participant and instructor motivation and goals; (d) culture of the group; and (e) degree of openness and trust, as well as participants' modes of thinking (Dieckmann, Gaba, & Rall, 2007). These are important considerations for nurse educators during the process of selecting or designing simulations. The patient's story in the scenario and the objectives for the simulation become part of the fidelity or realism of the experience and help to socialize the student to the role of the nurse.

Moulage is another aspect of fidelity that nurse educators can consider for simulation learning with manikins and other simulation modalities. Moulage incorporates the use of makeup, dress, and wigs to enhance the patient story, and wax, latex, artificial fluids, and simulation enhancers to simulate injury, disease, aging, and other physical enhancements to the manikin (Smith-Stoner, 2011). Adding moulage to the simulation increases realism for the student and can make the simulation experience more authentic for holistic learning.

Fidelity in simulation is intended to immerse the student in a realistic learning experience that represents a clinical setting or patient care situation. Attention to having realistic equipment, creating a representative physical environment, has an impact on the believability of the simulation experience for many students and can affect clinical learning. Low-, moderate-, and high-fidelity simulations can be valuable learning environments when they are incorporated into the curriculum and learning objectives for nursing students.

STANDARDIZED PATIENTS

A standardized patient (SP) is an individual who is trained to portray a patient with a specific condition and is able to play that patient consistently during every simulation (Association of Standardized Patient Educators [ASPE], 2011). During a simulation, an SP provides a consistent answer to questions asked by the learner and has been trained prior to the simulation not to go off script, embellish the response, or provide additional information that was not asked by the learner. To do this, the SP must rehearse the role with the faculty to ensure that each learner experiences the same patient portrayal in each and every simulation. Sometimes an individual is enlisted to role-play a part in a simulation with little or no training. In this case, this individual is not an SP, as there is no assurance that the role will be played in the same manner for each simulation.

SPs might be further subdivided according to the objective of the simulation and role they play. Within the simulation, they can portray patients but can also function as either teacher or evaluator. A female who is specifically trained to teach and provide feedback to the learner who is conducting a gynecologic exam is called a gynecology teaching associate (GTA), whereas a male who instructs a learner on how to conduct a urogenital and rectal exam is called a male urogenital teaching associate (MUTA; ASPE, 2011). SPs are often used to teach and evaluate other physical examination skills, such as a head-to-toe assessment. Certain SPs obtain further education and training to evaluate the student in either formative or summative evaluation experiences, including high-stakes simulation. Objective structured clinical examinations (OCSE) are a series of stations in which students care for a variety of patients according to a predetermined, time-limited schedule for each station. SPs are used to portray these patients and at times also participate in the evaluation of the student.

Simulations may be enhanced by the use of SPs, particularly in simulation scenarios that teach and evaluate communication skills (Ryan, Walshe, Gaffney, Shanks, Burgoyne, & Wiskin, 2010). Many prelicensure nursing programs use SPs for psychiatric mental health simulations, whereas advanced practice nursing programs use SPs to teach and evaluate history-taking skills. Other uses of SPs include simulations involving interprofessional education (IPE) teams, ethical and cultural competencies, safety, and patient education. SPs are also used as unannounced patients to evaluate providers, similar to secret shoppers who evaluate customer service.

Incorporating SPs within a simulation program requires planning and sufficient funds to hire and train them. Additional manpower may be required to coordinate the SP program within the school of nursing; however, most programs who use SPs believe that the experience is valuable (May, Park, & Lee, 2009).

VIRTUAL SIMULATION AND GAMING

Virtual simulation is an innovation in which learners access Internet-based, three-dimensional simulated environments for an educational experience (LeFlore et al., 2012).

Some virtual simulations have been built on Second Life® and may be used for teaching and learning or for evaluation. Although expensive to develop, there is some evidence that suggests that this type of simulation may be superior when compared with traditional lecture method or interaction with a SP (LeFlore et al., 2012; Wendling, Halan, Tighe, Le, Euliano, & Lok, 2011).

Gaming has also been incorporated within simulation. One nursing program found that high-fidelity simulation along with an experiential gaming experience enhanced the curriculum on end-of-life care (Kopp & Hanson, 2012). Another innovative simulation experience involved the use of a fictitious registered nurse (RN) blog to describe challenges during her first year of practice (Thomas, Bertram, & Allen, 2012).

The simulation learning objectives should dictate the type of simulation that will allow the student to accomplish the desired clinical outcomes. Regardless of the type of simulation selected, it is important to clearly identify how it will provide the realism necessary for the learner to fully engage in the simulation. To accomplish this objective, a detailed simulation scenario should include the type of HPS to be used, along with the patient condition and corresponding physiologic parameters throughout the simulation. Any additional equipment needed to either more accurately replicate the clinical setting or that should be used by the learner to accomplish the objectives of the simulation should also be included in the experience.

INTEGRATION OF SIMULATIONS INTO THE CURRICULUM

High-fidelity simulations offer a rich opportunity to improve student learning and achieve desired outcomes throughout a nursing curriculum. Simulations can be used in a variety of ways by faculty to meet different learning goals ranging from knowledge acquisition to application of a theoretical concept, professional role development, and evaluation of student competency.

Perhaps the most obvious use of high-fidelity simulation is creating a clinical experience for students. This experience can supplement or replace clinical hours or a clinical day for any type of experience in a nursing curriculum. Simulation allows all students in a program to experience patient care situations deemed critical for professional practice that cannot be guaranteed in a clinical setting. For example, it might be considered important for all new nurses to know how to assess and care for a diabetic patient with significant hypoglycemia. While all students could be assigned a diabetic patient in a clinical setting, there is no guarantee that they would all provide care for a patient with hypoglycemia. Yet, this experience can be granted to every student using simulation. Simulations can also create clinical experiences that are rare in clinical practice, but that are potentially life threatening in real life, and that require prompt recognition and intervention. Clinical simulations can be created to provide students with a practice setting or a type of experience that is difficult to provide due to a variety of factors such as limited clinical sites, lack of qualified faculty in a specialty area, or geographic remoteness. For example, it can be difficult to place all of the students in labor and delivery. Inpatient pediatric units can also be difficult to locate. In those cases, simulation can be used to meet the learning needs of students to care for children of all ages and to provide experiences that are difficult to provide consistently for students.

There are several possible ways to provide simulation experiences for students in remote locations where significant travel is needed to reach the school or an appropriate clinical agency. For example, a live simulation with a small group of students could be broadcast to a satellite location where there is no simulation laboratory. Simulations could be integrated completely online, whereby a recording of the simulation is posted, and then debriefing occurs via an asynchronous discussion. Or, students could be assigned to view an online video clip of a simulation or interact with a live telehealth simulation, followed by synchronous or asynchronous discussions. Simulation can help to develop critical thinking, clinical reasoning, team building, communication skills, and other professional attributes needed in a graduate nurse. Through simulation, the student acts in the role of the nurse caring for patients, interacting with other health care providers, acting independently on physician orders, and documenting care, because it is a safe learning environment.

Simulations should be leveled throughout the curriculum, building in complexity and ambiguity. When selecting or writing simulations, faculty should create experiences that help students develop competencies to meet national goals for professional practice, such as patient safety or quality goals. Faculty should also consider what content and skills students have found difficult to master and incorporate those into simulations.

High-fidelity simulation, in addition to its use in clinical courses, can be incorporated into traditional theory courses. This incorporation assists students in linking the theory to practice. For example, a didactic presentation could present information about a myocardial infarction and standard care of these patients. Following this classroom presentation, students could participate in a simulation that allowed them to apply that knowledge to assessment and care of a simulated patient with a myocardial infarction. Using another approach, the content could be presented first via the simulation, in which the students are given materials to prepare for the experience with the goal that knowledge would be attained through the simulation.

A mechanism of introducing increasingly complex simulations into a curriculum is to use an unfolding case. In an unfolding case, students are introduced to a particular patient repeatedly at different points in the care continuum within a simulation, throughout a course, or throughout the curriculum. The patient scenario becomes more complex and requires different assessment skills or interventions on the part of the nurse. For example, in a psychiatric mental health course, the students could be introduced to a patient with depression. Later in the semester, the students might meet the same patient, but this time the patient is suicidal. The students might encounter the same patient yet again at a later date in a different course, such as community health, when making a home health visit, and could observe the patient interacting with his or her own family.

Another way to add complexity to a simulation is to repeat the exact case but use a modified version. This could occur in one course where, after debriefing a simulation, the students switch roles and repeat the simulation. This time the scenario progresses in a slightly different way. For example, the first scenario might have the postpartum patient with normal vaginal discharge after delivery. When the simulation is repeated, the patient develops signs and symptoms of a postpartum hemorrhage, and the nurse needs to identify the differences and the appropriate nursing actions. Each of these simulations offers different opportunities for teaching and learning.

Simulation can play an important role in developing professional roles and behaviors in nursing students. In addition to learning to think and act like a nurse, students need to learn how to work with other health care professions. IPE has been nationally promoted as critical to providing high-quality and safe patient care (Institute of Medicine, 2003). Interdisciplinary simulations can represent basic to complex interactions in patient care. For example, beginning medical and nursing students might be involved in a simulation in which a patient has an abnormal laboratory value. The nurse would be responsible for identifying the problem, contacting the physician, and receiving and acting on new medical orders. The physician would be responsible for evaluating the data presented by the nurse, making a diagnosis, and providing appropriate medical orders. With more advanced students, the interdisciplinary simulation might reflect a difference of opinion as to best care or an ethical dilemma related to possible care and treatment options. Team members that should be incorporated include physical therapists, respiratory therapists, nutritionists, social workers, pharmacists, and others.

In IPE simulations, students typically portray roles within their own profession. They learn about other professions by observing others portraying their role in the simulation and through the discussion in debriefing. There might be occasions when it is valuable to switch roles. A variety of simulation experiences can be used to help students understand other health care provider roles and responsibilities and to create some empathy for what the other professions experience.

Simulation can also be used as a method to evaluate student knowledge and abilities. In introductory courses, students might have to identify normal or abnormal heart or breath sounds, and in more advanced courses might demonstrate competency, for example, recognizing deterioration of a patient's status and taking appropriate action. Faculty members need to reach a philosophical consensus when using simulation as an evaluation tool. Is the desired outcome to bring all students to a certain level of ability prior to allowing them to progress in the curriculum? This concept suggests that students would have multiple opportunities to attempt the simulation, with assistance to improve as needed. Or, is the desire to evaluate and grade performance in the simulation to certify competency and allow progression of only those students who can demonstrate a certain level of ability? This approach suggests that students would have only one opportunity to pass the simulation. Is there a grade associated with the simulation? If the simulation contributes to a grade in a course, a grading rubric is needed. Faculty should also reach a curricular consensus as to how to evaluate a simulation. At this time there is no standard recommendation as to how to most effectively evaluate student performance in a simulation.

When students need to achieve a certain level of performance during a simulation or else fail a course, or be unable to graduate, the simulation is termed *high stakes*. Cordeau (2010), in her study of students' perceptions of clinical simulation, provides several insights relevant to high-stakes simulations, which should be considered by nursing faculty. First, students have increased anxiety when simulation is used for testing or summative evaluation. Second, anxiety is experienced in all phases of the simulation from presimulation to the debriefing process. Though a small amount of anxiety can sharpen performance, high anxiety impairs performance. Student anxiety needs to be at a manageable level for students to be successful in meeting the outcomes of the clinical simulation. Third, adequate student preparation is needed to overcome anxiety and foster success. Students should be oriented to the simulation environment and given adequate information about the simulation experience prior to the start. Prebriefing should include information about the simulated patient similar to the nursing report that is shared before a nurse assumes the care of a patient. In addition, practice sessions and appropriate cues and fidelity in a simulation can help students to be successful and demonstrate their best performance during the simulation.

The National Council of State Boards of Nursing is developing competency assessments using standardized simulations to assess postlicensure competence (Hinton et al., 2012). Decker, Utterback, Thomas, Mitchell, and Sportsman (2011) contend that assessment of continued competency must be considered a shared responsibility by the individual nurse, professional organizations, regulatory agencies, and employers. As these assessment simulations are developed, it is likely that they will be added as a component for determining prelicensure competency.

IMPLEMENTATION OF SIMULATIONS

Once simulation experiences that are needed in the curriculum, and the faculty have identified the best methodology of presenting them, implementation can commence. Exhibit 5.1 provides a checklist to guide implementation of simulations. For simulations to be most effective as a learning experience, teachers must plan carefully all aspects relevant to running the simulation. Using simulation as a teaching method cannot be done successfully as a spur-of-the-moment decision.

EXHIBIT 5.1 Checklist for Implementation of a Simulation

- Create or select the simulation scenario and objectives.
- Determine your resources.
  - Number of manikins or SPs available
  - Number of simulation rooms available
  - Number of faculty available to assist in running simulation
- Determine the time needed to run scenario and debriefing.
- Determine the time needed to allow all students to participate in simulation.
  - Number of student groups
  - Include time to rotate groups
- Determine the date(s) and time(s) the simulation will run.

The first step is the creation or selection of the simulation scenario. These might be done with several content experts writing and reviewing a draft of the simulation, after consulting the literature to ensure that current guidelines for evidence-based practice are met. A template is helpful to provide a standardized structure for the simulation and to guarantee that key aspects are not overlooked. Specific learning objectives and student outcomes need to be identified. They should accurately reflect what students can actually accomplish in the allotted time, given their skills and abilities. A detailed description related to staging the scene should include factors such as:

- How the manikin or patient should "look"
- What equipment needs to be in the room
- What supplies the student needs to perform in the simulation
- What props are needed to add realism
- What information needs to be in the patient's medical record
- How the patient should respond (verbally, physiologically) to interventions made by the nurse

All of these details must be considered, planned, and written into the simulation scenario.

An alternative to writing simulations is using premade or purchased scenarios. These have the advantage that the content, in most circumstances, has been determined to accurately reflect current standards of practice. Premade or purchased simulations might need to be adjusted to meet local differences in care practices or to level the simulation based on the learner's abilities at a given point in the curriculum. For teachers learning to use simulation, this simplifies the process of incorporating simulation into the curriculum.

The remainder of planning and implementing simulations into a course involves practical issues of running a simulation. A primary consideration is how much time will be needed for the simulation and debriefing. This is not a simple question—many times scenarios run 10 to 30 minutes, and historically the debriefing takes at least twice the time of the scenario. However, these are generalizations, and many factors go into the timing decisions, including the complexity of the simulation, level and roles of the learners, and outcomes of the experience. It is also important to take into account the total number of students participating in the simulation and the amount of time that is available.

Consider this example. A basic simulation of 10 minutes also has 20 minutes of debriefing time. Therefore, it will take 30 minutes for each group of students to complete the simulation. If there are 50 students, they are to participate in the simulation in groups of 5. Each group needs 30 minutes for the simulation and debriefing so it will take 5 hours to run the simulation if there is only one manikin or SP to use at a time. Teachers should also consider how much time they have available. Is the class time during which the simulation is being implemented, for example, a 50-minute time slot? This amount of time is not sufficient to run the simulation twice. At least 60 minutes are needed to run it twice, plus time is needed to rotate students and reset the room for the next group.

In addition to time, there are other resources that should be considered. An important variable is the number of simulation rooms and manikins or SPs that can be used at a single time. Another consideration is the number of educators who are familiar with the pedagogy and technology and who are available to assist with facilitating the simulation. Teachers need to plan thoroughly for a simulation experience and consider all aspects needed to run the simulation smoothly. Sufficient time needs to be allotted to design, plan, and implement simulations into the curriculum. When the simulation runs without issues, the teacher is less stressed, and students experience a more positive learning experience.

DEBRIEFING

Debriefing is an important component of student learning in simulation. Typically, debriefing immediately follows a simulation as an opportunity for students and teachers to review the experience and learn from what occurred (Arafeh, Hansen, & Nichlos, 2010; Decker, 2007; Dreifuerst, 2009; Fanning & Gaba, 2007). During debriefing, teachers can guide students to reflect on, analyze, and discuss their thoughts and feelings about the experience. Debriefing also provides time to review carefully the actions and clinical decisions that occurred during the simulation and discuss options and alternatives to improve nursing care or patient outcomes (Rudolf, Simon, Raemer, & Eppich, 2008). Because of the sensitive nature of the discussion, debriefing should take place in a comfortable, private area away from the actual simulated patient environment (Wickers, 2010). Although there are many ways to debrief, it is common for teachers and students to focus the discussion on what went right, what went wrong, and what should be done differently during the next simulation experience or similar patient encounter (Dismukes, Gaba, & Howard, 2006; Dreifuerst & Decker, 2012; Flannagan, 2008).

Because debriefing is a constructivist, reflective teaching strategy, it typically involves an interactive discussion among the students who were directly involved in the simulation scenario, the students who observed the simulation, and the teacher (Cantrell, 2008; Dreifuerst, 2009; Shinnick, Woo, Horwich, & Steadman, 2011). These lively discussions often use the intended learning objectives for the experience to discover what was done correctly, what was done incorrectly, and what could be done differently the next time.

Debriefing in this format then becomes a type of formative feedback, which is intended to change thinking and behaviors when the student encounters similar issues in clinical practice (Decker, 2007; Rudolf et al., 2008).

Providing feedback is only one component of the role of the teacher as debriefing facilitator. The facilitator typically guides the debriefing experience by acting as a mentor, coach, teacher, or peer, depending on the situation, students, and simulation outcomes. The facilitator's role in the debriefing process can vary because it is dependent on the skill level of the participants, how much guidance is needed to keep the discussion flowing, and the objectives of the simulation (Rudolph, Simon, Raemer, & Eppich, 2008). Teachers generally are more active facilitators when the students are novices and new to simulation or when there has been an emotional experience on the part of one or more of the participants. Likewise, the teacher can guide the discussion to provide additional support when a negative simulation outcome or poor student performance has occurred (Dreifuerst, 2009; Fanning & Gaba, 2007). As the students gain experience and knowledge, they assume a more active role in the discussion, and the teacher becomes more of a guide and less of a facilitator.

Guiding the discussion can involve the use of many communication strategies by the teacher. These include incorporation of open-ended questions, active listening, Socratic questioning, restating, rephrasing, and leading questions. These techniques might require training and practice for the teacher prior to the actual simulation experience (Dreifuerst, 2012; Fanning & Gaba, 2007). Continuing education opportunities to learn evidence-based debriefing practices and strategies are available from a variety of venues including formal education sessions and informal peer coaching. These are also opportunities to learn new ways and methods that can be used to debrief students.

There are many debriefing methods and strategies, which are used in different health care disciplines and simulation environments (Exhibit 5.2). Although many share similar practices in the way debriefing occurs, each has unique attributes that support different learners and environments (Overstreet, 2010). Reflection is an essential component of debriefing regardless of the method (Dreifuerst, 2009; Shinnick et al., 2011). Revisiting the events of the simulation is important to understand the student's

EXHIBIT 5.2 Debriefing Methods

- Plus Delta
  - What went right
  - What would you change
- Debriefing for Meaningful Learning
  - Reflection in action
  - Reflection on action
  - Reflection beyond action
  - Clinical reasoning and thinking
- Advocacy-Inquiry
  - Statement of advocacy or assertion
  - Request for clarification
- Gather-Analyze-Summarize
  - Pull together pertinent information
  - Discuss details of what went well and what did not
  - Review all aspects of the experience in the context of the debriefing discussion

behaviors, decision making, and impact on patient outcomes. Reflecting also solidifies learning from the experience, particularly when attention is paid to reflecting-in-action, reflecting-on-action, and reflecting-beyond-action (Dreifuerst, 2009; Schön, 1983). There are many debriefing methods that can be used to guide the reflective process. Some of the more common debriefing methods include Plus Delta, Debriefing for Meaningful Learning©, Advocacy-Inquiry, and Gather-Analyze-Summarize.

Variations of the Plus Delta debriefing method are popular in interdisciplinary health care simulations. This method emphasizes what went well ("Plus") and what could be done better or differently ("Delta," the Greek symbol for change). This is accomplished by soliciting reflective responses from the students involved in the simulation (Fanning & Gaba, 2007). This method is not difficult to learn, and it is adapted easily to many different types of simulations and learners.

Debriefing for Meaningful Learning is a structured method that incorporates clinical teaching with debriefing to emphasize reflection in action, reflection on action, and reflection beyond action; clinical reasoning; and thinking like a nurse (Dreifuerst, 2009; Schön, 1983; Tanner, 2006). A premise of this method is that the facilitator needs to be a clinician or clinical teacher with knowledge about the patient population, who can guide the reflective process of uncovering the students' thinking that underpinned their actions and decisions during the simulation (Dreifuerst, 2012).

In the Advocacy-Inquiry debriefing method, which comes from the Debriefing With Good Judgment model (Rudolf et al., 2007), the teacher focuses the debriefing on a particular component of the simulation because the student involved in the experience has done something unexpected or unanticipated. The discussion begins with a statement of advocacy or assertion about what was observed from the teacher's perspective, followed by a nonthreatening question or request for clarification about student thinking and actions (Rudolf et al., 2007).

The Gather-Analyze-Summarize method uses a three-step process for debriefing (American Heart Association, 2010). Teachers guide the students to integrate or gather all of the pertinent information about the simulation experience, including what occurred, the decisions that were made, and the outcomes. Next, the participants and facilitator analyze the information that was gathered, using the objectives for the simulation and what went right and what did not. Finally, everything that has been discussed is summarized to reinforce learning (Exhibit 5.2).

Regardless of the method, debriefing that includes reflection and revisiting of the events and actions to understand behaviors, decision making, and the effects on patient outcomes are an essential part of simulation learning (Dreifuerst, 2009; Shinnick et al., 2011). Debriefing should include the objectives of the experience and recall of the events of the simulation. Students should be actively involved in the discussion and have an opportunity to have clarified anything that is uncertain during debriefing. Teachers who use simulation should feel comfortable facilitating debriefing as an important component of student learning.

SIMULATION EVALUATION

Simulation activities offer educators and researchers unique opportunities for evaluation. Similar to clinical evaluation, simulation evaluations often focus on participant performance. However, many view simulation as a highly adaptable alternative to traditional clinical experiences and may consequently hold simulation to higher evaluation standards. This is true because, when there was no alternative to evaluating performance in the clinical setting, there was little reason to question how well it worked.

However, with the advent of simulation, the teacher should examine the efficacy of both clinical and simulation teaching and learning more carefully. Simulation evaluations focus not only on participant performance, but also on design characteristics, educational practices, participant satisfaction, how learning in the simulation occurs and subsequently transfers to the clinical arena, and ultimately the impact of simulation on patient outcomes.

The first step in planning an effective simulation participant evaluation is to identify the purpose and focus of the evaluation. Questions to ask at this stage include: What type of data will be gathered and what will they be used for? Should the evaluation reflect individual or group performance? At this stage, it is also important to decide whether the evaluation is formative or summative. Next, it is important to identify the ideal simulation modality for the evaluation. For example, if the evaluation is meant to reflect participants' intravenous insertion skills, a task-trainer might be the most efficient simulation modality. However, if interpersonal communication skills need to be evaluated, an SP might offer the most realism and opportunities for valid evaluation.

Selecting or developing an appropriate evaluation instrument, with validity and reliability, is the next key step in the evaluation process. From this point, carefully selecting and training raters to complete the evaluation are important activities to help ensure valid and reliable results. This can be as simple as identifying an individual, or as complex as selecting and training a group of raters and assessing important criteria such as interrater reliability. With these decisions made, it is finally time for collecting, interpreting, and reporting evaluation data. More details about assessment and clinical evaluation are provided in Chapters 10 and 12.

CATEGORIZING SIMULATION EVALUATION STRATEGIES

In recent years there has been a proliferation of simulation evaluation instruments (Kardong-Edgren, Adamson, & Fitzgerald, 2010) and articles about simulation evaluation in nursing (Davis & Kimble, 2011; Yuan, Williams, Fang, & Ye, 2012) and the health sciences (Bray, Schwartz, Odegard, Hammer, & Seybert, 2011; Kogan, Holmboe, & Hauer, 2009). Simulation evaluation can be categorized into three basic phases: preimplementation, implementation, and outcomes. The Simulation Design Scale (SDS) and Educational Practices Simulation Scale (EPSS; Jeffries & Rogers, 2012) are examples of resources that can be used for evaluation during the preimplementation and implementation phases to evaluate the quality of simulation activities. The quality of simulation activities, in turn, influences the outcomes of the activities. Most simulation evaluations focus on student outcomes.

Kirkpatrick (1998) described four levels of outcomes that are helpful for categorizing evaluation strategies (Table 5.1). Here are the levels as they apply to simulation evaluation:

Level 1: Participants' reactions to the simulation activity
Level 2: Participants' learning from the simulation activity
Level 3: Changes in participants' behavior as a result of the simulation activity
Level 4: The long-term results that take place in practice because of the simulation activity

The category of learning (Level 2) can be further divided using the three domains of learning: cognitive, affective, and psychomotor. While the goal of many simulation evaluations is to cover multiple levels and learning domains, using Kirkpatrick's language helps to describe the focus (or foci) of the particular strategy.

TABLE 5.1 Different Levels of Evaluation According to the Kirkpatrick Model

Level of Evaluation	Example	Reference
Level 1: Reaction	National League for Nursing Participant Satisfaction and Self-Confidence in Learning Instruments	Adamson, Jeffries, and Rogers (2012)
	Emergency Response Confidence Tool	Arnold et al. (2009)
Level 2: Cognitive learning	Paper-and-pencil test questions	Hoffman, O'Donnell, and Kim (2007)
	Observation-based simulation evaluation instruments such as the Sweeny-Clark Simulation Performance Evaluation Rubric	Clark (2006)
Level 2: Affective learning	Interpersonal Communication Assessment Scale (ICAS)	Klakovitch and Dela Cruz (2006)
	Assessment of aspects of communication and the nurse/patient relationship	Framp, McAllister, and Hitchen-Holmes (2009)
Level 2: Psychomotor learning	Skills checklists such as that of the American Heart Association performance evaluation rubrics (e.g., for cardiopulmonary resuscitation)	American Heart Association (n.d.)
Level 3: Behavior	Clinical performance of students who attended simulations and students who had not yet attended simulations, compared using scores from Likert-type tool	Meyer, Connors, Hou, and Gajewski (2011)
	Multiple measures to investigate thinking and behaviors related to the care of a heart failure patient	Shinnick and Woo (2012)
Level 4: Results	Measure of cost savings resulting from simulation-based training on central venous catheters and blood infections	Cohen et al. (2010)
	Measures related to improved management of neonatal shoulder dystocia that resulted from simulation-based training	Draycott et al. (2008)

From Kirkpatrick (1998).

Evaluations become increasingly difficult, but potentially more meaningful, as they progress from Level 1 (reaction) to Level 4 (results). For example, it is much easier to ask participants to rate their level of satisfaction with a simulation activity

(Level 1: reaction) or assess participant knowledge before and after a simulation activity (Level 2: learning [cognitive]) than it is to determine whether a simulation activity has an impact on how participants perform in the clinical environment (Level 3: behavior) or changes patient outcomes (Level 4: results). However, the effort to produce higher level evaluations is commensurate with their potential impact. The information provided by Level 3 and 4 evaluations has more potential impact than the information provided by the lower levels of evaluation (Levels 1 and 2). Figure 5.1 is an adaptation of the Kirkpatrick Model.

FIGURE 5.1 The Kirkpatrick Model.

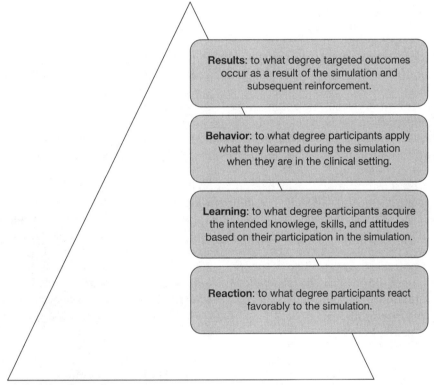

Based on the Kirkpatrick Model. Copyrighted by Kirkpatrick Partners, LLC, 2010–2012. Reprinted by permission, 2013.

PARTICIPANT PERFORMANCE EVALUATION

Many of the characteristics of clinical evaluation discussed in Chapter 12 are relevant to simulation participant evaluation. However, simulation offers evaluation opportunities that might not exist in traditional clinical settings. These include, but are not limited to, the ability to (a) create and standardize scenarios to isolate and elicit specific participant skills and behaviors, (b) allow multiple participants to engage in a given scenario or an individual participant to engage in a specific scenario multiple times, and (c) allow a participant to make errors without endangering a patient.

Simulation has enormous promise for participant evaluation beyond augmenting assessment in the clinical environment (Benner, Sutphen, Leonard, & Day, 2010). In the future, these evaluations can be implemented as an alternative or adjunct to the current tests used for academic progression and licensure or can be employed simply for formative evaluation of participant performance. Thoughtful planning and a focus on higher levels of evaluation that reflect learning, behavior, and results from simulation training are important to the development of simulation pedagogy.

BEST EVIDENCE AND RESEARCH IN SIMULATION

Simulation has been shown to be an effective educational method. In a recent, systematic review and meta-analysis of technology-enhanced simulation for health professional education, knowledge, skills, and behavior outcomes were consistently associated with large effect sizes (> 0.80). Furthermore, patient-related outcomes had a moderate effect size (0.50) when compared with no intervention (Cook et al., 2012). When compared with other active educational modalities, such as lecture, small group discussions, and video training, technology-enhanced simulation was associated with moderate positive effects for learner satisfaction (ES = 0.59); quality of skills (ES = 0.66); patient care behaviors (ES = 0.56); and small positive effects for knowledge (ES = 0.30), skill time (ES = 0.33), skill efficiency (ES = 0.38), and patient outcomes (ES = 0.36) (Cook et al., 2012). All of this means that simulation pedagogy has a positive impact on the teaching-learning process.

Over the past decade, researchers have identified 12 best practices that lead to effective learning in simulation (McGaghie, Issenberg, Petrusa, & Scalese, 2010). These are summarized in Exhibit 5.3.

The most important practice for simulation learning is to provide feedback. In most cases, feedback is given within the debriefing period to identify and correct performance gaps observed during the simulation. Although further research is needed to identify specific models for feedback, the Debriefing for Meaningful Learning method, which was presented earlier in the chapter, has been shown to improve clinical reasoning and judgment scores when compared with usual debriefing methods (Dreifuerst, 2012; Mariani, Cantrell, Meakim, Prieto, & Dreifuerst, 2012). Research is also needed on evidence-based strategies for debriefing that address the structure of debriefing, faculty demeanor, environment, types of probing and cuing questions, and the timeliness of debriefing (Neill & Wotton, 2011).

EXHIBIT 5.3 Best Practices of Simulation-Based Medical Education

1. Feedback
2. Deliberate practice
3. Curriculum integration
4. Outcome measurement
5. Simulation fidelity
6. Skill acquisition and maintenance
7. Mastery learning
8. Transfer to practice
9. Team training
10. High-stakes testing
11. Instructor training
12. Educational and professional context

From McGaghie et al. (2010).

Deliberate practice, another best practice within simulation, is a method used to assist the learner to master a clinical skill or behavior (Ericsson, 2008). This method requires well-defined objectives that guide engaged learners to improve their ability to perform a skill through repetitive practice with feedback, error correction, mastery, and advancement to the next level (Figure 5.2). Simulation that incorporates deliberate practice is associated with a large effect size (ES = 0.71) when compared with traditional clinical education, and it has been shown to be superior to traditional education in achieving acquisition of clinical skills such as advanced cardiac life support, cardiac auscultation, and central venous catheter insertion (McGaghie, Issenberg, Cohen, Barsuk, & Wayne, 2011).

FIGURE 5.2 Nine elements of deliberate practice.

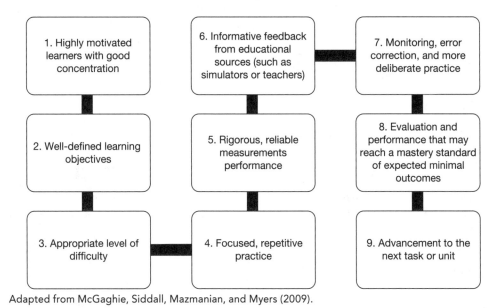

Adapted from McGaghie, Siddall, Mazmanian, and Myers (2009).

Although simulation as an educational method has been shown to have a positive effect on learning when compared with other educational modalities, more research is needed in several areas. First, there is a lack of valid and reliable evaluation instruments to measure simulation outcomes (Kardong-Edgen, Adamson, & Fitzgerald, 2010). Evaluation tools need to be developed and tested to ensure that the tool is measuring the outcomes of simulation, whether formative or summative, and improved patient outcomes are attributed to simulation learning. If simulation is to be used for high-stakes testing, such as at the end of a nursing program, further research is needed to determine the type of simulation scenarios and ensure reliable and valid tools that measure the outcomes (Bensfield, Olech, & Horsley, 2012; Rizzolo & Willhaus, 2012). Finally, there is much interest in determining whether using simulation in a nursing education program will have a positive effect on quality and safety in the health care setting. To that end, there is a move to use simulation as a method of evaluating competence of health care providers on the public's behalf (Decker, Utterback, Thomas, Mitchell, & Sportsman, 2011; Hinton et al., 2012).

Nurse educators who are interested in simulation research should search for opportunities to work collaboratively with other nursing and health care colleagues to build on current knowledge and expand the scholarship of simulation. There is a call for more large-scale multisite national studies to better evaluate the effect of simulation in nursing and health care. Simulation will have an increasingly important role in shaping the future of nursing education (Institutes of Medicine, 2011). In response to widespread questions about the use of simulation as an adjunct or replacement to traditional clinical experiences, the National Council of State Boards of Nursing embarked on a national, multiyear study to help guide the current and future use of simulation in nursing education (Hayden, 2010; Kardong-Edgren, Willhaus, Bennett, & Hayden, 2012). Findings from this research will guide integration of simulation in the nursing curriculum.

The science of simulation also continues to develop with Standards for Best Practice (International Nursing Association for Clinical Simulation and Learning, 2011) and certifications in simulation education (Society for Simulation in Health care, 2012). These credentials will define and recognize achievement of best practices in simulation pedagogy. Finally, simulation holds promise for increasing the validity of nursing licensure and the credentialing processes through incorporation of standardized testing practices involving simulation. Internationally, simulation is used for interdisciplinary health care professional licensure examinations and can play a future role in such processes within the United States (Holmboe, Rizzolo, Sachdeva, Rosenberg, & Ziv, 2011).

SUMMARY

The importance of the development of simulation pedagogy in nursing education cannot be underestimated. The rapid infusion of the innovative technology associated with high-fidelity manikins, sophistication of gaming, and impact of the use of SPs have contributed to the rise in simulation use in nursing education today. Despite this increased use, there is continued need for research to establish best practices for integration of simulation in the nursing curriculum and evaluation of simulation use and impact on health care practices of the future.

REFERENCES

Adamson, K., Jeffries, P., & Rogers, K. (2012). Evaluation: A critical step in the simulation practice. In P. Jeffries (Ed.), *Simulation in nursing education* (2nd ed., pp. 131–162). New York, NY: National League for Nursing.

American Heart Association. (2010). *Structured and supported debriefing*. Retrieved from http://npsc.us/acls/structured-and-supported-debriefing-aha?device=desktop

Arafeh, J. M., Hansen, S. S., & Nichols, A. (2010). 2 Debriefing in simulated-based learning: Facilitating a reflective discussion. *Journal of Perinatal & Neonatal Nursing, 24*, 302–309. doi:10.1097/JPN.0b013e3181f6b5ec

Arnold, J. J., Johnson, L. M., Tucker, S. J., Malec, J. F., Henrickson, S. E., & Dunn, W. F. (2009). Evaluation tools in simulation learning: Performance and self-efficacy in emergency response. *Clinical Simulation in Nursing, 5*(10). doi:10.1016/j.ecns.2008.10.003

Association of Standardized Patient Educators. (2011). *Terminology standards*. Retrieved from http://www.aspeducators.org/terminology-standards

Benner, P. E., Sutphen, M., Leonard, V., & Day, L. (2010). *Educating nurses: A call for radical transformation*. San Francisco, CA: Jossey-Bass.

Bensfield, L., Olech, M., & Horsley, T. (2012). Simulation for high-stakes evaluation in nursing. *Nurse Educator, 37*, 71–74. doi:10.1097/NNE.0b013e3182461b8c

Bray, B. S., Schwartz, C. R., Odegard, P. S., Hammer, D. P., & Seybert, A. L. (2011). Assessment of human patient simulation-based learning. *American Journal of Pharmaceutical Education, 75*(10), Article 208. doi:10.5688/ajpe7510208

Cantrell, M. A. (2008). The importance of debriefing in clinical simulations. *Clinical Simulation in Nursing, 4*(2), e19–e23. doi:10.1016/j.ecns.2008.06.006

Clark, M. (2006). Evaluating an obstetric trauma scenario. *Clinical Simulation in Nursing, 2*(2), e75–e77. doi:10.1016/j.ecns.2009.05.028

Cohen, E. R., Feinglass, J., Barsuk, J. H., Bernard, C., O'Donnell, A., McGaghie, W. C., & Wayne, D. B. (2010). Cost savings from reduced catheter-related bloodstream infection after simulation-based education for residents in a medical intensive care unit. *Simulation in Healthcare: Journal of the Society for Simulation in Healthcare, 5*(2), 98–102. doi:10.1097/SIH.0b013e3181bc8304

Cook, D. A., Brydges, R., Hamstra, S. J., Zendejas, B., Szostek, J. H., Wang, A. T., ... Hatala, R. (2012). Comparative effectiveness of technology-enhanced simulation verses other instructional methods. *Simulation in Healthcare: Journal of the Society for Simulation in Healthcare, 7*(3), 308–320. doi:10.1097/SIH.0b013e3182614f95

Cordeau, M. A. (2010). The lived experience of clinical simulation of novice nursing students. *International Journal for Human Caring, 14*(2), 9–15.

Davis, A. H., & Kimble, L. P. (2011). Human patient simulation evaluation rubrics for nursing education: Measuring the essentials of baccalaureate education for professional nursing practice. *Journal of Nursing Education, 50*, 605–611. doi:10.3928/01484834-20110715-01

Decker, S., & Dreifuerst. K. T. (2012). Integrating guided reflection into simulated learning experiences. In P. Jeffries (Ed.), *Simulation in nursing* (2nd ed., pp. 91–104). New York, NY: National League for Nursing.

Decker, S., Utterback, V., Thomas, M., Mitchell, M., & Sportsman, S. (2011). Assessing continued competency through simulation: A call for stringent action. *Nursing Education Perspectives, 32*, 120–125.

Dieckmann, P., Gaba, D., & Rall, M. (2007). Deepening the theoretical foundations of patient simulation as social practice. *Simulation in Healthcare: Journal of the Society for Simulation in Healthcare, 2*(3), 183–193. doi:10.1097/SIH.0b013e3180f637f5

Dismukes, R. K., Gaba, D. M., & Howard, S. K. (2006). So many roads: Facilitated debriefing in Healthcare. *Simulation in Healthcare: Journal of the Society for Simulation in Healthcare, 1*(1), 23–25.

Draycott, T. J., Crofts, J. F., Ash, J. P., Wilson, L. V., Yard, E., Sibanda, T., & Whitelaw, A. (2008). Improving neonatal outcome through practical shoulder dystocia training. *Obstetrics and Gynecology, 112*(1), 14–20. doi:10.1097/AOG.0b013e31817bbc61

Dreifuerst, K. T. (2009). The essentials of debriefing in simulation learning: A concept analysis. *Nursing Education Perspectives, 30*, 109–114.

Dreifuerst, K. T. (2012). Using debriefing for meaningful learning to foster development of clinical reasoning in simulation. *Journal of Nursing Education, 51*, 326–333. doi:10.3928/01484834-20120409-02

Dreifuerst, K. T., & Decker, S. (2012). Debriefing: An essential component for learning in simulation pedagogy. In P. Jeffries (Ed.), *Simulation in nursing* (2nd ed., pp. 105–130). New York, NY: National League for Nursing.

Ericsson, K. (2008). Deliberate practice and acquisition of expert performance: A general overview. *Academic Emergency Medicine, 15*, 988–994. doi:10.1111/j.1553-2712.2008.00227.x

Fanning, R. M., & Gaba, D. M. (2007). The role of debriefing in simulation-based learning. *Simulation in Healthcare: Journal of the Society for Simulation in Healthcare, 2*(2), 115–125. doi:10.1097/SIH.0b013e3180315539

Feinstein, A. H., & Cannon, H. M. (2002). Constructs of simulation evaluation. *Simulation & Gaming, 33*, 425–440. doi:10.1177/1046878102238606

Flannagan, B. (2008). Debriefing: Theory and techniques. In R. H. Riley (Ed.), *Manual of simulation in Healthcare* (pp. 155–170). New York, NY: Oxford University Press.

Framp, A., McAllister, M., & Hitchen-Holmes, D. (2009). Exploration of the value of using U3A volunteers as standardized patients in a nursing programme. *Clinical Simulation in Nursing, 5*(Suppl. 3). doi:10.1016/j.ecns.2009.03.168

Hayden, J. (2010). Use of simulation in nursing education: National survey results. *Journal of Nursing Regulation, 1*(3), 52–57.

Herrmann, E. K. (2008). Remembering Mrs. Chase. *NSNA Imprint, February/March,* 52–55. Retrieved from http://www.nsna.org/Portals/0/Skins/NSNA/pdf/Imprint_FebMar08_Feat_MrsChase.pdf

Hinton, J., Mays, M., Hagler, D., Randolph, P., Brooks, R., DeFalco, N., & Weberg, D. (2012). Measuring post-licensure competence with simulation: The nursing performance profile. *Journal of Nursing Regulation, 3*(2), 45–53.

Hoffman, R., O'Donnell, J., & Kim, Y. (2007). The effects of human patient simulators on basic knowledge in critical care nursing with undergraduate senior nursing students. *Simulation in Healthcare: Journal of the Society for Simulation in Healthcare, 2*(2), 110–114. doi:10.1097/SIH.0b013e318033abb5

Holmboe, E., Rizzolo, M. A., Sachdeva, A. K., Rosenberg, M., & Ziv, A. (2011). Simulation-based assessment and the regulation of Healthcare Professionals. *Simulation in Healthcare: Journal of the Society for Simulation in Healthcare, 6*, S58–S62. doi:10.1097/SIH.0b013e3182283bd7

INASCL Board of Directors (2011, August). Standard I: Terminology. *Clinical Simulation in Nursing, 7*(4S), s3–s7. doi:10.1016/j.ecns.2011.05.005

Institute of Medicine. (2003). *Health professions education: a bridge to quality.* Retrieved from http://www.iom.edu/Reports/2003/Health-Professions-Education-A-Bridge-to-Quality.aspx

Institute of Medicine. (2011). *The future of nursing: Leading change, advancing health.* Washington, DC: National Academies Press.

International Nursing Association for Clinical Simulation and Learning. (2011). Standards of best practice: Simulation. *Clinical Simulation in Nursing, 7*(4), s3–s19.

Jeffries, P., & Rogers, K. (2012). Theoretical framework for simulation design. In P. Jeffries (Ed.), *Simulation in nursing education* (2nd ed., pp. 25–43). New York, NY: National League for Nursing.

Kardong-Edgren, S., Adamson, K., & Fitzgerald, C. (2010). A review of currently published evaluation instruments for human patient simulation. *Clinical Simulation in Nursing, 6*(1), e25–e35. doi:10.1016/j.ecns.2009.08.004

Kardong-Edgren, S., Anderson, M., & Michaels, J. (2007). Does simulation fidelity improve student test scores? *Clinical Simulation in Nursing, 3*(1), e21–e24. doi:10.1016/j.ecns.2009.05.035

Kardong-Edgren, S., Willhaus, J., Bennett, D., & Hayden, J. (2012). Results of the national council of state boards of nursing national simulation survey: Part II. *Clinical Simulation in Nursing, 8*(4), e117–e123. doi:10.1016/j.ecns.2012.01.003

Kirkpatrick, D. L. (1998). *Evaluating training programs: The four levels* (2nd ed.). San Francisco, CA: Berrett-Koehler.

Klakovich, M. D., & Dela Cruz, F. A. (2006). Validating the interpersonal communication assessment scale. *Journal of Professional Nursing, 22*(1), 60–67. doi:10.1016/j.profnurs.2005.12.005

Kogan, J. R., Holmboe, E. S., & Hauer, K. E. (2009). Tools for direct observation and assessment of clinical skills of medical trainees. *Journal of the American Medical Association, 302*, 1316–1326. doi:10.1001/jama.2009.1365

LeFlore, J., Anderson, M., Zielke, M., Nelson, K., Thomas, P., Hardee, G., & John, L. (2012). Can a virtual patient trainer teach student nurses how to save lives–Teaching nursing students about pediatric respiratory distress. *Simulation in Healthcare: Journal of the Society for Simulation in Healthcare, 7*(1), 10–17. doi:10.1097/SIH.0b013e31823652de

MacGregor, C., O'Donnell, M., Haley, A., Martini, M., Robinson, J., & Vozenilek, J. (2012). Melanoma trainer using simulation back skin. *Simulation in Healthcare: Journal of the Society for Simulation in Healthcare, 7*(4), 251–254. doi:10.1097/SIH.0b013e31824b80aa

Mariani, B., Cantrell, M., Meakim, C., Prieto, P., & Dreifuerst, K. (2012). Structured debriefing and students' clinical judgment in simulation. *Clinical Simulation in Nursing, Vol*(X),e1–e9. doi:10.1016/j.ecns.2011.11.009

May, W., Park, J., & Lee, J. (2009). A ten-year review of the literature on the use of standardized patients in teaching and learning. *Medical Teacher, 31*, 487–492. doi:10.1080/01421590802530898

McGaghie, W. C., Issenberg, S. B., Petrusa, E. R., & Scalese, R. J. (2010). A critical review of simulation-based medical education research: 2003-2009. *Medical Educator, 44*(1), 50–63. doi:10.1111/j.1365-292009.03547.x

McGaghie, W. C., Siddal, L., Mazmania, P., & Myers, J. (2009). Lessons for continuing medical education from simulation research in undergraduate and graduate medical education. Effectiveness of continuing medical education: American College of Chest Physicians evidence-based educational guidelines. *Chest, 135*(Suppl. 3), 62S–68S. doi:10.1387/chest.08-2521

Meyer, M. N., Connors, H., Hou, Q., & Gajewski, B. (2011). The effect of simulation on clinical performance. *Simulation in Healthcare: Journal of the Society for Simulation in Healthcare, 6*, 269–277. doi:0.1097/SIH.0b013e318223a048

Neill, M., & Wotton, K. (2011). High-fidelity stimulation debriefing in nursing education: A literature review. *Clinical Simulation in Nursing, 7*(5), e161–e168. doi:10.1016/j.ecns.2011.02.001

Norman, G., Dore, K., & Grierson, L. (2012). The minimal relationship between simulation fidelity and transfer of learning. *Medical Education, 46*, 636–647. doi:10.1111/j.1365-2923.2012.04243.x

Overstreet, M. (2010). E-chats: The seven components of nursing debriefing. *Journal of Continuing Education in Nursing, 41*, 538–539. doi:10.3928/00220124-20101122-05

Owen, H. (2012). Early use of simulation in medical education. *Simulation in Healthcare: Journal of the Society for Simulation in Healthcare, 7*(2), 102–116. doi:10.1097/SIH.0b013e3182415a91

Rizzolo, M., & Willhaus, J. (2012). Simulation for high-stakes evaluation: Letter to the editor. *Nurse Educator, 37*(5), 1. doi:10.1097/NNE.0b013e318262eb43

Rudolph, J. W., Simon, R., Raemer, D. B., & Eppich, W. J. (2008). Debriefing as formative assessment: Closing performance gaps in medical education. *Academic Emergency Medicine, 15*, 1010–1016. doi:10.1111/j.1553-2712.2008.00248.x

Rudolph, J. W., Simon, R., Rivard, P., Dufresne, R. L., & Raemer, D. B. (2007). Debriefing with good judgment: Combining rigorous feedback with genuine inquiry. *Anesthesiology Clinics, 25*, 361–376. doi:http://dx.doi.org/10.1016/j.anclin.2007.03.007

Ryan, C., Walshe, N., Gaffney, R., Shanks, A., Burgoyne, L., & Wiskin, C. (2010). Using standardized patients to assess communication skills in medical and nursing students. *BMC Medical Educator, 10*(24), 1–8. doi:10.1186/1472-6920-10-24

Schön, D. A. (1983). *The reflective practitioner: How professionals think in action.* New York, NY: Basic Books.

Shinnick, M. A., & Woo, M. A. (2012). The effect of human patient simulation on critical thinking and its predictors in prelicensure nursing students. *Nurse Education Today.* 2012 May 5. [Epub ahead of print]. doi:10.1016/j.nedt.2012.04.004

Shinnick, M. A., Woo, M., Horwich, T. B., & Steadman, R. (2011). Debriefing: The most important component in simulation? *Clinical Simulation in Nursing, 7*(3), e105–e111. doi:10.1016/j.ecns.2010.11.005

Smith-Stoner, M. (2011). Using moulage to enhance educational instruction. *Nurse Educator, 36*(1), 21–24. doi:10.1097/NNE.0b013e3182001e98

Tanner, C. A. (2006). Thinking like a nurse: A research-based model of clinical judgment in nursing. *Journal of Nursing Education, 45*, 204–211.

Thomas, C., Bertram, E., & Allen, R. (2012). Preparing for transition to professional practice: Creating a simulated blog and reflective journaling activity. *Clinical Simulation in Nursing, 8*(3) e87–95. doi:10.1016/j.ecns.2010.07.004

Wendling, A., Halan, S., Tighe, P., Le, L., Euliano, T., & Lok, B. (2011). Virtual humans versus standardized patients: Which lead residents to more correct diagnosis? *Academic Medicine, 86*, 384–388. doi:10.1097/ACM.0b013e318208803f

Wickers, M. P. (2010). Establishing the climate for a successful debriefing. *Clinical Simulation in Nursing, 6*, e83–e86. doi:10.1016/j.ecns.2009.06.003

6

Teaching in Online Learning Environments

CAROL O'NEIL

Teaching online is not the same as teaching in a classroom. The focus of this chapter is on the differences between teaching in the traditional classroom and teaching online. The role of the facilitator and the student are discussed in relation to pedagogy, course content, teaching strategies, reconceptualizing and designing online learning environments, interacting online, and using technology to teach and learn.

The original purpose of the web was to communicate and to share information. Using the web to teach was a natural progression of its original purpose. Web-based teaching and learning means using the web to impart information and to learn. Using the web reduces the time and space barriers to learning: learning can take place any time and anywhere. An entire program, a course, or selected parts of a course or program can be taught via the web.

In online learning environments, the instructor acts as a moderator and facilitates learning. Students should be self-motivated and self-directed. The content material can be presented with text, videotapes, audiotapes, films, links to websites, charts, graphs, statistics data, and case studies, among others. Interaction takes place online, and this happens in three ways: from the instructor to the student, from the student to the student, and from the content to the student. Interaction can be synchronous (real time) or asynchronous (delayed). Synchronous interaction is having a discussion by typing or talking or meeting online. Asynchronous interaction is delayed and entails leaving messages at a specific posting site that others in the learning environment can read at their convenience (O'Neil, Fisher, & Newbold, 2009).

DEFINITIONS

Several definitions need clarification. *Distance learning* is the term used to describe any learning environment in which the teacher and student are separated by time and geography (Williams, Paprock, & Covington, 1999). If the entire learning opportunity is online, the learning is termed *web-based*. If part of the learning opportunity is online and part is face-to-face, the learning is termed *hybrid* or *blended*.

ADVANTAGES AND DISADVANTAGES OF ONLINE LEARNING

The advantage of online learning environments is that course material and activities are accessible 24 hours a day and seven days a week, anywhere with Internet access. The use of the Internet allows for access to resources and links on the web. Learning is student centered, and there are opportunities for high-quality dialogue (Table 6.1). Some considerations are that learners need to be computer literate in an online course, and they need hardware and software that are compatible with the online learning systems; there may be failures that prevent the system from functioning properly. Learning online is one type of learning style. If the student's learning style does not match the online style, the student may not learn effectively and efficiently (O'Neil et al., 2009).

TABLE 6.1 Advantages and Disadvantages of Online Learning

Advantages	Disadvantages
• Time barrier is reduced	• Needs typing skills
• Space barriers are reduced	• Needs technology competence
• Learning takes place any time and anywhere	• Learning away from the classroom
• Learning is flexible	

PREVALENCE OF ONLINE COURSES

The Sloan Consortium® conducts an annual survey of online education. Their 2012 Survey of Online Learning estimated that over 6.7 million students were taking at least one online course in the fall 2011 term (Allen & Seaman, 2013). It is estimated that one-third of all college students take at least one course online. Enrollment in online courses differs among institutions of higher education and among majors within an institution (Allen & Seaman, 2013).

Other key findings of this annual report include the following:

- The number of students enrolled in higher education increased by 2.6%, and the number of students enrolled in online courses increased by 9.3%.
- Online courses and face-to-face courses are thought to yield the same outcomes in student learning and satisfaction, and online courses are an important part of learning in higher education.
- As for academic leaders, 77% believe that the learning outcomes in online education are the same or superior to those in face-to-face courses. The majority also report that the lower retention rates for online courses are a barrier to the growth of online instruction (Allen & Seaman, 2013).

Massive open online courses (MOOCs) are courses offered by college and university faculty that are online and usually free. Examples of these courses can be found at the Coursera® website (www.coursera.org). In the most recent Sloan Consortium survey, only a small segment of higher education institutions are experimenting with MOOCs, although a larger number of such courses are in the planning stages (Allen & Seaman, 2013). The impact of MOOCs on teaching and learning remains unclear.

Online courses and programs are offered by colleges and universities as part of their curriculum. For example, the University of Maryland School of Nursing offers core undergraduate and graduate courses, both online and face-to-face. In addition to online courses, there also are online universities, such as Penn State Online (www. worldcampus.psu.edu), and virtual universities, such as the California Virtual Campus (www.cvc.edu). There are online professional organizations and journals such as EDUCAUSE® (www.educause.edu) and The Sloan Consortium (sloanconsortium.org). Faculty can learn the best practices in teaching online through courses, certificates, and program offered through these organizations and others.

SUCCESSFUL ONLINE COURSES

The American Association for Higher Education (AAHE) created the Principles of Good Practice in Undergraduate Education for teaching in the classroom in 1987. Chickering and Ehrman (1996) used the AAHE principles and developed a new set of principles for incorporating technology into teaching. The principles for good online teaching practice are listed in Exhibit 6.1 and examples of each are described below.

1. *Good practice encourages contact between students and faculty.* Teachers can contact students before the course starts with a welcoming text or video greeting sent by e-mail to each student; they should begin the course with a warm welcome in the form of an announcement. Teachers as facilitators conference with students via media chat or Skype and by asynchronous communication in a discussion board. Having a question and answer forum allows for interaction through student questions and faculty responses.
2. *Good practice develops reciprocity and cooperation among students.* Students interact with each other via postings on the discussion board. Students enter a course and are directed to a forum to introduce themselves. They are assigned to chat rooms where they can complete assignments in discussion groups and have asynchronous or synchronous discussions with the teacher and their peers.
3. *Good practice uses active learning techniques.* Students need to be actively involved in their learning through the use of active teaching strategies. Some of the strategies that can be used online are discussions, debates, concept maps, and case studies.
4. *Good practice gives prompt feedback.* Feedback provides students with specific information about how they are doing in the course. The teacher develops a schedule for feedback, communicates this to the students, and follows it. Feedback should be standardized, and this can be accomplished by using rubrics. Quizzes help students identify how they are mastering the content and expected outcomes.
5. *Good practice emphasizes time on task.* Taking a course online does not necessarily mean more or less work. Course work should be comparable with the credits of the course. It can be estimated that the student will spend about 2 to 3 hours of time per credit in the course per week. A 3-credit course, therefore, would suggest that students spend between 6 and 8 hours a week on the course.
6. *Good practice communicates high expectations.* At the beginning of the course, teachers should provide students with a list of rules and policies for online learning. This information is usually found in the course syllabus. For courses with face-to-face and online sections, and for which the syllabus cannot be changed, the teacher should create a manual for the online section of the course that includes the policies. For example, the manual might include a definition of the items on menus, netiquette, the day of the week that the modules start, and the expectations for the student and teacher. Expectations for participation and posts should be clearly delineated, and students should be held accountable for following the policies. If they are not followed, the student should obtain feedback detailing expected changes in behavior.

7. *Good practice respects diverse talents and ways of learning.* Each person in the course is an individual with unique knowledge, experience, and strengths. The course should include experiences that reflect these differences among students. Some strategies are to ask broad and open-ended questions; develop evaluation methods that can be completed using different formats, such as a paper, video, or presentation; and consider group assignments that have several components and allow each student to choose the component most suited for them.

EXHIBIT 6.1 Principles of Good Practice in Online Teaching

1. Good practice encourages contact between students and teachers.
2. Good practice develops reciprocity and cooperation among students.
3. Good practice uses active learning techniques.
4. Good practice gives prompt feedback.
5. Good practice emphasizes time on task.
6. Good practice communicates high expectations.
7. Good practice respects diverse talents and ways of learning.

From Chickering and Ehrmann (1996).

SUCCESSFUL ONLINE STUDENTS

Online students typically work full-time and have families, and many are traditional college students. The Illinois Online Network (ION) identified strategies for students learning online to be successful (ION, 2010b). These are described in Exhibit 6.2.

EXHIBIT 6.2 Strategies for Students' Success When Learning Online

1. Online students should be open-minded about sharing life, work, and educational experiences as part of the learning process.
2. Online students need to communicate by writing and typing, and it is helpful to enjoy engaging in these activities.
3. Online students need to be self-motivated and self-disciplined, and develop a set schedule and keep to it.
4. Online students need to be willing to "speak up" if problems arise. If the student believes there is a problem, the sooner the teacher knows about it, the faster it can be resolved.
5. There is a weekly time commitment, and online students need to schedule this into their lives.
6. Online students need to meet the requirements for the course.
7. Students should acknowledge that learning online will include high-level thinking and decision making.
8. Online students need to have the required hardware and software.
9. Online students should be willing to think through ideas before responding.
10. Online students should value online learning.

Adapted from ION (2010b).

There are many assessment tools that are available online to guide students in deciding whether online learning is a good option for them. Questions focus on the need and time for online learning, learning style, self-motivation, and experience with technologies. Results of the self-assessment indicate whether distance education would work for the student and whether changes in schedule and study habits might be needed for success.

Another resource is YouTube, which has videos available to help students decide whether online courses are appropriate for them, considering their learning styles and circumstances. Some of these videos present student views of online courses and include information about time management, motivation, writing skills, computer skills, and learning style. These videos are a resource for students who are making the decision about whether to take an online nursing course or program.

O'Neil and Fisher (2008) compared the differences between online and traditional classroom courses by examining learning goals and preferences, interaction, assessment and measurement (of learning outcomes), instructional media and tools, and learner support and services. The same course was offered online and face-to-face with the same content, activities, and assignments. The two groups were compared using both qualitative and quantitative measures. Based on the findings, four questions were developed for students to assess whether they would be successful learning online:

1. By what means do you learn best?
2. Do you learn through interacting with others?
3. Do you focus on the process or the outcome of learning?
4. What are your computer skills?

O'Neil and Fisher (2008) found that successful online students prefer learning from others and being involved in the process of learning for personal and professional growth, rather than focusing on the outcome (their grades). Successful students were also computer savvy.

SUCCESSFUL ONLINE FACILITATORS

The ION described the role of the teacher in an online course as an educator who facilitates learning (ION, 2010a). This role requires a unique set of characteristics, which include:

- Facilitators need a broad-based knowledge, not only of the content, but of the real world.
- They should project an online presence characterized by "openness, concern, flexibility, and sincerity."
- As with online students, the facilitator should communicate clearly in writing.
- Facilitators should value teaching online and facilitating learning.
- Facilitators should guide students in the critical thinking process so they can relate knowledge to the real world.
- Facilitators should have expertise in the content.
- They should be knowledgeable and skilled in teaching online. (ION, 2010a)

The facilitator is the "guide on the side." The teacher in the role of facilitator guides students in connecting and applying the knowledge to the real world. Table 6.2 summarizes the characteristics of successful online students and teachers.

TABLE 6.2 Characteristics of Successful Online Students and Faculty

Characteristics of Successful Online Students	Characteristics of Successful Online Faculty
• Is self-motivated	• Is a facilitator of learning
• Is self-directed	• Communicates clearly in writing
• Is open-minded	• Has broad knowledge base
• Likes to communicate in writing	• Has an area of clinical expertise (if practice-related course)
• Meets minimum online requirements	• Is skilled in teaching online

LEARNING THEORY

The pedagogy associated with online learning is social learning theory related to constructivism. Constructivism allows for the construction of meaning by using a process of action and reflection. New knowledge is built from past experiences and, thus, learning is authentic and represents real life. Learning is active and interactive: the active component is enhanced with technology, and the interactive component is enhanced with the use of discussion boards and videoconferencing. Figure 6.1 provides a model of the stages and process of creating an online learning environment, which includes learning theory and technology as one of the components.

FIGURE 6.1 Stages and process of creating an online learning environment.

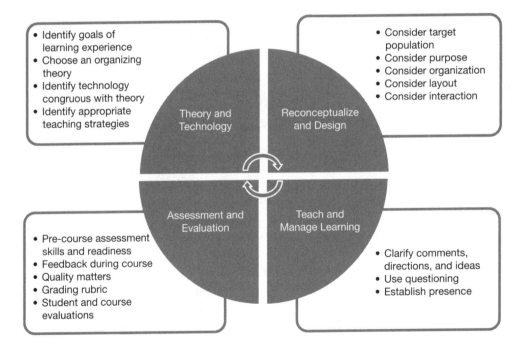

TECHNOLOGY AND LEARNING

Technology is chosen for a learning experience because it is appropriate for the objectives of the teaching session and is the most effective method of helping students learn the content and meet those objectives. Technology is a tool that is used to support knowledge construction. It allows students to share knowledge and experiences and build mental models. Students can use web-based resources and databases for increasing knowledge that supports learning. Technology supports learning through active strategies, such as simulations and case studies, so students can encounter real-world problems in a safe and supportive environment. Technology is a social medium that supports student learning by conversing; it is an intellectual partner that supports learning by reflecting and provides learners with ways to articulate and represent what they know (O'Neil et al., 2009).

TECHNOLOGY IN ONLINE LEARNING

Content is delivered to the student through systems such as Blackboard® (2013) and Moodle™ (2013), among others: these systems are called course management systems. A course management system has management capability, such as student enrollment monitoring; in addition it has a set of tools that can be used to create and manage the course. The tools can include discussion boards, quizzes and tests, videoconferencing, and learning modules.

An online learning environment needs a set of specific components. It needs places for the syllabus and course content, and the ability to submit and retrieve assignments and to share ideas about the content in synchronous or asynchronous ways. These places are organized to form a course learning platform.

Blackboard

Blackboard has an assortment of software within its package that the school or teacher can choose to use (Blackboard, 2013). Because the software is within the package, Blackboard is called a closed-source system. Some of the features of Blackboard include tools for course management, assessment and grading, and collaboration and student engagement.

Moodle

Moodle is a course management system that can be accessed for free online (Moodle, 2013). It is modular, allowing the faculty member to add to and modify the software. When using Moodle, assistance with instructional design and technology may be needed by the teacher.

When an instructor is making the decision as to which course management system to use, there are comparisons available online.

TECHNOLOGY REPORTS

There are two important reports on the use of technology in teaching. One of these is the Campus Computing Survey, which is conducted annually. These surveys and others are part of the Campus Computing Project,™ a continuing study of the role of information technology in American higher education. The second source of information is the NMC Horizon Report, which is an annual report about emerging technologies that will most likely have an impact on teaching (Johnson, Adams, & Cummins, 2012). The technologies are grouped into three categories: (a) those that will have an impact on teaching in the next 12 months, such as mobile applications and tablet computing, (b) technologies to watch, over the next 2 to 3 years, such as game-based learning and learning analytics, and (c) over the next 4 to 5 years, such as gesture-based computing.

The 2013 Horizon Report explored the use of flipped classrooms (a blended course in which the content is online and the learning activities are in the classroom), MOOCs, mobile applications, tablet computing, and augmented (blended) reality (Johnson et al., 2013). In the next 5 years, Web 2.0 will expand for use in teaching as well as Web 3.0. Devices will be smaller and more powerful, and there will be a widening gap between student and faculty perceptions of technology (Johnson et al., 2012).

OVERVIEW OF ACCESSIBLE TECHNOLOGY

Online learning needs to be active, and technology should actively involve the student in the learning process. Lemley and Burnham (2009) investigated the use of Web 2.0 tools in nursing and medical schools and found that 53% of nursing schools used them. The most commonly used tools were blogs, wikis, videocasts, and podcasts.

A blog is an online journal that is useful for an individual student or groups of students. Blogs can be public or private. Entries are saved in reverse chronological order, and students can view entries of their peers. Interaction can be enhanced by using the blog for case study discussions or answering discussion questions (Grassley & Bartoletti, 2009).

A wiki is space on the web that allows for sharing and collaboration. Students can share their ideas on a single website. New ideas are added, and old ideas are saved, thus collecting and expanding on ideas. Grassley and Bartoletti (2009) developed ways to enhance student collaboration using blogs and wikis. They used blogs for discussion forums and a group of students used wikis to develop thematic analysis. Each student had a journal blog and a research proposal wiki. They concluded that these technologies were useful in enhancing active and collaborative learning online.

Podcasting is the process of making audio files and publishing them to the Internet. Videocasting is using podcasts with video. The most frequent use of podcasting and videocasting is for the faculty to record lectures and publish them for students to have access to the content in this format. Podcasting and videocasting allow for repeated viewing at the student's convenience.

Communication is a necessary part of an online course; it is enhanced by the technologies just discussed. Interaction is between the teacher and student, among the students, and between the student and content. Interaction between the teacher and student can be enhanced by using e-mail, online office hours via videoconferencing, and question and answer forums on the discussion board. Student-to-student interaction can be facilitated by using blogs and wikis, and student-to-content opportunities can be enhanced with podcasting and videocasting.

HOW TO CREATE ONLINE LEARNING ENVIRONMENTS

If you have taught a course in the traditional classroom and now want to offer that course online, how do you do that? The classroom material cannot merely be placed online. Online is a different learning environment, and content must be reconceptualized because what works in the classroom may not be appropriate or successful online. The teacher first reconceptualizes the course and then designs the learning environment.

RECONCEPTUALIZE

To reconceptualize means that the content is reviewed in the context of the goals of the institution, available technology, and expertise of the faculty and students. The end products of the reconceptualization process are the decisions about how the course, and modules (or units) within, will be organized and how the content will be presented.

One consideration is the projected reach of the course, for example, in terms of where students are located. The larger the reach, the more likely that the content should be placed online. A statewide program with potential students who live at a great distance from the school would be better online than delivered face-to-face. Another variable is how long the information will be offered. The longer it is offered to students, the more amenable it is to online access. For example, a statewide program repeated throughout the year is best provided online.

Many schools of nursing offer large classroom courses with a hundred or more students enrolled. Online courses, however, are most successful when there are a smaller number of students. This emphasizes the need for the support of administration and financial considerations. Do online learning environments fit into the mission and vision of the school? Does the administration view online learning as important for the institution? Online courses typically have fewer students in them than large lecture-type courses; will the school of nursing support one faculty member for 25 or 30 students rather than or in addition to one faculty member for 100 students in a face-to-face course? If the administration and budget support online learning, these courses can be successful. The last institutional variable is resources. Nursing faculty considering online courses should assess the school's resources and support, both people and material. Some resources include a course management system such as Blackboard, technical support, instructional designers, faculty who are technologically competent, and ability to successfully market online courses and programs. It is important for nursing faculty to build resources before beginning development of online courses.

The second variable in reconceptualizing a course is assessing the available technology. The two main questions are these: What hardware and software are available, and how will the online courses be maintained? Having appropriate technology and support is important in creating an environment for success in online teaching.

The third variable is faculty. Faculty members in the school of nursing need to learn how to teach online. They should be mentored and provided with the knowledge and technological and educational skills to be successful online facilitators. They should know about pedagogy, online theory, learning and managing online courses, and evaluation of students and the course. Faculty orientation can be offered online or in a computer laboratory. One method of faculty development is to place the orientation material and learning activities in an online course and provide an orientation similar to how a student would take the course. As part of faculty development, teachers should learn to use different online teaching methods such as PowerPoint with voiceover narration, video clips, methods for online group work, and others, and have an opportunity to discuss the advantages and disadvantages of each for their own courses. Faculty should participate in synchronous and asynchronous learning activities and be guided in assessing and grading assignments in an online environment. For ongoing development, faculty members who are teaching online can form a group to meet regularly to discuss issues and explore alternate approaches to use.

The next consideration is students. Do students have the hardware and software essential for online learning, and do they have the support needed to take a course online? Students also need an orientation to online learning, advisement to help them determine if an online course is best for them, and support services.

Once the first set of decisions is made, the next decisions relate to how the course will be organized. The teacher should develop a course that will meet the needs of most of the learners and for which the teacher has skills (O'Neil et al., 2009).

Example of Reconceptualizing a Course

I was given a WebCT course management system to create a course in an RN-to-BSN program. I was assigned an instructional technologist, and our team of two was going to create this course. Based on the considerations discussed earlier, I had institutional support, a course management system, and an instructional technologist. I also knew how to use PowerPoint with voiceover narration and that there were students ready for an online course by verbal requests to me. My first attempt at reconceptualization was dividing the traditional classroom course into modules. The classroom course was organized by weeks and discrete content was delivered each week. Online modules, however, do not have a set time for learning, and their content can be mastered over one or several weeks, or even longer. I decided that each module would have a title, objectives, content in the form of a mini-lecture with PowerPoint with voiceover, learning activities, and a formative quiz.

I found that it required about 15 hours to create a module, and I had five of 12 modules completed when the course began. When all 12 modules were complete, I became aware that every module looked the same, and the only differentiating factor was the title. On the webpage listing the modules, I typed 12 times "title, objectives, content, activity, and quiz," rather than identifying the content or focus of each module. I realized then that the content needed to be reconceptualized. The first several modules, which provided an introduction to community/public health nursing and the role of the nurse, became my first *chunk* of content. A chunk is a group of modules that have something in common; it is one word that represents several topics and becomes a mental model for the course. This chunk was called "History." Another was "Tools," which included such content as epidemiology, and the third was "Practice," which referred to nursing care. Students were introduced to the reconceptualized course as having three concepts, or mental models, and within these concepts were the modules.

Reconceptualizing is making decisions about the type and structure of the course as well as thinking about the mental models that connect the course and modules. Reconceptualizing results in a course that is organized and logical to the learner, so the objectives, content, interaction, and assessments fit with one another.

HOW TO DESIGN ONLINE COURSES AND MODULES

Design means how the teacher develops the course and its components to achieve its objectives or outcomes. The component parts of an online course are the target population, purpose and objectives, course organization, navigation, page layout, and interaction (O'Neil et al., 2009).

The target population is the learner. An assessment of students' knowledge and learning styles is needed. What do the learners know and not know about the topic, and how will they best learn? A learning-style inventory might be used for this assessment; examples of these are in Exhibit 6.3. When designing a module, the teacher should consider students' different styles of learning and include multiple strategies. In addition to learning styles, students may differ in age, computer experience, socioeconomic status, motivation, and other characteristics. When planning technology, the teacher should consider using technology that meets the students' needs and is appropriate for the majority of students in the course.

EXHIBIT 6.3 Examples of Learning-Style Inventories

- VARK® Questionnaire (www.vark-learn.com/english/index.asp)
- Learning-Style Inventory (auditory, visual, or tactile learner; www.personal.psu.edu/bxb11/LSI/LSI.htm)
- Multiple Intelligences (www.thirteen.org/edonline/concept2class/mi/index.html)

The purpose and objectives of the course must be considered in the design. If this is a didactic learning environment, it would be designed differently from a seminar course. If there are skills to be learned, the laboratory experience might need to be arranged differently from when the course is offered face-to-face. If the course has a clinical component, the clinical experiences need to be organized with considerations that might differ from a more traditional course offering.

The organization of the course is its flow. Can the student get from one section of the online course to another with ease? Students should locate what they need within three clicks of the mouse. Each module should appear the same in terms of structure, so students know from module to module where to find information.

In creating the page layout, you should make lines clean and crisp. The font size should consider the needs of the target population, and all the fonts should be the same. There should be headers that divide the material, which are different fonts and colors from that of the general content. The teacher should use colors that facilitate reading and are pleasing to look at.

Interaction can be synchronous or asynchronous. Synchronous interaction can include videoconferencing, which can be used for office hours, student conferences, student group or individual projects, and seminars. As this type of interaction is live, the day and time need to be scheduled so students can plan to attend. There should be a purpose and an agenda for each session. The purpose is for face-to-face communication; synchronous interaction can be used for sharing, teaching, or evaluation. Asynchronous interaction strategies include discussion boards, blogs, and wikis. The purpose of these is to share ideas and provide feedback to students. There can be open or closed discussions for individual students or groups.

THE QUALITY MATTERS RUBRIC AND ITS USE IN DESIGNING ONLINE COURSE

Quality Matters (QM) is a faculty-centered and peer review process designed to assess and certify the quality of online and blended courses (MarylandOnline, 2010). QM has three components: the QM rubric, peer review process, and professional development. When designing a course, the teacher should begin by reviewing the QM rubric. The rubric is a table of characteristics of a high-quality online course that should be considered in designing nursing courses. The rubric, which was presented in Chapter 4, has eight standards: a course overview and introduction, learning objectives and competencies, assessment and measurement, instructional materials, learner interaction and engagement, course technology, learner support, and accessibility.

Although the QM rubric is used for assessment of an online course, the standards should be considered when designing the course. For example, the first standard in the rubric indicates that the instructions are clear as to how to get started and where to locate the course components. One way of accomplishing this clarity is to include a welcome message for students as they enter the course. A sample welcome message is presented in Exhibit 6.4.

EXHIBIT 6.4 Sample Welcome for Students in an Online Course

Welcome to the introduction to this course, and I am glad that you found us. This is the place to start, and your beginning steps will be outlined here. Go to the Course Information section and find the course syllabus and online material. Open each and read them. The syllabus will tell you about the content, and the online material will tell you about the technology. Remember to print both, because if there is a power outage, and a paper is due, it is too late to look for my phone number. When you have completed this task, go to the discussion board and type "I did it" in the "I did it" forum. Then go to the Introduction section and tell us about yourself.

If all of the courses in a nursing program are taught online, the faculty can include the QM rubric in the course syllabus. When a course is taught both online and in a traditional classroom setting, it would not be appropriate to include online specifications in the syllabus. By following the standards in the rubric, the teacher can identify information that should be included in the syllabus and as part of the online material.

Meeting the QM standards is a measure of the structure of the course, not of the teacher's effectiveness. Faculty peer review within the school of nursing determines the quality of teaching. QM outlines the characteristics of a high-quality online course. This means that instructions are present, and the purpose of the course is clear. There are learning objectives that match the purpose, and the assessment and measurement validate whether students have met the objectives. The instructional materials are accessible. How students interact with each other, with the content, and with the faculty, and what technology is used to facilitate the learning process are described for students. The students need to know where to go for support, and the course needs to be accessible to all students who can take it (Quality Matters Program, 2011).

HOW TO TEACH AND MANAGE ONLINE LEARNING ENVIRONMENTS

Faculty members are facilitators of learning, and thus managing learning is the process of guiding the student to achieve the learning objectives. Prior to beginning the course, the syllabus and online expectations should be available to students, and they should read them and become familiar with the course site. One strategy is to make the course available to students, "open the course," a few days before the first module. A scavenger hunt is a way of encouraging students to access different parts of the course and become familiar with them. For example, the teacher can ask how many students are enrolled in the course, and students can navigate to the roster to locate this information. Orientation to the course management system should be included as a reference for students who may be taking an online course in the nursing program for the first time. Netiquette should be discussed, and acceptable online behavior should be stated clearly for students.

Ragan (2007) identified principles of best practice for online teachers. These include:

- Show up and teach (interact with students and guide them through the learning experience).
- Practice proactive course management strategies (such as monitoring assignment submissions and reminding students of upcoming deadlines).
- Establish patterns of course activities (establish and communicate a course pace and pattern of work).
- Plan for the "unplanned" (have a strategy in place for informing students of unexpected situations).

- Expect and require responses (provide timely feedback to students and responding promptly).
- Think before you write (be clear and concise in written responses to students to avoid misinterpretation).
- Help maintain forward progress of students (ensure timely return of assignments and test scores).
- Maintain a safe and secure learning environment (use an institutionally supported course management system, which provides security and confidentiality).
- Remember that quality counts (establish strategies for addressing the quality of the online course).
- Confirm the technological infrastructure for offering the online course.

There are several functions of the online teacher during the course, and the first and foremost is to correct errors. For example, when the discussion board opens, the teacher should enter the course and review what is posted. If the first student who posts a comment in the discussion board has not understood the assignment, other students might continue to make that same error. Or, a student may provide inaccurate information on a discussion board, which the teacher should correct immediately. Students need to know that faculty members are reading the postings and assessing the accuracy of the information posted.

A second function of the online teacher is to clarify the points the student makes and relate them to the module objectives or outcomes. To do this, the teacher can start a reply with the phrase, "I think you are saying that ..." and then summarize the key points of the student. Students can provide examples from their clinical practice, or the teacher can include scenarios that apply the concepts learned in the module to practice.

Questioning is an effective technique to raise the level of student thinking. One technique is called the "sandwich": it starts with positive reinforcement of the student's answer, followed by another question to extend thinking about other possibilities. For example, the teacher might pose this series of questions using the "sandwich" approach: "You have made some valid and important points. What might be the impact of this idea on the budget? I appreciate your rethinking this." Asking "what if" questions is another way of encouraging higher level thinking among students.

Telling a story is a strategy for enhancing the teacher's online personality. One idea is to create a folder for the course with files for modules. In the appropriate module, the teacher can save a story that relates to the content of the module and, when appropriate, copy and paste that story into the module discussion.

Presence is a concept that means that the students know you are in the course and actively involved with their learning. One way is through posting to the discussion board, but this is not the only way. Other ways of letting students know you are present is through announcements, adding a humorous comment related to the content being learned, and moving the order of the modules at the course site. For example, if students are working on module 8, the teacher might move modules 1 to 7 to the bottom of the list, indicating he or she is present in the course.

ASSESSMENT AND EVALUATION

Traditional classroom evaluation measures are neither comprehensive nor appropriate for online learning. Some reasons are that students need to assess their skills, and they desire to enroll in an online course. Students need continued feedback about how they are progressing through the course. An online course should be created and ready to be implemented before the students enter it. The course needs to be reviewed before it goes live, and links need to be tested and updated, which would not occur in a face-to-face course. To accommodate the differences in evaluation, O'Neil et al. (2009) developed a model of evaluation for online courses. The model is based on student assessment and course evaluation, each conducted in three phases. Students should be assessed before the course begins, during the learning experience, and at the end of the learning experience. The course should be evaluated before it goes live, during the learning experience, and at the end of the learning experience.

Examples of student assessment before the course begins include surveys of computer skills, pretests, and readiness surveys. During the learning experience, students can keep logs or journals, take formative quizzes, and post answers to the discussion board. Student learning at the end of selected modules and the course itself can be assessed by examinations, presentations, or papers, among other methods.

Grading rubrics should be used for the assessment and grading of student assignments in an online course, similar to a rubric for face-to-face courses. Shipman, Roa, Hooten, and Wang (2012) suggested rubrics provide meaningful and consistent assessment of assignments. Nursing faculty members can create their own rubrics or can use rubrics posted in a public gallery (Rcampus™, 2012). In the Rubric Gallery, faculty can develop, assess, and share rubrics with others. Further discussion and examples of rubrics for assessment in nursing courses are in Chapter 10.

Courses should be evaluated before they go live, allowing the teacher to resolve any problems or issues with the course before the students begin taking it. An excellent tool for evaluating an online course is the QM rubric, discussed earlier in the chapter (MarylandOnline, 2010). Schools can join the QM organization and learn about evaluating their courses through workshops and consultations.

Continuous feedback is necessary throughout the course, because with most online courses, the teacher does not "see students" or take attendance. One example of formative evaluation is the "pulse check." This should be done several times during the course. In an announcement the teacher can ask students to "Stop a moment and take your pulse. Is it strong and bounding, weak and thready, or another combination? E-mail me your assessment and tell me what I can do to help you be successful." The teacher can post a summary announcement if the feedback will assist the group (O'Neil et al., 2009). Summative evaluation is assessment of the modules and course, typically at the end. Surveys may be sent to students and faculty members, asking questions pertinent to course evaluation such as student satisfaction with the course content, instructional methods, assignments, and other areas (O'Neil et al., 2009).

SUMMARY

Teaching online is different from teaching in a classroom because the students cannot be seen and different technology is used. The advantage to students of learning online is the flexibility of learning anytime and anywhere. The disadvantage is often the technology and learning alone. The pedagogy differs in that students learn from each other. Interaction with the teacher as facilitator, the content, and other students is essential. Learning in an online environment is reflective and active. Online learning requires administrative support for the technology, and choices need to be made about course management systems. Learning modules are designed before the students enter the online course. A module includes objectives, content, learning activities, strategies for interaction, and resources for learning. Once the students are in the course, the role of the teacher is to guide them through the learning experience, assess the outcomes of student learning, and evaluate the course.

Learning in online environments has an important role in nursing education, and the learning environments must be of high quality. Technology continues to influence online courses and programs, and learning online will become more accessible, portable, and mobile in the near future.

REFERENCES

Allen, E., & Seaman, J. (2013). *Changing course: Ten years of tracking online education in the United States*. Retrieved from http://sloanconsortium.org/publications/survey/changing_course_2012

Blackboard Inc. (2013). *Blackboard*. Retrieved from http://www.blackboard.com

Chickering, A. W., & Ehrmann, S. C. (1996). Implementing the seven principles: Technology as lever. *AAHE Bulletin*, 3–6. Retrieved from http://www.tltgroup.org/programs/seven.html

Grassley, J. S., & Bartoletti, T. (2009). Wikis and blogs: Tools for online interaction. *Nurse Educator*, 34, 209–213. doi:10.1097/NNE.0b013e3181b2b59b

Illinois Online Network. (2010a). *What makes a successful online facilitator?* Retrieved from http://www.ion.uillinois.edu/resources/tutorials/pedagogy/instructorProfile.asp

Illinois Online Network. (2010b). *What makes a successful online student?* Retrieved from http://www.ion.uillinois.edu/resources/tutorials/pedagogy/StudentProfile.asp

Johnson, L., Adams, S., & Cummins, M. (2012). *The NMC horizon report: 2012 higher education edition*. Austin, TX: The New Media Consortium.

Johnson, L., Adams Becker, S., Cummins, M., Estrada, V., Freeman, A., & Ludgate, H. (2013). *NMC horizon report: 2013 higher education edition*. Austin, TX: The New Media Consortium.

Lemley, T., & Burnham, J. F. (2009). Web 2.0 tools in medical and nursing school curricula. *Journal of the Medical Library Association*, 97(1), 50–52. doi:10.3163/1536-5050.97.1.010

MarylandOnline. (2010). *Quality matters program*. Retrieved from http://www.qmprogram.org

Moodle. (2013). *Moodle*. Retrieved from https://moodle.org/

O'Neil, C. A., & Fisher, C. (2008). Should I take this course online? *Journal of Nursing Education, 47*, 53–58. doi:10.3928/01484834-20080201-04

O'Neil, C. A., Fisher, C., & Newbold, S. (2009). *Developing online learning environments in nursing education* (2nd ed.). New York, NY: Springer Publishing Company.

Quality Matters Program. (2011). Quality Matters™ Rubric Standards 2011–2013 Edition with Assigned Point Values. MarylandOnline, Inc. Retrieved from https://www.qualitymatters.org/rubric

Ragan, L. C. (2007, May 15). The 10 commandments of effective online teaching. *Distance Education Report 11*(10), 3.

Rcampus. (2012). *Rubric gallery*. Retrieved from http://www.rcampus.com/rubricshellc.cfm?sms=publicrub&sid=35&

Shipman, D., Roa, M., Hooten, J., & Wang, Z. (2012). Using the analytic rubric as an evaluation tool in nursing education: The positive and the negative. *Nursing Education Today, 32*, 246–249. doi:10.1016/j.nedt.2011.04.007

Williams, M. L., Paprock, K. E., & Covington, B. (1999). *Distance learning: The essential guide*. Thousand Oaks, CA: Sage Publications.

7

Learning Laboratories as a Foundation for Nursing Excellence

CAROL F. DURHAM AND DARLENE E. BAKER

Skills acquisition is an important component of nursing education beginning early in the curriculum and continuing throughout the nursing program. Learning laboratories provide a safe environment for initial psychomotor skills acquisition while offering opportunities to socialize students into the professional role of a nurse. The phrase *learning laboratory* used in this chapter refers to what might frequently be termed a resource center, learning center, or skills laboratory. The phrase is used to allow for a broader understanding of the function and purpose of this environment, which may encompass a wide range of learning activities, processes, supplies, and equipment to enhance clinical reasoning and provide for deliberate practice prior to applying knowledge, skills, and attitudes in patient care.

The learning laboratory is designed to simulate the clinical setting and to be a non-threatening space for the development of knowledge, skills, and attitudes that are foundational to clinical practice. Students enter learning laboratories excited about becoming nurses, and they often envision the psychomotor skills taught there as being *what* nurses do. The challenge for laboratory personnel is to assist students to understand that acquisition of psychomotor skills is foundational and important but is only one component of being a nurse. Educators in laboratory settings are charged with encouraging the development of a strong foundation of learning so students can advance in their understanding of the depth and breadth of the art of nursing.

This chapter provides practical strategies embedded in educational pedagogy of skills acquisition. It is understood that students' ability to perform skills is essential to safe and high-quality patient care. Acceptable competence of clinical skills is a prerequisite to developing a professional expert competency. Professional performance of psychomotor skills is not simply automated but requires sound judgment, careful planning, critical thinking, and decision making to ensure safe and effective patient care. This knowledge is integral to the successful implementation of psychomotor skills, and it represents a critical cognitive component of skill mastery. It is critical that learners not only *understand* the skill and the rationale for the skill but also be able to *perform* it. Educators and learners have to understand that knowing and doing are two different things. As an example, memorizing the skills checklist for evaluation does not prepare a learner to perform the skill in the dynamic context of patient care.

SKILL DEVELOPMENT: ESSENTIAL CONCEPTS

A solid understanding of the skill and ability to perform it enables learners to develop their competence and confidence as practitioners, allowing them to consider the clinical situation in a broader context. Diers (1990) early on provided a succinct description of the complexity of skills acquisition that can be shared with students as they begin learning in the laboratory and embarking on their nursing career:

> Skills are thought to be the rudiments of more complicated things, and therefore rote, unchanging, mechanical. But the acquisition of skill is neither easy nor automatic. Once learned, however, a skill is absorbed into the banks of memory and the fibers of the nervous system so it can be called up and counted upon with instant reliability. Carefully learned skills free the mind for analysis, for decision making, for innovation and choice. Skill implies mastery, but skill mastery does not define excellence in practice. It is only one of the spring boards from which a leap to excellence becomes possible. (p. 66)

The automation of basic skills mentioned by Diers allows the learner to examine what is going on with the patient at a higher level. However, reflecting on Ericsson's (2004) deliberate practice, discussed below, it is important not to move too quickly to automation of nursing skills.

In the learning laboratory, teachers should understand that they are working with novice learners, defined by Benner (1984) as "beginners [who] have had no experience of the situations in which they are expected to perform" (p. 20). Because "novices have no experience of the situation they face, they must be given rules to guide their performance" (p. 21). Students' experiences in the learning laboratory have an important role in developing their understanding of skills in a contextual framework. Students are embarking on a career with its own language and set of skills and applications that are unique in the health care field. Often educators expect learners to be expert in skill performance prior to beginning clinical rotations. However, they have been introduced only to skills, and they have minimal competence in their performance. Clinical and laboratory educators have to create opportunities for students to continue developing their skills. For example, when designing laboratory experiences, nurse educators can teach some skills early, such as donning sterile gloves and universal precautions. As students progress through subsequent laboratories, they can be held accountable for the skills of sterile gloving and universal precautions.

This scaffolding of learning is essential for moving learners toward expert skill development. Benner (1984) suggested that an expert "no longer relies on an analytic principle (rule, guideline, maxim) to connect her or his understanding of the situation to an appropriate action" (p. 31) because the expert nurse has "an enormous background of experience" (p. 32). Only through practice and experience can students advance in their skills development. This enormous amount of experience takes time. Some suggest that it may take approximately 4 hours of practice per day for 10 years to achieve a level of mastery for more complex knowledge and professional skills (Colvin, 2008; Ericsson, 2008; Levitin, 2006). Therefore, it is important for educators to establish an expectation of acceptable performance early on with the understanding that skills development continues throughout a professional career.

The importance of solid skills development cannot be underestimated for the patient, nurse, or employer. Patients equate excellence in care with the ability of their nurse to perform the skills necessary for their care. The confidence of nurses is intertwined with their ability to competently perform those same skills. The employer relies on nurses to deliver excellent care, which requires high levels of knowledge and psychomotor skills development. If this important foundation is not established properly, early in the curriculum, then the students will continue to struggle with skills and will adopt poor practices that can have a negative impact on the quality and safety of nursing practice.

PHASES OF SKILL DEVELOPMENT

Fitts and Posner (1967) described three phases of skills development: cognitive, associative, and autonomous. The *cognitive phase* requires a lot of attention and is focused on understanding the skill, how best to implement the skill, and the evaluation of the skill. The *associative phase* is devoted to refining the skill so the performance is more consistent with less variability. The *autonomous phase* is more habitual and automatic, requiring less attention and freeing the learner for higher level thinking. Students in learning laboratories are in the cognitive phase and may begin to move to the associative phase near the end of their laboratory experience, depending on the amount of practice and instructor feedback they obtain. It is more likely that the associative and autonomous phases will occur in professional practice, where certain skills such as washing hands, introducing self, and environmental surveillance will become second nature. These automatic abilities require initial skill learning, followed by practice and then repeated performance in a variety of patient care scenarios, both simulated and real. For example, we want to equip learners with the ability to automatically implement skills, such as taking blood pressure for a rapidly deteriorating patient, without having to think about the sequence of steps needed to take the blood pressure.

DELIBERATE PRACTICE

However, automation of all skills is not the end goal for expert performance. To facilitate the journey to expert performance, it is helpful to consider deliberate practice. Ericsson (2004) defined deliberate practice as "engaging in practice activities with the primary goal of improving some aspect of performance" (p. S73). He delineated the steps as first identifying an area for improvement for a well-defined task, then receiving immediate feedback, and finally problem-solving for improved performance through repetition of the task (Ericsson, 2004). Ericsson (2008) cautioned, however, that those who are trying to achieve expert performance must work to counteract automaticity by striving for continual improvement. For example, students arrive at the school of nursing with hand washing automated from years of washing their hands. However, in health care, we need them to be more deliberate not only in the technique of hand washing but also in the frequency and timing of hand washing. Educators are not trying to automate the *task* but are trying to automate the *expectation* that hand washing will be done on entering the patient's room and prior to patient care.

For high-risk patient safety skills such as medication administration, it is important that they not be automated because of the required concentration and careful attention to detail for accuracy. Ericsson (2008) suggested that with careful evaluation of the procedure as it occurs and with concurrent problem-solving for potential areas of improvement, skill development can be enhanced. Many agencies and nurses are reflecting on the practice of medication administration, considering methods to improve the skill of medication administration, and implementing "do not disturb zones" for the medication administration nurse. Faculty members should instill in their learners an expectation that they should personally as well as within the profession continually reexamine how skills are performed and explore ways to improve patient care, using deliberate practice instead of settling for acceptable performance.

DEVELOPMENT OF PROFESSIONAL CONFIDENCE

The learning laboratory is also essential for establishing the professional confidence that graduates need to begin their nursing career. It can be the milieu where students begin to develop the *therapeutic use of self* (Kardong-Edgren, 2012) and to provide patient-centered care. Cronenwett and associates for the *Quality and Safety Education for Nurses* (QSEN) competencies define patient-centered care as "[recognizing] the patient or designee as the source of control and full partner in providing compassionate and coordinated care based on respect for [the] patient's preferences, values, and needs" (Cronenwett et al., 2007, p. 123). Assisting students in learning how to approach patients with respect and dignity, being responsive to their individual needs, being sensitive to cultural differences, and collaborating with the patient as well as with other members of the health care team in the delivery of safe and quality care are a few of the overarching goals of socialization into the nursing profession. As educators design experiences for students, it is important not to overlook these core values of good nursing care. Oermann (2011) stated that leaners need the opportunity to practice cognitive as well as motor skills. Educators can embed skills in patient care scenarios to teach these concepts.

ROLE OF FACULTY, STAFF, TEACHING ASSISTANTS, AND PEER MENTORS

The type of nurse educator chosen to teach in a learning laboratory varies based on the objectives and academic considerations. Laboratory teachers should be nurses and can include faculty members, staff, or graduate nursing teaching assistants, based on staffing needs. Undergraduate peers may also be used with qualified nursing oversight. All teachers, regardless of position or experience, require training on the content of each laboratory to promote consistent teaching and demonstration of skills, to enable teachers to effectively communicate rationales and evidence-based practice (when available), and to permit them to adequately and consistently assess student performance during evaluation. Training sessions should be held at the start of the academic term and regularly throughout the semester or quarter. These sessions should be structured to allow review of previously taught material as needed, discussion of upcoming skills to be learned, and demonstration of skills. Teachers may practice the skills and received coaching on skills demonstration as needed. At the end of the term, a wrap-up session should occur to discuss opportunities to refine the teaching plan and improve educational practices.

Faculty members provide supervisory oversight of all activities, including learning module development, laboratory scheduling, and coordination of laboratories with clinical courses, and represent the laboratory on nursing school curriculum and other committees. In addition, faculty members should be capable of teaching skills in an interactive and engaging manner and of facilitating simulation experiences.

Full- or part-time staff members who engage in direct teaching of nursing skills should be nurses. The educational background required to work in a learning laboratory is based on standards and policies established by the state board of nursing. Staff members might be nurses who work at local health care facilities or might be employed solely by the school of nursing. Apart from teaching in the laboratory or simulation settings, staff members might be responsible for laboratory operations, such as ordering and maintaining supplies and equipment, supervising the setup and breakdown, and tracking student progress through learning modules and simulation experiences. Staff members might also complete administrative work, such as copying, entering grades, scheduling student evaluations and practice sessions, and rescheduling any missed laboratories or evaluations. Some of these administrative duties can be assigned to nonnursing personnel.

Part-time teaching assistants might be graduate nursing students or practicing nurses. If graduate students are available, they provide a great resource for staffing laboratories because they typically bring current clinical expertise to their teaching and benefit from being mentored into the educator role. Many teaching assistants seek the position because they desire to become nurse educators. Because it is likely that teaching assistants can earn more working per diem in a health care agency, recruitment for the position requires an appealing package that includes financial compensation, tuition reimbursement, and health insurance coverage. In addition, work schedules must coordinate with academic schedules. To provide teaching assistants with a more holistic understanding of the laboratory environment beyond teaching content and skills, they should also be trained to assist with the laboratory setup and breakdown and routine cleaning tasks, and to input data to monitor student attendance.

If a peer-mentored environment is desired, students in upper levels of the nursing program can be recruited to provide additional practice for beginning students. Peer mentoring not only allows additional time for deliberate practice of psychomotor skills but it also allows for informal mentoring of students. The peer-mentored system needs to have established guidelines and expectations of the mentors and identified benefits for the students who participate in it.

EXPECTATIONS FOR LEARNERS IN A LABORATORY

To encourage development of the professional nurse role, students should be given a written overview of guidelines and rules for laboratory attendance and preparation that parallels behaviors they will be expected to demonstrate in their role as professional nurses in the clinical setting. This information should be given with or before their first exposure to the learning laboratory. Students should learn about behavioral expectations, which emphasize the importance of personal accountability, patient and nurse safety, and compliance with the Health Insurance Portability and Accountability Act (HIPAA) and Family Educational Rights and Privacy Act (FERPA) standards. In addition to written guidelines, teachers should role-model the expected clinical behaviors during laboratory sessions. Students should learn to clean up the bedside work area after patient care and ensure proper disposal of all supplies and equipment according to Occupational Safety and Health Administration (OSHA) and agency guidelines, which parallel the expectations of their behavior in a patient care environment.

Students should be required to dress in a professional manner while performing patient skills in the laboratory, following established guidelines regarding necklines, hemlines, and footwear, which would be appropriate to a working patient care environment. Some schools of nursing ask students to dress for laboratory experiences, including simulation sessions, in their clinical uniforms. This approach is supported by the work of Adam and Galinsky (2012), who describe the basic principle of "[enclothed cognition as having a] co-occurrence of two independent factors—the symbolic meaning of the clothes and the physical experience of wearing them" (p. 922). Their research suggests that donning a laboratory coat as a physician increases the person's attentiveness and carefulness. This can be transferrable to nursing students wearing their uniforms in laboratory settings, affecting their psychological perception of being and acting like a nurse. What they wear in the laboratory might have an influence on how they begin to build confidence in their role as nurses. Consequences of violating expectations of dress and appearance should be clearly outlined in the laboratory guidelines.

INTEGRATION OF LABORATORIES INTO CURRICULA

A successful learning laboratory is one that is integrated throughout the curriculum, allowing students regular, repetitive opportunities for deliberate practice. It is important for skills acquisition to provide a psychologically safe environment in which the learner "is able to behave or perform without fear of negative consequences to self-image, social standing, or career trajectory" (Ganley & Linnard-Palmer, 2010, p. e2). The climate of the learning laboratory is that of collaboration. Achievement of acceptable psychomotor skills demonstration (a designated level of performance, determined by nurse educators using evidence-based practice and best standards of practice) and attainment of related knowledge is the joint responsibility of the students and teacher. Students are responsible for participating in designated learning activities to attain knowledge and promote acceptable skills acquisition. Oermann (2011) suggested that although students might be able to perform a skill at the time of assessment, skills can be retained only with practice. Educators are responsible for providing opportunities for practice, feedback, and repeated practice at regular intervals, not only in the laboratory but also in the clinical setting.

Many learning laboratories include not only psychomotor skills acquisition but also simulation experiences using computerized manikins, standardized patients, virtual reality, and case-based scenarios. These provide an opportunity for students to apply what they are learning in the laboratory to patient care scenarios that simulate clinical practice. Simulation can be integrated throughout the curriculum beyond content for adult health, pediatrics, and obstetrics courses to include leadership, community health, mental health, and interprofessional experiences. Chapter 5 discusses the pedagogy of simulation in the learning laboratory.

TYPES OF LEARNING LABORATORIES

A variety of laboratories associated with both clinical and nonclinical courses might be offered throughout the prelicensure program and in graduate nursing programs. Schools of nursing vary in the sequencing of skills across the curriculum, usually beginning with basic foundational skills and advancing to more complex skills. There is no consensus on what constitutes a complex skill; however, hand-washing is a basic skill, whereas central line care is a complex skill. Grouping of skills should be a deliberate decision by faculty to meet the learning needs of their students as they move from laboratories to practice settings. The established flow of clinical experiences in a nursing program will also influence how skills are grouped. Beyond beginning with foundational skills and building to complex skills, there is no consensus about the sequence in which skills should be taught (Table 7.1). In the graduate curriculum, laboratories can be offered for advanced health assessment, diagnostic reasoning, and various content-specific learning experiences. Additional laboratories that interface with other professions or service organizations can promote interprofessional education.

Table 7.1 provides an example of typical laboratories offered in a nursing program, listed by course and purpose, examples of skills taught for each course, and necessary preparation by students and laboratory personnel. The table includes prelicensure laboratories and also more advanced laboratories that might be offered, such as a laboratory in a Diagnostic Reasoning course for graduate students in nurse practitioner programs and an interprofessional education laboratory to provide essential immersive environments for interprofessional learners to develop essential skills in communication, collaboration, and teamwork.

TABLE 7.1 Types of Learning Laboratories

Learner Groups

- Scheduled laboratory groups (can be based on clinical assignments, arbitrarily assigned, or self-selected)
- Small group for deliberate practice (students self-select attendance days and times)
- One-to-one skills review and/or deliberate practice (completed at the request of students or faculty/staff)
- Small simulation sessions (tabletop exercises such as problem-based learning and patient care scenario-based case studies)

Course and Purpose	Sample Skills Focus Areas	Preparation
Fundamentals Skills Laboratory/Basic Medical Surgical Skills Laboratories (can bridge across several clinically oriented courses or be contained in one fundamentals nursing course) Learn, practice, and refine: • Communication skills • Bedside psychomotor nursing skills • Increase students' confidence in the clinical setting	Basic to advanced patient care skills based on course requirements. Generally encompass aspects of: • Microbial safety and vital signs • Personal care • Immobility interventions • Safe patient handling and movement • Medication administration techniques for various nonparenteral routes • Injections • Intravenous therapy • Wound care • Elimination • Respiratory interventions • Gastrointestinal (GI) intubation • Postmortem care • Central venous access devices • Venipuncture	Provide learning modules in advance for student review prior to the laboratory session. Set up supplies, equipment, and charts specific to the skills to be taught in each laboratory.
Health/Physical Assessment Laboratories Learn, practice, and refine: • Communication and interviewing skills • Body system assessment skills • Documentation skills	Conduct body system assessment specific to each session's content. Provide regular practice, integrating the systems learned each week into a cohesive patient assessment.	Provide learning modules in advance for student review prior to the laboratory session. Online format: No room laboratory resources needed Classroom format: Laboratory setup Provide a private space with appropriate diagnostic equipment for the body systems reviewed in each session.

(continued)

TABLE 7.1 Types of Learning Laboratories (*continued*)

Course and Purpose	Sample Skills Focus Areas	Preparation
		Set up additional learning resources such as simulators and anatomical models.
Advanced Medical Surgical/Capstone Laboratories Refresh previously learned communication and psychomotor skills. Increase students' confidence with psychomotor skills.	Basic to advanced patient care skills based on course requirements. Generally encompasses aspects of: • Medication administration: oral, injectable, intravenous, gastrostomy, central line flushes • Sterile dressing changes • Tracheostomy care • Catheterization • Health/physical assessment • Venipuncture • Equipment review	Provide learning modules in advance for student review prior to the laboratory session. Set up supplies and equipment for: • Applicable medication administration routes • Selected beside clinical skills • Health/physical assessment review
Pharmacology Competency Laboratories Synthesize content from multiple courses (health/physical assessment, fundamentals, pharmacology). Integrate pharmacologic knowledge with medication administration procedures.	Interpretation of laboratory values Use of pharmacologic references Medication administration includes: • Recognizing and/or averting medication errors • Medication administration skills: oral, topical, eye, ear, injectable, intravenous Health/physical assessment skills pertinent to each scenario Effective communication with health care team	Provide learning modules in advance for student review prior to the laboratory session Instruct students to perform a focused review of content: • Applicable medication administration procedures from fundamental skills training • Selected drug classifications and categories, including but not limited to the drug agents found in the scenarios • General health assessment skills Set up supplies, equipment, and charts for each patient care scenario.
Pediatric and Family Health Laboratories Review previously learned skills in a pediatric and family-oriented context. Practice patient-specific skills and interventions for the pediatric population	Generally includes practice in: • Medication administration: oral, injectable, intravenous • Use of infusion devices • Infant bathing, feeding, and diapering	Provide learning modules in advance for student review prior to the laboratory session. Instruct students to review required modules prior to laboratory.

(*continued*)

Course and Purpose	Sample Skills Focus Areas	Preparation
Review equipment.	• GI intubation: insertion, feedings, medications, removal • Urinary catheterization and specimen collection • Ostomy care as applicable to area • Tracheostomy care as applicable to clinical setting	Set up supplies, equipment, and charts for: • Medication administration • Infant care skills • Bedside procedures
Maternal and Newborn Health Laboratories Review previously learned skills in the context of a labor patient, a newborn, and a postpartum patient. Practice patient-specific skills and interventions for the maternal/newborn population. Review equipment.	Generally includes practice in: • Labor support techniques and interventions for the patient and family • Fetal heart monitoring • Postpartum assessment checklist • Newborn assessment and medication administration • Practice counting newborn heart rate and respiratory rate	Provide learning modules in advance for student review prior to the laboratory session. Set up supplies, equipment, and charts specific to the skills to be reviewed.
Public/Community Health Laboratories Review previously learned skills in the context of a community setting. Develop and practice patient education and intervention skills in a community-oriented context.	Generally includes review of: • Vital signs: use of manual and/or nonelectronic equipment • Glucometer use • Basic wound care Use of patient education materials: posters, supplies, equipment, models:	Provide learning modules in advance for student review prior to the laboratory session. Set up supplies, equipment, and charts specific to the skills to be reviewed.
Diagnostic Reasoning Laboratories (Graduate Student Nurse Practitioner laboratories for various specialty areas) Practice and refine body system assessment skills. Refine communication and interviewing skills with a provider-oriented focus.	• Body system assessment specific to each session's content. • Regular practice integrating systems learned each week into a cohesive assessment.	Provide learning modules, case studies, and integrated clinical scenarios as required. Provide a private space with appropriate diagnostic equipment for the body systems reviewed in each session. Set up additional learning resources such as simulators and anatomical models. Set up audio or video equipment as required based on scenario needs and objectives.

(continued)

TABLE 7.1 Types of Learning Laboratories (*continued*)

Course and Purpose	Sample Skills Focus Areas	Preparation
Interprofessional Education Laboratories Learn, practice, and refine: • Interprofessional communication skills • Principles of teamwork and collaboration Practice skills and procedures within interprofessional teams.	• Basic to advanced patient care skills and assessment techniques based on patient care scenarios	Provide learning modules in advance for student review prior to the laboratory session. Set up supplies, equipment, and charts specific to the skills to be reviewed.
External Clients Nursing skills refresher for skills development laboratories • Practice specific skills and procedures • Improve communication skills. Videotaping education offerings	• Basic to advanced patient care skills and assessment techniques based on course requirements	Provide learning modules in advance for student review prior to the laboratory session. Set up supplies, equipment, and charts specific to the skills to be reviewed.

Copyright Education-Innovation-Simulation Learning Environment, School of Nursing, The University of North Carolina at Chapel Hill, 2013. Reprinted by permission, 2013.

SAMPLE LEARNING MODULE

Teaching materials and instruction guides pertaining to each specific laboratory taught should be standardized across content to promote consistency in teaching among individual teachers. To assist the reader in understanding how the learning laboratory environment for a content area can be operationalized, the Central Venous Access Device (CVAD) learning module is used as an exemplar throughout the chapter. The materials included in Appendix A can serve as sample templates in the development and revision of learning laboratory documents in the reader's own institution. Appendix A provides the reader with ten documents for the CVAD laboratory: (1) how to set up a laboratory room (including specific manikin preparation), (2) a setup and breakdown guide for the laboratory teacher, (3) a lesson plan, (4) a teaching box supply list, (5) the standardized learning module overview, (6) specific module content (key concepts and skill procedure), (7) a provider's order sheet, (8) a medication administration record, (9) a parental nutrition order form, and (10) a skill evaluation checklist (Appendices A.1–A.10).

LABORATORY ORGANIZATION

INSTRUCTOR-TO-STUDENT RATIO

The instructor-to-student ratio in laboratory is determined based on several criteria and can vary based on the intent of each laboratory. Several laboratory groupings are suggested at the top of Table 7.1. Room size, number of staff available to teach, availability and amount of equipment and supplies, student level in the program, and technical difficulty of skills in a particular laboratory all influence the instructor-to-student ratio. The evolving learning styles of students should also be considered. Ratios can range from 1:8 or 1:10 to mimic the clinical setting, or can be 1:12 or higher with a large group focus. Because skills acquisition requires more than theoretical knowledge, students need the opportunity to practice with timely feedback, which can be difficult to offer in laboratories with a high student-to-faculty ratio.

STUDENT ASSIGNMENT

Students can select their laboratory section through a registration process, which allows for individual preferences, or might be placed in laboratories based on pre-determined criteria such as clinical group assignments. Teachers can be assigned to specific laboratory groups for the term or to laboratory sections on a rotational basis. Assigning educators to a specific laboratory section across the term provides them an opportunity to become familiar with the students in that section and to better understand the students' learning styles. It can also establish an atmosphere of trust and collegiality. However, rotating teachers between laboratory groups can provide learners with an opportunity to experience diverse teaching styles and to learn strategies for working within contingency teams, an arrangement that parallels staffing patterns in clinical practice.

STAGING AREA

Organization of the laboratory is essential to the success of the laboratory and nursing program. The need for organization cannot be overestimated, and when done well, organization makes the laboratory environment seem to run effortlessly. The learning laboratory requires a lot of consumable supplies, durable equipment, staff, and logistical systems to manage both staff and the flow of large numbers of students. Because supply and equipment management is essential to a well-run laboratory, the laboratory requires a staging area. The staging area is more than a storage room. In fact, if called *storage*, facility management committees might be tempted to move the laboratory storage area to an inconvenient location, making it challenging to access. If the focus of the space is on *staging*, the space is recognized as being an integral component of the laboratory operations. The staging area is the center of activity of the learning laboratory.

Functionality of the staging area is dependent on appropriate building infrastructure and a high level of organization and tidiness to allow for accessibility of equipment and supplies when needed. It needs to be equipped with at least one sink for cleaning and resetting equipment, such as intravenous (IV) fluids and suction canisters. A sink is also essential to prepare supplies for laboratories that require simulated liquids, such as IV fluids; parenteral nutrition (PN); blood, urine, and gastrointestinal fluids; and fake stool samples. The staging area also needs adequate shelving and power sources to store supplies and equipment, flat work areas for assembling and packing, and appropriate carts for item transport. A variety of cleaning supplies should be readily available to assist in harvesting used supplies. It is helpful to have various adhesive removers to use for removing adhesive residue from tubing, manikins, and other surfaces. Basic office supplies, from scissors, tape, and markers to printers and label-making equipment, should be accessible if they are not maintained in the staging area.

LABORATORY ACTION PLAN

Standardization of room setup across simultaneously occurring laboratories promotes consistent educational experiences among separate laboratories. To promote standardization, it is helpful to create a room setup guide outlining how to prepare the space and/or manikins for student learning and practice. Appendix A.1 provides the *How to Set Up* guide for the CVAD learning module as a sample template.

Appendix A.2 provides a sample laboratory supply/equipment setup and breakdown guide for this same learning module. It includes instructions for distributing supplies for the laboratory session and for resetting the supplies to prepare for the next laboratory. This guide should be reviewed by each laboratory teacher prior to beginning the laboratory to ensure familiarity with the setup supplies and equipment.

In addition to the room and laboratory setup guidelines, there should be a lesson plan that both outlines the content to be covered and indicates the amount of time to be spent on each topic. Recommendations for possible teaching strategies such as observation, participation during the teacher's demonstration (round table practice, discussed further later in the chapter), and practice after observation should be included on the lesson plan for consistency among educators. Appendix A.3 provides an example of a laboratory lesson plan.

To enhance efficiency and consistency in each laboratory and among rooms, a teaching box can be created for each module (Figure 7.1). A teaching box is prepared for each learning laboratory and restocked after completion of the laboratory. If there are laboratories running simultaneously, it is helpful to create one teaching box per laboratory room, and these can be stored in the staging area ready for the laboratory (Figure 7.2). Module-specific equipment and supplies are placed in the teaching box, along with a list of contents. Items that are necessary for the laboratory but do not fit into the teaching box also can be listed, along with the storage location of those items. The content list should indicate where to obtain replacement supplies if needed. Appendix A.4 provides the laboratory teaching box supply list for the CVAD learning module as an example.

LEARNING MODULES

Students should enter each laboratory experience with a basic understanding of the content to be covered in that laboratory. Each learning module should start with a standardized overview of expectations for student preparation, required supplies, laboratory objectives, required and recommended readings, and a list of the skills to be covered in the laboratory. The learning module overview for the CVAD module is found in Appendix A.5 as an example.

Specialized module content should include the key theoretical concepts and outline the procedures for the skills to be covered, giving students a standardized baseline from which to start skills acquisition. Providing students with the key concepts underlying individual skills is a component of teaching any skill. Learning the theoretical underpinnings and patient care application of skills assists the learner to understand how the knowledge can be used in practical clinical situations. Making the connections between acquiring and using knowledge is what Benner, Sutphen, Leonard, and Day (2010) refer to as *teaching for a sense of salience* (p. 94). This sense-making assists students to understand the nuances of skills, their application to patient care, and how skills acquisition affects their professional development as a nurse.

Learning modules can vary from locally prepared documents to ones obtained from commercial publishers and nursing organizations. They should be available for either printing or downloading to meet different reading and learning styles. Faculty

FIGURE 7.1 Teaching boxes from side and top views.

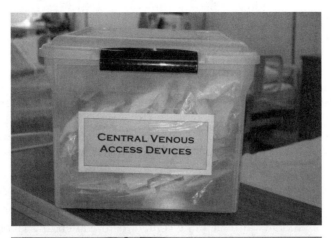

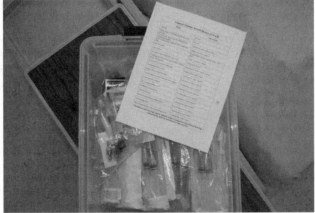

Copyright Education-Innovation-Simulation Learning Environment, School of Nursing, The University of North Carolina at Chapel Hill, 2013. Reprinted by permission, 2013.

FIGURE 7.2 Teaching boxes stacked in a laboratory staging area.

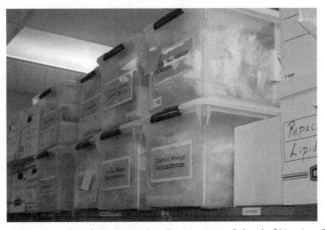

Copyright Education-Innovation-Simulation Learning Environment, School of Nursing, The University of North Carolina at Chapel Hill, 2013. Reprinted by permission, 2013.

members should ensure that content found in the course textbook and learning resources matches the laboratory modules. These documents need to be revised each year to stay current with practice, the books, and other resources used in the course. If learning module content differs from these resources, that fact should be noted in the module, with a rationale for the difference. Appendix A.6 provides a sample template for laboratory learning module content for the skill of administering PN from the CVAD module.

In addition to learning modules, an audio file (MP3 file as a podcast) can be provided to deliver standardized key theoretical or procedural content, eliminating the possibility of inconsistent coverage of material in laboratory. The podcast allows students who are auditory learners an alternative method for acquiring the content. Students read the module and have the option of listening to a podcast of the content prior to attending laboratory.

LEARNING LABORATORY SESSIONS

It is important for students to review the content before attending laboratory to avoid spending a significant amount of time during the laboratory discussing key concepts and to allow more time for practicing skills. To encourage student review and a basic level of preparation, a quiz might be administered as the first component of the laboratory before teaching begins. The frequency of these quizzes can vary from each laboratory session to be given randomly throughout the course. The aim of these quizzes is to assess preparation for the laboratory and understanding of key concepts, not to assess skill application.

Ideally, all students will have an opportunity for supervised practice of all skills (either by the teacher or by a fellow student observing using the procedure guide). Another option is to have students view video recordings that demonstrate the skills and include evidence-based practice. Students can then use laboratory time to apply what they have learned around case-based scenarios. A third approach, referred to previously as *round-table practice*, is used when students move through the steps of a skill together. As an example, students can arrange the over-bed tables in a half circle as the teacher demonstrates and walks the students through a skill (such as donning sterile gloves) in a step-wise manner. Students continue to practice while the teacher walks around the room to critique technique and offer feedback. The best approach depends on the learners, content, space and time constraints, and expertise of the teacher. During the laboratory sessions, students should have practice time, with feedback after skills are demonstrated, to allow them the opportunity for deliberate practice to improve performance. Some skills can be practiced outside the laboratory setting, but others require specialty laboratory equipment and supplies, for example, tracheostomy suctioning; adequate time in the laboratory environment is an important consideration. Regardless of where skills are practiced, it is important to provide specific criteria to facilitate accurate practice.

REALISM

Realism in the learning laboratory enhances preparation of students for actual patient care. Realism should be enhanced as much as possible within the constraints of the learning laboratory to encourage students to immerse themselves in the patient care scenario. There are many ways to promote a realistic environment, from setting up simulated hospital rooms with patient records and manikins in the beds to obtaining the actual equipment and supplies available at local facilities.

Cost is always a consideration when determining how realistic a laboratory can be. The school of nursing needs to make a decision whether to purchase or make some of the items necessary for teaching, such as call bells and medication labels. For example, call bells can be made from pictures downloaded from the Internet, which are then laminated or affixed to a surface and attached to a cord. The cord can be a purchased electrical cord or a cloth or cable that is made to represent a hospital call bell cord. Simple computer software found free on the Internet can be used to simulate medication labels, or labeling systems can be purchased from a vendor. Items such as protective disks for CVADs can be purchased from hospital supply vendors or can be created using foam board and a cutting instrument (Figure 7.3). Learning laboratory personnel need to constantly balance educational needs and funding constraints.

FIGURE 7.3 Sample of crafted protective disks for central venous access devices.

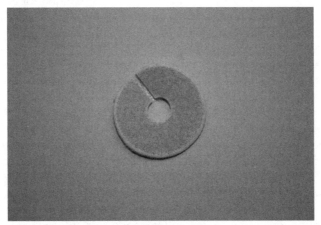

Copyright Education-Innovation-Simulation Learning Environment, School of Nursing, The University of North Carolina at Chapel Hill, 2013. Reprinted by permission, 2013.

Another way to create realism is to provide paperwork that the student will need when performing the skill and for documenting when completed. For medication administration in a laboratory, a provider's order sheet, medication administration record, and other pertinent documentation forms should be available for the specific laboratory content. The forms can be hard copies or in an electronic charting format. In the interest of patient safety and to clearly differentiate simulated documents from actual patient care documents, it is important to label these forms and documents "For Educational Use Only—Not For Actual Patient Care." Appendix A.7 provides a sample template of a Provider Order Sheet from the CVAD learning module. Appendix A.8 is the Medication Administration Record, and Appendix A.9 is the PN Order Form, both from the CVAD learning module.

SUPPLY BAGS

Supply bags provide students with a specified list of supplies for skill development. Bags can be purchased for a specific nursing course or periodically throughout the program to meet specialized clinical requirements. The contents of each bag will reflect the skills that the faculty consider most important for students to gain competency in performing. Supply bags can be charged for as a fee that students pay in addition to other course costs, or they can be provided internally using student fees. Supply bags can promote student responsibility while providing all students with the same level of supplies, either new or used. Providing supplies up front to students can decrease the amount of supplies needed in laboratories, which has implications for space utilization and storage. Decisions should be made about the specific contents to offer in the supply bag, such as whether to supply needles and syringes for practice, and appropriate disposal or recycling of used supplies at the end of training.

PRACTICE LABORATORIES

Practice laboratories allow for deliberate practice of skills taught in laboratories and can enhance student performance. Practice laboratories can be regularly scheduled or can occur on an as-needed basis, depending on the requirements of the specific course and nursing program. Practice laboratories can be open to general practice of any skill requiring refinement, or they can be geared toward preparation for an upcoming performance evaluation with a focus on the set of skills to be evaluated. Practice laboratories for evaluation should not be considered a time to reteach laboratory content, but rather a time for skill refinement using deliberate practice. These laboratories do not have to be tied to a specific clinical course, but they can be offered to any student who needs to refresh skills or who requires remediation.

Staffing decisions for practice laboratories depend on the availability of resources, both personnel and physical. Ideally, all practice laboratories should be staffed with a qualified teacher, and the ratio of students to teachers should be low to allow for more direct supervision of and feedback to students as they practice skills. If the decision is made to offer practice laboratories without a teacher present, space access and accountability issues need to be addressed. Practice laboratories should occur with the same room setup as the one in which skills were taught, which can result in competition for space and faculty. Decisions also have to be made about when to offer practice laboratories and what equipment and supplies will be made available to students during them. General practice laboratory policies and procedures should be in place and available for students, including cleaning and resetting the laboratory space for later students, timeliness and attendance requirements, and penalties for nonattendance. When students do not attend, they prevent other students from having the benefit of that laboratory practice.

INDIVIDUAL DELIBERATE PRACTICE

Individual deliberate practice sessions, which are also known as 1:1 teaching time, can benefit students who are struggling to grasp a specific skill or concept in the laboratory or group practice sessions or who want to improve their competence through practice. Individual practice sessions should not be used in place of initial teaching or group practice, but should be used as an adjunct to maximize resource utilization. Clear guidelines for the use of deliberate practice time have to be established to ensure the most equitable availability for all students who seek assistance. Consideration should be given to the frequency of deliberate practice time, the best-qualified teacher to guide learning in the session, and policies for determining the frequency of individual student access because of limited resources.

COMPETENCY EVALUATIONS

Demonstration of skills through competency evaluation provides visible evidence of the student's psychomotor skill learning. Competency in skill performance should be assessed in periodic performance evaluations throughout the term, but it can be assessed only at the end of the term. Designated levels of performance expected in clinical practice and determined by faculty are the traditional ways to constitute skills competence. Skills evaluation can be formative or summative. Formative evaluation judges students' progress in developing skills and is focused on diagnostic feedback, without assigning a grade to the evaluation experience. Summative evaluation, on the other hand, is end-of-instruction evaluation to determine what the student has learned. Summative evaluation provides a basis for grading and other high-stakes decisions (Oermann & Gaberson, 2014).

Formative skills competency evaluation occurs through an informal assessment of selected skills, such as when an evaluator observes a student performing a dressing change and provides real-time feedback about the student's technique and ability to perform the skill at a safe and competent level. A summative skills competency evaluation of the same dressing change skill is a formal assessment of the student's ability to perform the skill according to predetermined criteria on a checklist. Proceeding without feedback from the evaluator, the student attempts to perform the skill at a safe and competent level. At the end of the summative evaluation, the student receives feedback that counts toward a weighted evaluation of the skill demonstrated. Both types of evaluation are essential components in learning laboratories (Table 7.2). More in-depth discussion about formative and summative evaluation can be found in Chapter 10.

TABLE 7.2 Types of Competency Evaluations

Formative Evaluation	Summative Evaluation
• Skills to be evaluated can be randomly selected or preassigned	• Skills to be evaluated can be randomly selected or preassigned
• Informal assessment of selected skills	• Formal assessment of selected skills
• Uses skill procedure checklists	• Performance evaluation based on predetermined criteria (pass-fail or graded)
• Immediate feedback provided throughout procedure	• Feedback provided at end of evaluation
	• Can be partial or complete (e.g., demonstrate either a complete head-to-toe examination or a selected body system)

Decisions concerning the amount and type of feedback to be offered during skills performance have to be made, reviewed, and agreed on by all evaluators to promote standardized evaluation criteria. At the beginning of the term, provide an evaluation study guide for student reference. Students should refer to the guide when they are introduced to the skill in laboratory, while refining their technique in practice laboratory, and when preparing for the competency evaluation. Knowledge of the underlying cognitive components relative to skills is essential to skills acquisition and is evaluated through laboratory quizzes, course examinations, and competency evaluations.

Consistency in teaching skills is evident at the point of evaluation; inconsistency places the learner at a disadvantage for the performance evaluation. Students need to be assured they have been taught what is necessary to be successful, not only on the competency exam, but also for practice. Standardized evaluation checklists are important to enhance consistency among evaluators and can be developed based on the course material, based on a skills guide, or generated locally. Evaluations can be awarded a grade or a successful result can be considered a pass–fail requirement for a course. The importance of skills evaluation as a component for successful completion of the course needs to be outlined in the course syllabus. The selection of skills for evaluation can vary based on local agency and nursing program requirements.

Skills to be evaluated might be a predetermined set that all students complete, or they might be randomly assigned from the skills to be demonstrated. Evaluations can be documented on paper or in an electronic format. Electronic formats are easy to send to students for review after each evaluation is complete, and the teacher can upload the performance evaluation checklists into a secure student file. With an electronic format, the laboratory teacher can access the checklist at the time of the evaluation and then save it into the student file after the evaluation (Figure 7.4). Verbal feedback given at the end of the evaluation can be followed up with an e-mail attachment of the actual check- list documentation. This provides students the opportunity to review what was missed as they prepare for return demonstration of the skill at a later time. As with all testing instruments, information security concerning evaluation forms must be in compliance with established academic standards.

FIGURE 7.4 Faculty using an electronic form to record student performance evaluation.

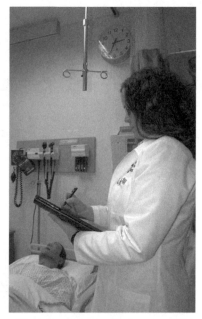

Copyright Education-Innovation-Simulation Learning Environment, School of Nursing, The University of North Carolina at Chapel Hill, 2013. Reprinted by permission, 2013.

When the instructor creates student evaluation checklists, it is helpful for both stu- dents and evaluators to know which critical steps are mandatory for successful completion of the skills. If there are critical patient or nurse safety elements that, when omitted, would require students to repeat the evaluation, both evaluator and student should be aware of those elements. However, students should not expect to pass skills if only the critical steps are completed, but other less critical but important steps are not demonstrated.

A star system is an example of a transparent evaluation system that triages the steps of skills into different levels. A star system, assigning one, two, or three stars to each step of the skill, encourages students to understand the critical steps in a skill, promotes patient and nurse safety, and reinforces the understanding that all steps have a rationale and degree of importance. If students omit or do not perform correctly a one-star step, they can be required to be reassessed for that skill, regardless of how well they perform the rest of the steps. If students omit or do not perform correctly two of the two-star steps, they need to be evaluated again, and so forth. Appendix A.10 provides a sample laboratory competency evaluation checklist for the skill of administering PN from the CVAD learning module.

Students should be able to review the evaluation results, especially if they will be required to be reassessed on those skills at a later date. When students do not perform a skill satisfactorily, they are usually evaluated again on the same skill. Students can, however, be required to perform a different skill in subsequent evaluations, based on local policy and depending on the importance of the skill or underlying concept. High-risk skills such as administration of an IV push medication would benefit from a second attempt at the same skill, possibly with a different medication.

Performance evaluation can contribute points to a course grade or be pass–fail. If evaluations are pass–fail, students might not attend to the important work of skills acquisition due to competing priorities. If points (even minimal points) are attached to skills performance, students might give higher priority to the laboratory content. The number of allowable reassessments should be incorporated into the course syllabus to avoid a situation in which students continually fail performance evaluations but still pass the course. The consequences of not obtaining a satisfactory pass after the established number of allowable attempts need to be determined and communicated to students at the beginning of the course.

LOGISTICS

SCHEDULING

Scheduling is a key consideration when running a learning laboratory. The need for multiple student interactions requires careful scheduling to avoid conflict and meet staffing requirements. Regularly scheduled teaching laboratories, practice laboratories, evaluations, opportunities to be on reassessed on the performance of skills, and remediation sessions have to be coordinated around the students' class and clinical schedules. Laboratories and simulation experiences for students in different terms of the nursing program have to be interwoven because of competition for space and staffing. The schedule should be developed and maintained centrally in the learning laboratory to minimize conflicts and accidental overbooking.

SIGN-UP TOOLS

Scheduling students for practice laboratories, evaluations, and individual practice time can be accomplished in different ways. Students can be allowed to sign up independently, or they can be scheduled for activities by laboratory personnel. If students are allowed to sign up on their own, the method chosen must be accessible to all students. They should be notified in advance when the sign-up will be available. Guidelines should be in place for determining how many times students can sign up for recurring activities, when sign-up will open and close, how students notify learning laboratory personnel if they cannot attend a scheduled laboratory, and any penalties for nonattendance.

INVENTORY TRACKING

An inventory system for tracking equipment needs to be in place in the learning laboratory. Personnel should be able to track equipment purchases, schedule and complete maintenance, and check out equipment to students, staff, and faculty members. The inventory tracking system can be hardcopy or electronic, but it must include a labeling system to track each individual piece of equipment. Regular inventory checks should be accomplished to ensure all equipment is available and tested for usability. Equipment needing an upgrade can be noted in the inventory for future purchasing opportunities.

BUDGET AND PURCHASING

The budget for learning laboratories varies across schools of nursing and can range from minimal to substantial. It can come from different sources, both internal and external. The budget for the learning laboratory should include recurring supply purchases, plans for one-time equipment purchases, and personnel salaries, if applicable. A purchasing and budget tracking system should be in place, using both hardcopy forms and electronic tracking processes. Information concerning warranties, recall notices, and items purchased via outside sources for the laboratory should be kept with purchasing and budget documents to facilitate continuity in equipment maintenance, planning, and utilization of funds.

The fiscal costs to run a laboratory include obtaining sustainable equipment and consumable supplies. Sometimes laboratories acquire used beds, over-bed tables, bedside tables, and other equipment when area hospitals are purchasing new items. Additionally, purchasing from companies that have refurbished equipment can lower costs, but it is recommended to complete a reference check to ensure that the equipment has been adequately refurbished. Laboratories lay out large financial investments in computerized simulation manikins, static manikins, and task trainers. As good stewards, learning laboratories need to care for these teaching aids to maximize longevity. Even with excellent care, equipment will eventually need to be replaced. Replacement considerations should be woven into annual fiscal planning for the laboratory.

Consumable supplies are a large expense for laboratories. If schools have the option to affiliate with a medical facility purchasing department to order supplies, it can be cost effective because of bulk ordering. Additional fees such as stocking fees charged by the medical facility need to be calculated into the budget. Outside vendors are also a viable resource for laboratory supplies. Often it is beneficial to have accounts with multiple supply vendors to allow for access to various products, competitive cost comparisons, and flexible shipping timelines.

EXTERNAL CLIENTS

Given the rich resources of a learning laboratory, there are often external clients who request utilization of the laboratory to equip their learners. External clients can include health care continuing education programs, local hospitals, emergency services, and researchers, among others. External clients benefit from having a laboratory located nearby to provide an easily accessible space for learner practice. Researchers can use a laboratory to properly train employees in such tasks as blood collection, vital signs, and administration of medications. Depending on legal requirements and local needs, a business contract outlining the details of staffing, funding, reimbursement, and purchasing should be established.

SUMMARY

Learning laboratories exist both to create meaningful learning experiences during skills acquisition and to nurture the development of professional nurses who can provide safe and quality care. For learning laboratories to function effectively, they should be integrated into the curriculum to provide students the opportunity to review skills and engage in deliberate practice, while applying skills across the patient care continuum. Although educators who work in the learning laboratory might come from a variety of backgrounds or hold varied positions, they should all agree on the importance of the learning laboratory in the greater context of nursing education. Teaching in learning laboratories can be a rewarding role because students enter the laboratory excited about learning psychomotor skills, and the teacher has the opportunity to encourage depth and breadth of professional competency.

When planning learning laboratory content, educators must consider staffing needs, training requirements for laboratory teachers, expectations of and by students, the teacher-to-student ratio, and the depth and breadth of student assignments and evaluations to be completed. Storage and staging of equipment and supplies, the action plan for laboratory setup and breakdown, type and quantity of supplies available to students, and efforts to promote realism in the laboratory setting also need to be considered within budgetary constraints. Laboratory content should be structured and presented in a timely manner, preferably at the same time as or as close as possible to the time when that applicable course content is taught. Careful development of learning experiences that provide consistent opportunities for all learners is an important consideration when determining the flow of laboratory content. The availability and frequency of psychomotor skills practice, including the amount of deliberate practice that can be provided, has to be interwoven with the need to present new content, evaluate skills acquisition, and provide simulation experiences. All of these factors, while challenging, contribute to making the learning laboratory an environment that is both rewarding and renewing with each new influx of students.

Learning laboratories should be vibrant, educational hubs for engaging learners to be immersed in deliberate practice to provide quality and safe patient care. Faculty members are responsible for providing creative learning experiences that move the learner from knowing about to implementing those skills, while considering how to provide optimal care in each unique patient situation. Laboratory teachers are privileged to be a guide for learners during this portion of their journey from novice to expert practitioner.

REFERENCES

Adam, H., & Galinsky, A. D. (2012). Enclothed cognition. *Journal of Experimental Social Psychology, 48*(4), 918–925. doi:10.1016/j.jesp.2012.02.008

Benner, P. (1984). *From novice to expert: Excellence and power in clinical nursing practice.* Menlo Park, CA: Addison Wesley Publishing Company.

Benner, P., Sutphen, M., Leonard, V., & Day, L. (2010). *Educating nurses: A call for radical transformation.* Standford, CA: The Carnegie Foundation for the Advancement of Teaching.

Colvin, G. (2008). *Talent is overrated: What really separates world-class performers from everybody else.* New York, NY: Penguin Group.

Cronenwett, L., Sherwood, G., Barnsteiner, J., Disch, J., Johnson, J., Mitchell, P., …. Warren, J. (2007). Quality and safety education for nurses. *Nursing Outlook, 55*, 122–131. doi:10.1016/j.outlook.2007.02.006

Diers, D. (1990). Learning the art and craft of nursing. *American Journal of Nursing, 90*(1), 64–66.

Ericsson, K. A. (2004). Deliberate practice and the acquisition and maintenance of expert performance in medicine and related domains. *Academic Medicine, 79*(10) Supplement, S70–S81. Retrieved from http://fournier.facmed.unam.mx/ib2/ut2/s11/AndersDeliberate-PracticeExpertPerformanceAcadMed.pdf

Ericsson, K. A. (2008). Deliberate practice and acquisition of expert performance: A general overview. *Academic Emergency Medicine, 15,* 988–994. doi:10.1111/j1553-2712.2008.00227.x

Fitts, P. M., & Posner, M. I. (1967). *Human performance.* Belmont, CA: Brooks/Cole Publishing Company.

Ganley, B. J., & Linnard-Palmer, L. (2010). Academic safety during nursing simulation: Perceptions of nursing students and faculty. *Clinical Simulation in Nursing,* e1–e9. doi:10.1016/j.ecns.2010.06.004

Kardong-Edgren, S. (2012). Non-technical skills vs therapeutic use of self: An observation. *Clinical Simulation in Nursing, 8,* e35. doi:10.1016/j.ecns.2011.12.003

Levitin, D. J. (2006). *This is your brain on music: The science of a human obsession.* New York, NY: Dutton.

Oermann, M. H. (2011). Toward evidence-based nursing education: Deliberate practice and motor skill learning. *Journal of Nursing Education, 50,* 63–64. doi:10.3928/01484834-20110120-01

Oermann, M. H., & Gaberson, K. B. (2014). *Evaluation and testing in nursing education* (4th ed.). New York, NY: Springer Publishing Company.

8

Clinical Teaching in Nursing

LISA K. WOODLEY

The clinical teacher plays a pivotal role in shaping the learning for nursing students in the clinical setting. Because of this, it is essential that clinical teachers exhibit effective teaching behaviors and best practices in teaching nursing, and that they inspire students. This chapter explains why effective clinical teaching is so critical, the process of clinical teaching, and how the clinical teacher should best address learning outcomes for students. Specific teaching strategies, such as how to create a learning climate that is inviting and supportive to students, how to foster effective relationships in the clinical setting, how to design an effective and inspirational clinical orientation, and how to choose best patient assignments for students are discussed. This chapter also describes other best clinical teaching practices, such as structuring and organizing the clinical day, creating clinical conferences and other learning activities that enhance student learning, and giving guidance and feedback to students in the clinical setting. The concepts and teaching strategies described in the chapter are applicable across clinical settings and other sites in which students have practice experiences. New models of clinical teaching, such as dedicated education units and other types of partnerships, are described in the next chapter, and clinical evaluation is discussed separately in Chapter 12.

THE IMPORTANCE OF EFFECTIVE CLINICAL TEACHING

The clinical experience has long been recognized as a significant and essential component of nursing education. Because of the importance of clinical learning experiences, and because resources are limited, clinical teachers need to optimize clinical practice opportunities. Clinical teachers have a responsibility not only to their students, but also to patients, families, and the nursing profession to identify and exhibit highly effective clinical behaviors.

Many clinical teachers, however, have had little formal preparation for this complex teaching role. New clinical teachers might have clinical competence and have completed a graduate program related to advanced practice nursing, but might have little to no experience or formal education in how to effectively teach students. Additionally, complex practice areas, increasing patient complexity, and acuity in patient conditions add to the challenges faced by clinical faculty (Hewitt & Lewallen, 2010; Spurr, Bally, & Ferguson, 2010). Highly specialized interventions, new and ever-changing technology, and a focus on nursing excellence and patient safety despite high patient turnover also contribute to the challenges faced by today's clinical teachers and highlight the importance of using effective and innovative teaching strategies (Phillips & Vinten, 2010). Shortages of faculty can make it challenging to hire and retain effective clinical faculty members with current expertise in the clinical area (Maguire, Zambroski, & Cadena, 2012).

Clinical teachers represent a pivotal component of the clinical experience for students. Consider a unit that has wonderful learning opportunities for students, rich patient experiences, and a helpful staff. If the clinical teacher working on that unit with students lacks teaching skills, students might have a negative learning experience. Conversely, students might be placed in a clinical setting with less optimal learning experiences, but when the teacher is highly effective and inspirational, students will likely have a positive learning experience. In essence, the clinical teacher can promote learning regardless of experiences available in the clinical setting, and can hamper learning despite valuable experiences being available (Gaberson & Oermann, 2010).

The clinical experience offers nursing students the opportunity to apply theory from the classroom setting into the practice setting. However, simply placing a student in the clinical area will not guarantee that this learning will occur. Without an effective clinical teacher, students might develop poor habits and disillusionment because they might view the classroom and clinical environments as two completely separate worlds. It is up to the clinical teacher to help students navigate the clinical setting and to assist students in merging these two environments. For instance, students might say that the dressing change materials in the hospital setting are "completely different" from the ones they practiced with in the laboratory setting of the school of nursing. It would be easy for the student in such a scenario to become frustrated. However, by pointing out the principles that govern this skill and helping the student see how to safely adapt the materials to comply with those skill-related principles, the clinical teacher can guide the student in merging the two worlds of clinical and classroom learning.

RESEARCH RELATED TO CLINICAL TEACHING

The literature suggests that for clinical teachers to be effective, they need to possess a variety of teaching behaviors. These behaviors fall into several categories, including knowledge and clinical judgment, teaching skills, interpersonal skills, personal characteristics, and evaluation skills (Knox & Mogan, 1985). Knowledge and clinical judgment refer to not only having extensive, up-to-date knowledge, but also the ability to clearly communicate that knowledge to students and facilitate their development of clinical judgment. Teaching skills include such activities as helping students organize their thoughts about patient problems and being well prepared and organized. Interpersonal skills are reflected in a clinical teacher's ability to display mutual respect; listen to students; and be supportive, and encouraging, yet challenging. Personal characteristics include being approachable and enthusiastic, being a strong role model for students, admitting mistakes, and having a sense of humor. Evaluation skills include the ability to provide feedback and evaluate students fairly, constructively, and in a manner that will facilitate learning (Knox & Mogan, 1985). Beginning and senior-level students emphasize the importance of similar clinical teacher behaviors, and note that clinical teachers need to possess behaviors in all five categories to be deemed effective.

Other research has emphasized the importance of a passion-centered philosophy of clinical teaching in nursing. Clinical teachers should have a passion for collaboration with students and for genuinely caring about individual students, including building a comfortable and supportive relationship with students. They should also demonstrate a passion for seeing students succeed and reach excellence, for the profession of nursing, and for the teacher-student relationship (Edgecombe & Bowden, 2009; Spurr et al., 2010).

Research on clinical teaching in nursing reflects that students experience a variety of stressors in the clinical practice area. These stressors range from fear of making mistakes that could harm patients to being unfamiliar with the clinical setting and clinical practices; experiencing different types and acuity of patient conditions; interacting with patients, staff members, and other health care providers; and interacting with/being observed by clinical faculty members. Some settings, such as pediatrics, are seen as creating more stress for students, presumably because of the vulnerability of pediatric patients and the frequent but potentially intimidating involvement of families in patients' care. It is essential for clinical teachers to be aware of how stressful the clinical experience can be for students, and to reassure students that the role of the clinical teacher is not just to evaluate, but rather to teach, mentor, and help students learn. Keeping clinical feedback instructional and not overly personal or critical can also reduce students' stress and increase student motivation to learn (Gaberson & Oermann, 2010).

It is important to note that the stress experienced by nursing students does not diminish as they advance through the program. Senior students who are about to graduate might be anxious about passing their licensing examination, fear whether they know enough to practice competently, and experience the anxiety of job hunting while they are completing their studies. The need for clinical teachers to role-model excellence in nursing and to support and guide senior students remain just as paramount as when working with beginning nursing students.

Stressors exist for clinical teachers as well. Clinical teachers report stress related to multiple demands and role expectations, balancing heavy teaching workloads with other activities, receiving less than desirable compensation, and feeling physically and emotionally drained at the end of the clinical day (Whalen, 2009). Working with students who are ill-prepared for the clinical experience, and working with borderline or failing students in the clinical setting are situations that are also stressful for faculty (Whalen). Developing teaching strategies for dealing with these issues can help the clinical teacher remain positive and cope effectively. Enjoying the personal satisfaction that develops as the result of being professionally competent can also counterbalance this stress for clinical faculty.

RELATIONSHIPS WITH STUDENTS AND STAFF

The clinical learning environment has a much more complex context than the more controlled classroom environment, and is essential in socializing students into the profession of nursing, through positive role modeling, encouragement, support, and quality feedback (Edgecombe & Bowden, 2008). It is important for clinical teachers and students alike to remember that the clinical learning environment is an established health care or community setting, and that students and clinical teachers are guests in that site. The clinical teacher's role, in addition to mentoring, guiding, planning for, and teaching students, is also to act as a culture broker or boundary spanner in this clinical setting (Gaberson & Oermann, 2010).

As much as possible, clinical teachers should have input into clinical site selection and should advocate for stability in their clinical site placements, so that relationships with staff and administrators can be forged and maintained. When staff get to know and can build a trusting, collaborative relationship with clinical faculty, a positive experience ensues for all involved. Staff nurses will often watch for additional opportunities for students to learn when a known and respected clinical teacher is present on the unit, and the teacher can feel confident in having students team up with staff for additional learning experiences, or tap into additional learning resources within the clinical area.

As a gatekeeper in the clinical setting, it is critical that the clinical faculty member keep lines of communication open between students and staff (Gaberson & Oermann, 2010). Keeping staff informed and up-to-date about the specific activities in which students will be engaging from week to week helps avoid confusion and frustration on the part of both students and staff. Patient safety is also maintained as a result of clear communication between faculty, students, and staff. Further discussion pertaining to the relationship between clinical teachers and students is woven throughout this chapter.

PROCESS OF CLINICAL TEACHING

Clinical teaching includes identifying the outcomes for learning, assessing student learning needs, planning clinical learning activities, guiding students, and evaluating their learning and performance (Gaberson & Oermann, 2010, p. 61). This chapter addresses outcomes for learning, assessing learner needs, planning clinical learning activities, and guiding students. Clinical evaluation is discussed in Chapter 12.

LEARNING OUTCOMES

Learning outcomes of the clinical experience can be intended as well as unintended. Intended learning outcomes for students relate to three domains of learning. Each of these domains of student learning can be fostered through effective clinical teaching behaviors and strategies, which promote learning and student confidence.

Cognitive learning reflects students' growing knowledge level, an ability to engage in clinical reasoning and problem solving, and the development of students' higher level thinking skills (Gaberson & Oermann, 2010). Faculty can promote the achievement of cognitive learning outcomes by engaging students as participants in patient-centered discussions, encouraging students to examine patient situations from multiple points of view, and engaging students in rigorous yet supportive questioning, thereby teaching students how to *think* rather than to memorize.

A second domain of learning, psychomotor learning, reflects students' skill acquisition, including the ability to perform skills in a safe, effective, accurate, and fluid manner over time (Gaberson & Oermann, 2010). Faculty can encourage psychomotor learning outcomes through careful patient selection, and by providing guidance, support and encouragement for students during skills and procedures. These learning outcomes can also be fostered by positive role modeling on the part of the clinical teacher and by encouraging students to use clinical resources effectively. Within this domain, students also need to learn organization, priority setting, and time management skills to function effectively in complex health care environments. Clinical nurse educators can teach students these skills using tools, group discussions, and role modeling.

Within the third domain of learning, the affective domain, students develop professional attitudes, beliefs, and values that form an essential part of nursing practice (Gaberson & Oermann, 2010). Faculty can provide clear expectations and directions, role-model professional behaviors, and use other teaching strategies to develop and challenge students within the affective domain of learning.

In addition to the intended learning outcomes noted above, students might also experience unintended learning outcomes as a result of the clinical experience. These unintended learning outcomes can be positive, such as the student considering the specialty area as a potential career choice and developing a passion for that area of nursing. Unintended outcomes, however, can be negative and long lasting, such as students losing self-confidence, becoming disengaged, being "turned off" to the clinical area, or even questioning their own ability to become nurses. All of these unintended learning outcomes hinge directly on the clinical teacher and the teacher's interactions with students in the clinical setting.

ASSESSING LEARNER NEEDS

Today's clinical teachers have the added challenge of working with multiple groups of students, each with the unique learning needs and diversity that these student groups bring. Faculty working in all types of nursing programs often teach a diverse student population, with differences in race, gender, age, work experiences, and life experience. Faculty working with undergraduate students might be working with an added layer of diversity: traditional baccalaureate students as well as accelerated second degree nursing students (those with at least a bachelor's degree in another field). The research on relationships between faculty and second degree students remains primarily descriptive and anecdotal, but it is apparent that accelerated second degree nursing students may present challenges and have a unique set of needs (D'Antonio et al., 2010). Second degree students appear to anticipate intellectual challenges in nursing programs, but also experience emotional challenges related to their tremendous workload (D'Antonio et al., 2010). In turn, some faculty members express unease when teaching those students, finding them driven and potentially intimidating, whereas others enjoy the challenges and rewards that come with working with accelerated students. Similarly, faculty members teaching in advanced practice nursing programs may have an equally diverse student population, with differences in prior work and life experiences. It is essential that discussions occur among *all* students and faculty members on a regular and ongoing basis about how individual students learn best, and how faculty and preceptors can foster that learning, so that congruent expectations can be achieved (D'Antonio et al., 2010).

Creating an effective learning experience with students in the clinical setting also begins with assessing individual learner characteristics and learning needs (Edgecombe & Bowden, 2008). Even before the clinical experience starts, faculty members can get to know students through learner assessments. Additionally, a carefully planned and orchestrated clinical orientation can help teachers assess students' learning needs, as well as establish a climate for nursing. Further discussion of learner needs is found in the section concerning clinical orientation in this chapter.

PLANNING CLINICAL ACTIVITIES

Creating an Effective Learning Environment

Planning clinical activities for students starts with shaping the clinical environment so that it will be a safe and enjoyable place in which to learn. Creating an effective learning environment for nursing students begins with the clinical teacher establishing a partnership with the clinical site even before the course begins. By orienting to the clinical agency, the faculty member gains familiarity with the clinical environment and patient population. This familiarity is essential in guiding students (Gaberson & Oermann, 2010). The clinical teacher might shadow a seasoned staff nurse, or work alongside staff for several shifts, home visits, or other experiences, before teaching begins in that site. During this time, the faculty member can also communicate clear expectations to staff and managers in the setting about the roles that the clinical teacher, students, and staff will take during the upcoming clinical course and establish collaborative relationships with staff. It is important to remember that in traditional clinical courses, teachers and students are typically guests within a larger, more stable health care setting and that interactions with staff reflect this. In partnerships, these roles vary, as discussed in the next chapter.

Establishing the Climate for Learning: Clinical Orientation

A well-thought-out student orientation is a key aspect of the clinical experience. It is essential that the clinical teacher take every opportunity during this critical time to establish a positive climate for learning. Consider, for example, the clinical faculty member who arrives late to orientation, does not have his or her materials ready, talks about the upcoming experience without eliciting students' input or responses, and makes little effort to learn about the students themselves. Students will likely be given the impression that the clinical teacher is disorganized, is intimidating, and does not care about them as individuals or partners in learning. In turn, these students are likely to become concerned about having to guess what the teacher wants, might "hide" when the faculty member is present, or might be afraid to ask questions. Because clinical time is so limited and valuable to student learning, it is important that faculty maximize every learning opportunity for students, and those opportunities begin with orientation.

The teacher should consider developing a folder for each student, to be distributed electronically to students or as hard copies within the first few minutes of clinical orientation. These folders can contain such documents as a clinical schedule; an outline of a typical day on the unit, in the clinic, in the home, and so on; descriptions of clinical assignments; documentation examples; and key resources that are site and specialty dependent. A folder (paper or electronic) made individually for each student provides a personal touch. It also provides concrete evidence that the faculty member cares enough about individual students to provide them with key materials to get them started in the course. This is a simple but effective way to begin building the student-faculty relationship. Students can be encouraged to add to these folders as they progress through the course, with relevant articles, policies and procedures, clinical assignments, and so forth. Through these actions, students learn the importance of building their own professional portfolio and developing a vehicle for evidence-based practice, professional growth, and life-long learning.

Clinical orientation provides an opportunity to get to know students individually, as well as an opportunity to establish the climate of the clinical group. By emphasizing that the clinical group will act as a team that will learn together and support each other in the clinical setting, the faculty member sets the expectation that students will assist each other and not compete with one another for faculty time or for learning experiences. This is another important concept to establish at the outset to prevent clinical groups from becoming competitive or polarized.

Clinical orientation can be an excellent time to introduce the use of analogies to inspire students. A sample analogy useful to share during clinical orientation related to professional growth, group teamwork, and the development of nursing competence in the clinical setting is found in Appendix B.1.

Additional key questions to ask students during orientation, to achieve the goals of establishing the climate for learning, might include the following:

- *What are students excited about as they begin this clinical course? What are they nervous about?* These types of questions encourage students to begin sharing and establish that the clinical group and setting is a safe environment in which to learn where students will be supported and stimulated. This kind of initial dialogue is also important for student engagement and underscores the importance of transparency in the clinical teacher-student relationship.

- *What are the students' expectations of the clinical teacher?* Students might be surprised to hear this question, as faculty typically spend a great deal of time discussing expectations of students. That question, too, should be discussed, but if students are *first* asked expectations of faculty, they can be put more at ease, and the *partnership* of learning can be established. By articulating what they expect from the clinical teacher, students invariably will reflect on what *they* also bring to the learning situation, including past learning experiences that have been positive or negative and why. This question also allows for a frank and open discussion about which student expectations might be easily met (for instance, that the faculty member is approachable) versus expectations that might be unrealistic (for instance, that they would prefer to observe care interventions prior to carrying them out themselves). Having an honest discussion of this nature is an excellent way to enhance group cohesiveness, clear up misconceptions before they have a chance to surface and, again, establish the learning climate as a partnership where both students and teachers share responsibility. This dialogue informs faculty about individual students' previous experiences as learners in the clinical setting, and makes it easier for faculty to avoid assumptions about the types of experiences that students might or might not have had. It also sets the stage for another, slightly different discussion—faculty expectations of students.

- *What are the clinical teacher's expectations of students in the clinical setting?* Once student expectations of faculty have been discussed, students are more receptive to hearing, understanding, and caring about faculty expectations of them. If students feel respected as adults and as individuals and understand that their clinical teacher is committed to the partnership of teaching and learning in the clinical setting, student motivation increases and so does students' commitment to learning. The open discussion of faculty expectations of students during clinical orientation provides students with clear guidelines. Students, as a result, do not have to spend valuable time during the clinical course itself guessing what the faculty member wants. Issues such as clinical preparation, when and under what circumstances teacher supervision is required, types of learning activities that will take place during the clinical experience, what student activities are appropriate during "down time," specific skills that students cannot engage in, and the progression of activities that will occur over the course are important topics to address within the context of faculty expectations of students.

Students cannot be expected to remember all the verbal details shared with them during orientation, as they are likely experiencing some degree of anxiety at the time, and there is often a great deal of information shared in orientation. Because of this, it is helpful for students to be given a written copy of key faculty expectations as a part of the orientation packet. This copy should be shared and reviewed with orientation, and they should be encouraged to keep this information with them during the clinical experience. These faculty expectations can be labeled "Clinical Guidelines" or a similar title. These clinical guidelines can include such information as where, when, and under what circumstances to contact the clinical teacher outside of the clinical setting, contact information, expected student behaviors, guidelines for submitting written work, directions for clinical preparation, and so forth. Additional information about the clinical site, the types of common patient and family problems, common interventions, and other information can also be shared in these clinical guidelines (Exhibit 8.1).

EXHIBIT 8.1 Sample Clinical Guidelines to Share With Students in Orientation

- Clinical teacher contact information (preferred method of contact, don't call after X pm, etc.)
- Clinical site contact numbers
- Clinical site information (short description of the clinical setting where students are practicing, including phone number, typical patient population, types of common patient and family problems, common interventions, typical staffing, etc.)
- What students should do if absent or late
- Preparing for clinical practice (process, student and teacher roles, clinical worksheets, preconferences, etc.)
- Expected student behaviors (important actions if unsure about care or have questions; need for communication and sharing pertinent information about patient with nurse, teacher, others; school dress code and why important; new orders and process; documentation; working as a team)
- Typical day in the clinical setting (hospital unit, in the clinic, during a home visit, etc. depending on type of clinical practice)
- Written assignments and submission information
- "Treasure hunt" or "list of supplies" (if hospital setting)

Additional topics to cover during clinical orientation should include the following:

- *What are the ways in which individual students in the clinical setting learn best?* By asking students this during the initial orientation session, teachers communicate that they care about each student individually and that students are respected as unique, adult learners. When students are required to articulate how they learn best, they need to reflect on their own learning styles, consider what has and has not worked well in the past, and take responsibility for themselves as learners. Establishing how individual students learn best sets the stage for the rest of the clinical experience and also allows the opportunity to have frank discussions. For instance, in response to students who indicate they learn best through demonstration, the clinical teacher has an opportunity to dispel any misconceptions about the clinical experience. It might be worthwhile to point out that although sometimes the opportunity to observe might be present, there might be other times in which unique clinical experiences present themselves. In the latter case, provided that the student has the requisite skills and knowledge, faculty can assert that they will not demonstrate first, but will rather support the students as they engage in the particular activity. By having this open discussion in orientation, expectations can be clarified and student anxiety can be diminished.
- *Are individual students visual, auditory, and/or kinetic learners?* This question can help guide clinical teachers in providing each student with a method of teaching that best matches individual student learning styles. Given that the clinical environment is fraught with anxiety for students, it makes sense for faculty members to minimize that anxiety in whatever way possible, and matching teaching to individual student learning styles is a small but powerful way to achieve this. There is no sense in teaching students in a way that they will not learn.

Consider the following scenario. A nursing student in the clinical setting has attention deficit hyperactivity disorder (ADHD) and cannot take her ADHD medications because she is pregnant. She is a student who articulated during orientation that she is a visual learner, who also benefits from using concrete directions. She is attempting to administer medications with a staff nurse who becomes very frustrated and approaches the clinical teacher, saying that the student is "ill-prepared and doesn't know what she is doing." The clinical teacher seeks out the student to gather more information and finds her crying in the medication room. After learning about the situation and calming the student, the clinical teacher reminds the student of her aptitudes, and issues a vote of encouragement to the student. She then has the student write down an appropriate medication ratio on a paper towel in the medication room, and further reviews key steps of the procedure in a written format. The student relaxes, takes a deep breath, and says "I've got it." She proceeds to carry out the skill without further difficulty. She later reflects on the experience, and realizes that her current situation makes her more emotional and also makes auditory learning particularly difficult for her. She reflects that when placed in the situation with a staff nurse who was trying to verbally explain the procedure, she blanked out and then panicked. The use of alternate methods of teaching and learning (e.g., visual learning through the use of the written math ratio; the use of concrete, step-by-step directions as a guide to follow; and giving encouragement to the student), allowed the student to relax, process the information, learn, gain confidence, and successfully engage in reflective practice. Because the clinical teacher asked key questions during orientation and remembered these details about the individual student, the faculty was able to effectively teach the student not just about the skill, but about herself as well.

- *What is at least one personal goal that each student has in terms of this clinical experience?* Involving the students in guiding their own learning within the clinical experience is critical for their personal and professional growth, and this should be done at the outset of the course, in orientation. Questions such as their personal goals of what they want to achieve in the course help students become personally invested in each clinical course. Students can be encouraged to use the acronym "SMARTER" when formulating their goals, whereby the goals are specific, measurable, attainable, relevant, and timely, and can be evaluated and reevaluated (Baird, 2008). Articulating these goals and putting them in writing can make students invest more personally into the clinical experience.
- *What are some good and bad experiences from previous clinical courses?* Asking students to share these with clinical faculty in private or through a writing exercise provides transparency for students and faculty alike, and it allows all to have a similar starting point. It might be difficult for some students to share openly, particularly if they have had a previously negative clinical experience. However, if trust is established with the teacher beginning with the first clinical day, and the message is sent that the teacher is asking this information to help students learn, then students can feel empowered.

Another topic that can be included in orientation to the clinical setting is the system used by the clinical agency for medical records and documentation; a treasure hunt can be planned for this learning, and an example is provided in Appendix B.2. Additional topics are professional dress, including what students should wear when they visit the clinical agency, home, or other setting, and what constitutes appropriate student identification; typical timeline of a clinical day; timeline of the course including when assignments are due; demonstrations of patient care-related equipment; and when and where to find agency policies and why doing so is important. The use of an analogy, as shown in Exhibit 8.2, emphasizes student accountability and responsibility for their own learning, clarifies expectations of both student and clinical teacher, and underscores the importance of a team approach where faculty and other students' time is considered.

EXHIBIT 8.2 Example Analogy for Communication of Student Expectations

A simple analogy of a baseball game can be helpful in discussing student responsibilities with respect to new nursing procedures and interventions, which require teacher or preceptor guidance, in the clinical setting. This analogy assumes that students have obtained the requisite knowledge in the learning laboratory, have been shown where appropriate documentation can be located in the clinical setting, where supplies and equipment are kept, and where they can find appropriate nursing policies.

Starting a baseball game requires communication among team members. Students need to communicate with their clinical teacher, the patient, and the preceptor/clinician with whom they are working that they are planning on carrying out a specific procedure. They also need to consider other members of their team (their peers and the need for students to have access to the clinical teacher or preceptor). Use of this baseball analogy allows for a more streamlined student–teacher interaction and allows the clinical teacher or preceptor to be available for other students.

- Getting to first base. Students can be expected to locate and verify the care provider's order for the skill. If the student has taken the time to verify the order, then he or she can effectively show it to the clinical teacher or preceptor and save valuable time searching through the medical records.

- Getting to second base. Students can also be expected to find and review the relevant nursing policy. The teacher or preceptor can then review key points of the procedure with the student and increase efficiency, rather than taking the additional time to *locate* the policy with the student.

- Getting to third base. Students should gather the equipment and supplies for the procedure.

- Getting to home plate. Students can now locate their clinical teacher or preceptor and begin a brief focused discussion of the steps of the procedure. Students gain in self-confidence and independence by doing this additional preparatory work prior to spending one-to-one time with the teacher or preceptor. Because the student has gone around the bases, he or she should be able to quickly identify the provider order to verify, show the teacher or preceptor the equipment and supplies gathered, be prepared to discuss why they were chosen (building problem-solving and organizational skills), and review key points of any relevant nursing policies. Use of this analogy also underscores the importance of nursing students using and thinking about agency policies, an important aspect to safe, professional nursing care.

Choosing Clinical Assignments

It is essential for faculty to keep the clinical objectives, or competencies, in mind when choosing patient assignments and other clinical activities. Specific patient assignments should be made purposefully, with the idea that, by caring for the patient or engaging in other types of activities, the students will work toward meeting the clinical objectives for the course. Specific goals for each week should be transparent to students and faculty, alike, and learning activities should provide opportunities for students to meet those goals. Although students might view a more simplified approach to patient selection, such as desiring the opportunity to engage in a particular psychomotor skill or interact with a parent in the clinic, clinical teachers should keep goals in mind and consider all types of learning opportunities for students. The potential to engage in a particular kind of communication with a patient or family member, chance to explore patient advocacy issues or ethical concepts with patients, and opportunity to be exposed to diversity all represent examples of valuable learning experiences for the students.

Keeping track of student experiences can assist the clinical teacher in ensuring that each student obtains a variety of learning opportunities during the course. Creating a simple table, reflective of essential learning activities, and tracking each student's activity over the course is an easy way to stay organized and ensure that students are exposed to a diverse set of learning experiences.

It is also helpful to obtain student input for patient selection and other learning experiences. By doing so, clinical teachers again convey that they care about the student as an adult learner and value student input in creating each student's own learning opportunities. For example, in pediatrics, students might be asked which patient ages they are most or least comfortable with. Faculty can then solicit student input as to whether they would rather be eased into new experiences, depending on their comfort level, or just "jump in" with teacher, preceptor, or clinician support. Each student will respond individually, and, by honoring those responses whenever possible, the teacher-student relationship deepens through collaboration and trust.

Patient assignments do not always need to take the traditional form, where one student is assigned to one patient. Clinical teachers should be encouraged to think creatively about patient assignments and various configurations for these assignments. For instance, two beginning students can be assigned to one more-complex patient, students may work collaboratively with staff nurses, and other models. Students can also be offered learning activities in the clinical setting that enhance professional behaviors. For instance, students can learn leadership skills by buddying with a team leader for an experience or learn management skills by working for a short time with a case manager or first-level or middle manager (Gaberson & Oermann, 2010).

In some clinical settings, teachers might use a form to record students' assignments for use by students and staff; these forms should be clear, specific, and individualized each week. Clarity on the assignment form can help avoid misunderstandings about who is responsible for what patient care when the students are in the setting. The form should include the teacher's contact information if staff need to contact the faculty member outside of the clinical hours. It should be specific about the starting and finishing times for the students and the activities in which each student will be engaged. In addition, it is important to be clear that the staff nurse remains the primary patient caregiver, so miscommunication is avoided.

Faculty must be intentional about how much information to give to students about their patients in writing. Patient privacy and confidentiality laws prohibit faculty from posting patient assignment forms in areas that might be visible to visitors and others, and assignment forms should not include identifying information about patients, such as full names or medical record numbers. Some clinical teachers post the same assignment form in several places on the unit; other teachers share the assignments electronically or orally with students. It is helpful if staff have access to a copy of the assignment form to avoid duplication of care and ensure all members of the health care team are working together. A sample patient assignment form that can be used when teaching in a hospital or long-term care setting is found in Exhibit 8.3.

In some states, the State Board of Nursing outlines specific skills that students might not perform under any circumstances. Clinical teachers in each state should be aware of this information so as not to put the student, patient, family, staff member, or themselves at risk.

Learning objectives should become more complex as students progress through a given clinical course and as they progress through the nursing program. Patient assignments and other clinical learning activities should reflect this increasing complexity of learning objectives. The clinical teacher needs to decide whether students will engage in certain activities during a given day. This can depend on the comfort and confidence

EXHIBIT 8.3 Sample Nursing Student Assignment Sheet

- School of Nursing
- Course Number and Name
- Clinical Teacher, Credentials
- E-mail Address and Contact Phone Number
- Dates of Care: _____
- Clinical Activities: Nursing students are responsible for the following activities: Basic care of the assigned patient including hygiene, assisting with patient nutrition, vital signs, etc. The assigned staff nurse remains the primary caregiver for the patient.
- Clinical Hours: x to x

Student Name	Patient Initials	Room Number

level of teacher and students, the acuity and needs of the patients, and other experiences that might be happening in the clinical area that day. This information should be communicated clearly to students and staff.

It is helpful to periodically ask students to identify their goals for learning. These goals can reflect course or clinical objectives or their personal goals and needs. The teacher can then use these to inform patient assignments and other clinical activities for the student. Students can be encouraged to use the SMARTER (specific, measurable, attainable, relevant, timely, evaluated, and reevaluated) acronym for their goals, as this process teaches students about professional growth.

GUIDING STUDENTS: KEY TEACHING STRATEGIES

There are a multitude of teaching methods that can be used to enhance student learning in the clinical setting. Some of these teaching methods are described below.

Organization for Faculty and Students

Being organized is paramount to having the clinical experience run smoothly. Clinical teachers have a great deal of responsibility: to students, patients, families, and staff nurses and other clinicians. Teaching in the clinical environment can be exhausting and stressful. Organization is a key strategy to not just survive, but to flourish as a faculty member.

Organizational strategies for faculty include being well-prepared for the clinical experience, carefully selecting patients and other learning activities for students so that specific learning outcomes are achieved, and learning about the patients to guide the questions asked of students. Clear directions are essential for students and staff as to what students will be doing and not doing and the times that the students will be in the setting. It is also helpful to provide structure for students regarding what activities they might engage in during "down time," for example, in an acute care setting when their patient is sleeping or in the clinic between appointments. Guidance for students in terms of how to access the faculty member and staff if they are not immediately visible on the unit is also helpful to discuss with students. The use of a pager system and texting the faculty member are strategies that can help with this and make the teacher's presence on the unit more apparent.

Specific learning objectives should also be shared with staff and students. By having clear directions provided to them, all parties are aware of the goals, and the students can function as an organized, cohesive unit. For example, faculty teaching beginning students might want to strategize whether all students will perform certain skills in a given clinical day or whether a controlled approach is more appropriate, such as a few students giving medications early in the day, and other students giving medications in the latter part of the day.

As simplistic as it sounds, the better organized and more prepared clinical teachers are for the clinical course, the more effective they will be as nurse educators. Faculty need to take the necessary time to review patient histories and problems to be able to ask students specific questions about them and to be familiar with each patient's *unique* health experience. It does not do the student any good for the faculty member to ask "blind" questions.

Structure Within the Clinical Day

The clinical teacher and preceptor, or other clinician with whom the student is working, are key in helping students organize their patient care. It is essential that students learn to practice patient- and family-centered care in the clinical setting, and not focus only on tasks (Forbes, 2010). This can be challenging in the face of the unpredictability of the clinical setting, and the fact that a patient's status often changes during the course of the clinical day, with new nursing actions as a result. Similarly, clinics, homes, and other settings in which students have clinical experience can be equally unpredictable. Teachers should collaborate with students to help them organize their day using patient-focused strategies (Forbes, 2010). For example, a student performing a task such as a dressing change might often focus only on the dressing change itself and have tunnel vision. As the teacher accompanies the student to the bedside and guides performance, the teacher can engage the patient in an individualized way. During the dressing change, the faculty member might talk with the patient about what is important, discuss patient-centered goals, or simply just get to know the patient better. In this way, the faculty member demonstrates the importance of considering the whole person while performing a skill and role models this for the student. At the same time, it is important for the clinical teacher to realize that considering the whole person while simultaneously performing a psychomotor skill is a developmental process for many students, and that the student will improve with time and practice and gain confidence. This same principle is applicable to guiding performance in other types of practice settings.

Teachers can provide students with tools to help them organize their patient care. Some clinical teachers provide students with course-specific tools for use in preparing for clinical practice, giving direction to the student as to what information they need to know about their patients prior to engaging in their care. In addition, other tools can be used, such as a time sequence plan, to give students structure with which to organize their day. Even though the clinical environment and the patient's status might change, having some beginning structure to the experience lessens student anxiety and gives students a framework from which to begin their care. As students become more comfortable in the clinical setting, they can be encouraged to develop their own tools for organizing nursing care. Examples of organizational tools are found in Appendices B.3 and B.4.

Clinical Conferences

Clinical conferences are essential to the learning and support of nursing students. They can provide an environment that facilitates learning, offer opportunities for brainstorming and problem solving, and allow the clinical teacher to gain knowledge about the students' understanding of the patient or patients for whom they will be caring. When structured carefully and intentionally, clinical conferences can underscore that the clinical environment is a safe place in which to learn, and can promote active learning among all student members of the group.

From the outset, during orientation, clinical teachers should establish the notion of the group working together as a team and that team members will support and learn from each other. The clinical group should form an environment where students are free to ask questions, challenge each other, and not always have to have the right answer. They should be free to debate a topic without becoming threatened, and learn to respect others' points of view. If the clinical faculty member emphasizes that questions can be asked freely, that debates and differences of opinions are celebrated, and that faculty are approachable, then students can relax and focus on learning, instead of feeling intimidated.

The literature suggests that clinical teachers spend much of their time in the clinical setting asking lower level questions and should try to use higher level questioning (Hsu, 2007). Group conference time is an ideal time to introduce higher level questioning. Done in a safe, nonthreatening, and supportive manner, higher level questioning can stimulate not only individual students, but the clinical group as a whole, where the group is challenged as a team to respond to faculty questions.

If students are struggling in response to higher level questions, it is helpful for the clinical teacher to rephrase questions and sequentially ask a lower level question. When students are able to successfully answer a lower level question, they gain confidence with their own knowledge base and skill level. This, in turn, increases their confidence at responding to higher level questions. Words of encouragement such as "you can do this" or "I know you know this" also remind students that faculty have faith in their abilities. This in turn boosts their self-confidence, making many students want to learn more.

McAllister, Tower, and Walker (2007) suggest that students need to "practice engaging in critical reflection, dialoguing, being sensitive to difference, being compassionate in caring, and using creative thinking" (p. 306). Clinical conference is one such arena in which faculty can employ strategies not only to get students to learn about patients and nursing care, but also to engage them in transformative learning. Teachers want students to pause for a moment and think critically beyond the tasks.

Clinical Preconference. One type of clinical conference is the preconference, which typically takes place prior to the students engaging in patient care, depending on the course and type of agency. Clinical preconferences can have several purposes. One important purpose is to provide an opportunity for the teacher to assess students' knowledge and understanding about their patients. During preconference, the teacher assesses whether students have the knowledge for caring for patients and areas in which they need further information and guidance.

Another purpose of a clinical preconference is to encourage students to think critically and creatively about their patients. To do this effectively, faculty members should feel comfortable and confident with information about the patient and clinical context to ask challenging and stimulating questions. The preconference, therefore, can provide the venue for teachers to ask a variety of lower- and higher level questions to develop students' thinking. For clinical courses in which the teacher has a group of students, a preconference also affords an opportunity for students to ask questions in a group setting, where the environment is safe, group members are supportive, and students learn from each other.

It can be helpful for teachers to ask pointed questions of the group, such as a question about a particular approach students might have to a challenging psychosocial situation. Questions such as "Tell me about your nursing priorities for the day," "What do you anticipate as expected outcomes for your patient today?," "What might be the worst case scenario for your patient, how would you recognize it, and what would you do about it?," and so forth allow students the opportunity to develop their thinking skills and apply theory to practice. Additionally, a focused discussion of students' patients and families allows students to compare individuals and situations, encourages them to learn about patients' experiences in differing stages of an illness, and helps them compare different interventions or treatments modalities. Students are able to compare the impact of family and culture on a patient's health trajectory and on how patients at different life stages cope. In this way, students learn about important nursing concepts across patients and situations.

Clinical preconferences can also serve to build relationships among students. For instance, assigning students buddies during preconference sets up a partnership among students for the rest of the day. A buddy system allows students to get to know more than one patient, affords students a fall-back person who can help them with care, and can also expose students to multiple approaches without having the additional responsibility of actually caring for that patient. Students can also gain additional learning experiences as they watch out for and interact with each other's patients.

During clinical preconferences, clinical teachers can provide students with an opportunity to briefly present their patient(s) to the rest of the group. This gives them practice at being concise and developing the skills needed later for handoff. In addition, the preconference offers a venue for faculty to discuss certain practical issues, such as any special learning activities planned for that day, reminders of what students can and cannot do, and other information.

Clinical Postconference. A second type of clinical conference, the postconference, provides different opportunities for student learning. It is important to note that postconferences do not have to take place at the end of the clinical day, although in many cases that can be the most opportune and convenient time for students and faculty to convene. Clinical teachers, however, should consider the best time for students to engage in postconference without being distracted by patient care and other activities.

An important component of clinical postconferences is the opportunity for students to debrief (Gaberson & Oermann, 2010; Hsu, 2007). Some students might have had a particularly trying experience with a patient, family member, or staff member. Strategies such as role-playing, active listening, having other students offer suggestions, and group discussion can make individual students feel supported and can stimulate further learning. Questions from clinical teachers such as, "If you could do anything different, what would it be and why?" or "What was particularly useful that you learned today that might influence your clinical practice next week?" can be useful in helping students learn reflection and reflective professional practice.

A clinical postconference can also augment student learning in other ways. Students can share perspectives of clinical situations, teach each other, gain self-confidence and appreciation for each other's contributions, and enhance the sense of teamwork among students. Postconferences can be used in other ways. Students can be given an assignment in which they need to present a patient to each other and compare the care they gave based on evidence. Students need preparation time to be successful at this activity. Student peers can be invited to ask higher level thinking questions of each other, thus allowing student presenters to hone their problem-solving skills as well as their confidence in oral skills. Since nurses often present and discuss patients with other members of the health care team, being able to articulate themselves successfully and confidently are essential skills for students to learn.

Clinical teachers should be free to use whatever creative strategies they can develop to enhance student learning in postconferences. "Pass the problem" is one such strategy to get other clinical group members involved. In this strategy, one student presents a clinical situation or problem that he or she encountered that day. The next student offers an analysis of that situation, and a third student then critiques this analysis. When done in a supportive and open manner, this is an excellent strategy to foster critical thinking, and it underscores the importance of having more than one solution to a clinical problem.

During postconference, students can also be asked to write a one-minute care plan in which they draw an algorithm pertaining to their patient, the nursing priorities they focused on, and where those priorities were at the end of the day (Gaberson & Oermann, 2010). Students can be creative and then share their ideas with their peers. Some faculty members use postconferences as an opportunity to enlist guest speakers, who can have their own topic area that they present. Though potentially effective, this type of conference should not be done frequently, as students' time might be better used in active engagement with each other, rather than listening to a minilecture.

Case Studies

Case studies can be helpful in assisting nursing students to develop advocacy and delegation skills in a safe and nurturing environment (Powell, 2011). Students can be given opening case scenarios, and then given additional patient information as they respond to the scenario. These cases can be an excellent platform for developing skills, enhancing group teamwork, and augmenting self-confidence of students. Case studies can also take the form of problem-based learning in the clinical setting, which can promote student-directed solutions, group work and dynamics, and cooperative learning (Oja, 2011).

Concept-Based Learning Activities

Concept-based learning activities, such as having students focus on a particular concept in a given day, can enhance critical thinking. Students can then be asked to compare this concept across the various patients that the group cared for during that clinical day (Lasater & Nielsen, 2009). For instance, in a pediatric setting, students might be asked to collectively analyze how the concept of fluid and electrolytes compared in some of the patients the group cared for that day, such as an infant with short bowel syndrome, an adolescent with Crohn's disease, and a toddler with leukemia.

Nursing Rounds

Conducting nursing rounds during the clinical day is another teaching strategy that can enhance nursing students' critical thinking skills and problem-solving abilities, as well as their confidence in communicating with other health care team members. During nursing rounds, one or two students per week present their patient and the care they have been engaged in to the clinical group, clinical teacher, staff nurses, and other available health care team members. This provides a valuable opportunity for students to learn to present their patients to other team members in a confident and concise manner, advocate for patients, ask questions of and collaborate with the health care team, consider multiple approaches to care, and so forth.

Student Presentations

Providing students with an opportunity to conduct a short presentation within their peer group is an additional teaching strategy that clinical teachers can employ to enhance student learning. Students might be asked to share a few key points about their patient from a previous week, focusing on one aspect of nursing care that intrigued them. They can then be asked to retrieve a nursing article related to evidence-based practice about that aspect of nursing care and compare the care they observed or engaged in with the article. Other students in the group can be asked to pose critical thinking questions to the presenter or, alternatively, the presenter can ask questions of the group. Opportunities such as these can boost students' thinking skills and self-confidence in communication.

Lab Blitzes

In addition to one-to-one discussions with individual students about their patients, in clinical courses in hospitals, or in outpatient or community settings, it can be helpful to use an occasional clinical conference for group discussions of key patient data, such as laboratory results that are often poorly understood by students. Teachers should use as many creative strategies as possible when conducting laboratory blitzes. For instance, sample laboratory results from one of the patients can be printed, with all patient identifying information removed. Students can then be asked to analyze these results, determine possible diagnoses for the patient, and identify nursing priorities based on these laboratory results.

Alternatively, students can be given pointers, such as Ten Key Questions to Ask Yourself About Your Patient, and laboratory values can be incorporated into these questions. As an example, students might be directed to look up the patient's potassium level for any patient receiving diuretics. This can, in turn, stimulate a rich discussion about the effects of some diuretics versus others, how these medications relate to their patient's unique health status, what other laboratory results in addition to potassium level might be affected by diuretics and why, and so forth. Laboratory blitzes are most effective if they are kept short, focused, and fun.

Short Written Clinical Assignments

Different types of written clinical assignments can be used, depending on the learning to be achieved in clinical practice. For an affective learning outcome, students might be asked to provide in a journal a short reflection about what went well and what did not go well in their experience with their patient, what they would change for next time, and events that had an impact on them during the experience. This activity can enhance students' critical thinking, and it also helps teachers understand challenges that the student faced that day that they might not have otherwise verbalized (Chan, 2013).

Cognitive learning can also be enhanced through short written clinical assignments (Gaberson & Oermann, 2010). Ideally, students are given guided questions within the assignment, specific to the clinical objectives. Examples of guided questions might include the following: How were the safety needs of your patient met? What were the developmental needs of your patient based on concepts of growth and development, and how did these developmental needs compare to those of the actual patient today? Did your perceptions about the patient and home environment change between this home visit and the prior one? In addition to encouraging the student to explore a select clinical situation, written assignments can enhance writing skills and the ability to convey ideas in a clear, succinct manner.

USE OF GUIDANCE AND FEEDBACK IN THE CLINICAL SETTING

Because the student-teacher relationship is critical to the learning and development of the student, feedback from the teacher needs to be consistent, specific, transparent, honest, and encouraging. Students respond well to the *feedback sandwich*, in which constructive feedback is placed between two pieces of "bread" (i.e., positive feedback). Rather than saying, "You were disorganized during that nursing procedure," the teacher can explain, "I liked how you were able to find the policy for that nursing procedure in the clinic. It seemed as though your organization needed improvement, because you forgot a few supplies, but you did an excellent job of engaging the patient during the procedure itself." It is important to remember that teacher observation is a major source of stress for many nursing students, so keeping feedback instructional versus punitive is key.

Also, teachers should be sensitive to how, where, and when feedback is delivered in the clinical setting. Feedback in front of the patient, peers, staff, or in a public area has potential for the student to feel criticized and should be avoided.

Guidance in the clinical setting can take many forms. When carrying out care, it is most helpful to students if the teacher provides guidance before student interaction with the patient. Students can be independent with the behind-the-scenes activities, for example, verifying a provider order and reviewing the agency policy and procedure. However, it is essential that the teacher review what students will do before they interact with patients, anticipate patient responses and challenges, prepare students for those, and elicit a brief self-evaluation by the student concerning what went well and what changes might be made for next time. This provides an opportunity for giving feedback to the student.

Formative written feedback should also be provided to students on a regular basis during the clinical course. Koh (2008) suggested that high-quality formative feedback enhances learning and student achievement. A running log of brief written faculty comments, shared electronically with students on a weekly basis, as well as the student contributions to a written clinical portfolio about the nursing care they provided ensures open communication between faculty and student—and that evaluation is a collaborative process. The provision of prompt, specific, and regular feedback, both verbal and written, is critical to the learning process, allowing the student opportunities to correct mistakes before they become patterns and to feel supported and mentored during the clinical experience. With this feedback, summative evaluations are fair, do not pose surprises for the student, and are less anxiety-producing. Examples of weekly feedback are found in Exhibit 8.4.

EXHIBIT 8.4 Sample Weekly Student Feedback

Student Name:	
Clinical Teacher:	
Dates of Clinical Practice:	
Week 1	Clinical orientation, introduction to the clinical area.
	You were self-directed in terms of your learning needs, asked thoughtful questions, and demonstrated therapeutic communication with your patient. You submitted a well-thought-out beginning clinical worksheet, which was complete and was supported by the evidence you summarized. A good start to this clinical course—keep up that energy and enthusiasm!

Week 2	You came well prepared for the clinical experience as evidenced by your clinical worksheet and participation in our preconference. You provided thorough basic care for your patient and were aware of her needs. You appear to be more comfortable with the electronic charting system, and your documentation was clear and specific about your patient's change in condition. Remember that a full assessment needs to be documented in the patient record by 0900; I would like to see you work on this more next week. Keep up the good work!
Week 3	You were astute in your care of your patient this week, identifying key changes in the patient's respiratory status, including changes to breath sounds, and communicating those to the staff nurse. Glad to see you following through on a thorough morning assessment—the fact that you did this allowed you to discover the patient's respiratory changes. Your organization needed some work this week with wound care—you reviewed the appropriate policy and understood the rationale but were missing several supplies. Make sure you gather all your supplies before you begin next time and review them with me. I'm impressed with your energy and passion for nursing.
Week 4	You demonstrated critical thinking and clinical judgment this week in your analysis of the relationships among your patient's pathophysiology, lab work, medications, and nursing interventions. This was evidenced by your participation in preconference and nursing rounds as we discussed the patient and discharge needs. You showed confidence and competence in caring for a patient with complex medical and psychiatric problems, and you demonstrated patient-advocacy skills.

SUMMARY

The clinical experience for nursing students is often brief, expensive to operationalize, and dependent on limited resources, and yet it is the environment in which students learn to apply theory to practice and become socialized into the profession. The effectiveness of the clinical teacher is pivotal to student learning. It is essential that clinical teachers in nursing be effective, inspirational, and motivational, and that they engage in best teaching practices.

Many clinical teachers in nursing have had little formal education on how to effectively teach students and on best teaching practices in the clinical setting. Other challenges also face clinical teachers, such as advanced technology in the clinical setting, patient acuity, and balancing multiple demands and a heavy workload in the clinical teaching role, among others. These factors can be sources of stress for clinical teachers. For clinical teachers to be effective, they need to have knowledge and clinical judgment, teaching skills, interpersonal skills, personal characteristics, and evaluation skills. Passion for nursing and teaching is paramount as well.

The process of clinical teaching includes identifying learning outcomes, assessing learner needs, planning clinical learning activities, guiding students, and evaluating students' learning and performance. Learning outcomes can be intended or unintended. Intended outcomes reflect cognitive, psychomotor, and affective domains; the clinical teacher can employ a variety of teaching strategies to facilitate learning in each of these areas. Unintended learning outcomes can range from being positive to negative, and they are closely tied to the effectiveness of the clinical teacher.

When assessing learner needs, clinical teachers need to recognize and honor the diversity of the student population with whom they are working and use best teaching practices accordingly. They also need to assess individual learner characteristics and learning needs.

Planning clinical activities begins with creating an effective learning environment. The clinical teacher can influence the learning environment before the students begin their clinical course, through establishment of collaborative teacher-staff relationships, becoming comfortable with the clinical practices in that setting, and clarifying teacher, student, and staff expectations and roles. A carefully planned and orchestrated clinical orientation for students also helps to establish a climate conducive to learning. Planning clinical activities involves the careful selection of learning activities, which will enhance learning and students' confidence levels. Patient assignments and selection of other clinical activities should be made thoughtfully and intentionally, and they should provide opportunities for students to achieve learning objectives as well as personal goals.

To effectively guide students in the clinical setting, the clinical teacher should use teaching methods that reflect best practices. Some of these methods include organizing the clinical experience, providing structure and clearly stated expectations for students, and conducting clinical conferences that are meaningful for students. Other teaching strategies that are helpful in guiding students include nursing rounds, student presentations, and short writing exercises. Guidance and feedback in the clinical setting also involve sharing feedback with students in a consistent, specific, and encouraging manner; balancing positive and constructive feedback; and providing formative written feedback regularly.

REFERENCES

Baird, K. (2008). *Raising the bar on service excellence: The healthcare leader's guide to putting passion into practice.* Fort Atkinson, WI: Golden Lamp Press.

Chan, Z. C. Y. (2013). A systematic review of critical thinking in nursing education. *Nurse Education Today, 33,* 236–240. doi:10.1016/j.nedt.2013.01.007

D'Antonio, P., Beal, M., Underwood, P., Ward, F., McKelvey, M., Guthrie, B., Lindell, D. (2010). Great expectations: Points of congruencies and discrepancies between incoming accelerated second-degree nursing students and faculty. *Journal of Nursing Education, 49,* 713–717. doi:10.3928/01484834-20100831-08

Edgecombe, K., & Bowden, M. (2009). The ongoing search for best practice in clinical teaching and learning: A model of nursing students' evolution to proficient novice registered nurses. *Nursing Education in Practice, 9*(2), 91–101. doi:http://dx.doi.org.libproxy.lib.unc.edu/110.1016/j.nepr.2008.10.006

Forbes, H. (2010). Issues in Nurse Education: Clinical teachers' approaches to nursing. *Journal of Clinical Nursing, 19,* 785–793. doi:10.1111/j.1365-2702.2009.03078.x

Gaberson, K., & Oermann, M. (2010). *Clinical teaching strategies in nursing* (3rd ed.). New York, NY: Springer Publishing Company.

Hewitt, P., & Lewallen, L. (2010). Ready, Set, Teach! How to transform the clinical nurse expert into the part-time clinical nurse instructor. *The Journal of Continuing Education in Nursing, 41,* 403–407. doi:10.3928/00220124-20100503-10

Hsu, Li-Ling. (2007). Conducting clinical post-conference in clinical teaching: A qualitative study. *Journal of Clinical Nursing, 16,* 1525–1533. doi:10.1111/j.1365-2702.2006.01751.x

Knox, J., & Mogan, J. (1985). Important clinical teacher behaviours as perceived by university nursing faculty, students, and graduates. *Journal of Advanced Nursing, 10*(1), 25–30.

Koh, L. C. (2008). Refocusing formative feedback to enhance learning in pre-registration nurse education. *Nurse Education in Practice, 8,* 223–230. doi:10.1016/j.nepr.2007.08.002

Lasater, K., & Nielsen, A. (2009). The influence of concept-based learning activities on students' clinical judgment development. *Journal of Nursing Education, 48,* 441–446. doi:10.3928/01484834-20090518-04

Maguire, D., Zambroski, C., & Cadena (2012). Using a clinical collaborative model for nursing education: Application for clinical teaching. *Nurse Educator, 37,* 80–85. doi:10.1097/NNE.Ob013e3182461bb6

McAllister, M., Tower, M., & Walker, R. (2007). Gentle interruptions: Transformative approaches to clinical teaching. *Journal of Nursing Education, 46,* 304–312.

Oja, K. (2011). Using problem-based learning in the clinical setting to improve nursing students' critical thinking: An evidence review. *Journal of Nursing Education, 50,* 145–151. doi:10.3928/01484834-20101230-10

Phillips, J., & Vinten, S. (2010). Why clinical nurse educators adopt innovative teaching strategies: A pilot study. *Nursing Education Perspectives, 31,* 226–229.

Powell, R. (2011). Improving students' delegation skills. *Nurse Educator, 36*(1), 9–10. doi:10.1097/NNE.0b013e3182001e2e

Spurr, S., Bally, J., Ferguson, L. (2010). A framework for clinical teaching: A passion-centered philosophy. *Nursing Education in Practice, 10,* 349–354. doi:10.1016/j.nepr.2010.05.002

Whalen, K. (2009). Work-related stressors experienced by part-time clinical affiliate nursing faculty in baccalaureate education. *International Journal of Nursing Education Scholarship, 6*(1), 1–18. doi:10.2202/1548-923X.1813

9

Partnerships With Clinical Settings: Roles and Responsibilities of Nurse Educators

GAYLE PREHEIM AND KATHERINE FOSS

Nursing is a practice discipline. The core of nursing education is the clinical education of nursing students. Academic-practice partnerships exist at several levels for the purpose of preparing the nursing workforce to meet nursing practice realities and contemporary health care challenges. Partnerships developed by nurse leaders in a nursing program and a clinical setting are defined as intentional relationships, based on mutual goals, respect, and shared knowledge (American Organization of Nurse Executives [AONE]-American Association of Colleges of Nursing [AACN], 2012b).

This chapter provides guidelines for establishing meaningful partnerships. Nurse educator roles and responsibilities relevant to school of nursing collaboration with clinical settings are explored. Specific examples are provided to illustrate concepts and strategies to improve the educational preparation of nurses and ultimately the quality and safety of patient care.

The purpose of this chapter is to present ideas about establishing and sustaining meaningful partnerships between education and practice to stimulate collaborative, contemporary models of clinical nursing education. The nature of education-practice partnerships is explored within the context of quality and safe patient care and excellence in clinical education. The chapter includes a discussion of the value and significance of academic-practice partnerships, characteristics of meaningful partnerships, roles and responsibilities of the nurse educator in establishing and sustaining effective partnerships, and relevant research and evidence for concepts underlying exemplar clinical education partnerships.

VALUE AND SIGNIFICANCE

EVOLUTION OF ACADEMIC-PRACTICE PARTNERSHIPS

Historically, academic-practice partnerships were established for a wide range of purposes relevant to advancing religious missions, delivery of patient care with physicians, government programs, and hospital initiatives. Hospitals and universities began forming alliances later to address the need for nursing care delivery and to prepare the future nursing workforce. The Institute of Medicine (IOM, 2003) established an over-arching expectation that health care professionals be responsible to ensure collaborative practice and education. Emphasis is placed on opportunities for students to provide patient-centered care as a member of an interprofessional team within a context of evidence-based practice, quality improvement, and informatics.

The looming nursing shortage, access to health care, the need for continuous quality care and improved patient safety outcomes illuminate shared interests among academic and health care service organizations. Community and regional workforce develop-ment initiatives and health care consumers are joining together to address the issues of preparing the future nurse. As a result, academic programs, service agencies, and regulatory or policy-making bodies are aligning and leveraging resources to meet the challenges of educating the health care workforce and building safer delivery systems (Joynt & Kimball, 2008).

CURRENT STATUS OF ACADEMIC-PRACTICE PARTNERSHIPS

The AACN *Essentials of Baccalaureate Education for Professional Nursing* (2008) recog-nize ongoing collaborative academic practice partnerships as a quality indicator for promoting student learning. Nursing schools and clinical agencies are challenged to determine capacity for optimizing clinical learning during times of expanding nursing programs and increasing enrollments. Ridenour (2009) and Broome (2009) highlight the value and significance of partnerships to impact the quality and effectiveness of nursing education by calling for support and collaboration among stakeholders. Collaboration is necessary to maximize use of limited resources and build capacity to educate more nurses. An additional impetus is the IOM report, *The Future of Nursing: Leading Change, Advancing Health* (2010), which recommends increasing the proportion of baccalaureate-prepared nurses to 80% by 2020.

The AONE and AACN provide evidence of support for the development of academic-practice partnerships. Nurse leaders participated in a task force to explore the nature of partnerships, including components and strategies that were deemed to be characteristic of good partnerships and effective in achieving desired outcomes. The purpose of formal academic-practice relationships is to advance nursing practice and to improve the health of the public (AONE-AACN, 2012b).

The *Summary of Literature Related to Academic-Service Partnerships*, compiled by the AACN-AONE Task Force (2010), suggests an abundance of recent examples of formal academic-practice partnerships and provides evidence of a proliferation of partner-ships. Partnerships are evolving in significance, purpose, structure, and expected out-comes. Examples of academic-practice partnerships focus on educating nurses, sharing resources, and undertaking projects focused on nursing student clinical education, evidence-based practice initiatives, and professional development or academic pro-gression programs. Additional examples reflect priorities for interprofessional educa-tion (IPE), increased use of clinical simulation to develop clinical competency, and the advancement of evidence-based practice initiatives. Efforts and outcomes are perceived to be mutually positive. However, following the extensive review of the literature over the past decade, the AONE-AACN Task Force concluded that the majority of reported partnerships were anecdotal, describing examples of specific efforts and providing little data-based evidence to support effectiveness or generalizability. Nonetheless, different types of partnerships provide examples of best practices that might be ben-eficial in developing a mutually beneficial relationship or shared goal. For example, a chief nurse officer and dean might identify key components or strategies relevant to achieve a specific shared goal. Joint faculty appointments, shared resources for preceptor training, participation in clinical agency evidence-based practice initiatives, or a nursing program curriculum committee might be mutually valued.

ESTABLISHING MEANFUL PARTNERSHIPS

PRINCIPLES AND PRACTICES

From reported initiatives, the AACN-AONE Task Force identified current evidence of four partnership themes: principles, types, benefits, and barriers. Understanding the concepts and strategies underlying these themes is critical to increasing effectiveness and the potential positive impact of academic-practice partnerships. Eight guiding principles identified and endorsed by AACN and AONE (2012b) provide a useful framework for nurse leaders in academic and practice settings for understanding the development and sustenance of meaningful relationships (Exhibit 9.1).

EXHIBIT 9.1 AACN-AONE Guiding Principles for Academic-Practice Partnerships

1. Collaborative relationships between academia and practice are established and sustained through
   - Formal relationships established at the senior leadership level and practiced at multiple levels throughout the organization
   - Shared vision and expectations that are clearly articulated
   - Mutual goals with set evaluation periods
2. Mutual respect and trust are the cornerstones of the academic-practice relationship and include
   - Shared conflict engagement competencies
   - Joint accountability and recognition for contributions
   - Frequent and meaningful engagement
   - Mutual investment and commitment
   - Transparency
3. Knowledge is shared among partners through mechanisms such as
   - Commitment to lifelong learning
   - Shared knowledge of current best practices
   - Shared knowledge management systems
   - Joint preparation for national certification, accreditation, and regulatory reviews
   - Interprofessional education
   - Joint research
   - Joint committee appointments
   - Joint development of competencies
4. A commitment is shared by partners to maximize the potential of each registered nurse to reach the highest level within his or her individual scope of practice, including
   - Culture of trust and respect
   - Shared responsibility to prepare and enable nurses to lead change and advance health
   - Shared governance that fosters innovation and advanced problem solving

(continued)

EXHIBIT 9.1 AACN-AONE Guiding Principles for Academic-Practice Partnerships (*continued*)

- Shared decision making
- Consideration and evaluation of shared opportunities
- Participation on regional and national committees to develop policy and strategies for implementation
- Joint meetings between regional/national constituents of AONE and AACN

5. A commitment is shared by partners to work together to determine an evidence-based transition program for students and new graduates that is both sustainable and cost-effective via

 - Collaborative development, implementation, and evaluation of residency programs
 - Leveraging competencies from practice to education and vice versa
 - Mutual/shared commitment to lifelong learning for self and others

6. A commitment is shared by partners to develop, implement, and evaluate organizational processes and structures that support and recognize academic or educational achievements:

 - Lifelong learning for all levels of nursing, certification, and continuing education
 - Seamless academic progression
 - Joint funding and in-kind resources for all nurses to achieve a higher level of learning
 - Joint faculty appointments between academic and clinical institutions
 - Support for increasing diversity in the workforce at the staff and faculty levels
 - Support for achieving an 80% baccalaureate-prepared RN workforce and for doubling the number of nurses with doctoral degrees

7. A commitment is shared by partners to support opportunities for nurses to lead and develop collaborative models that redesign practice environments to improve health outcomes, including

 - Joint interprofessional leadership development programs
 - Joint funding to design, implement, and sustain innovative patient-centered delivery systems
 - Collaborative engagement to examine and mitigate nonvalue-added practice
 - Complexity
 - Seamless transition from the classroom to the bedside
 - Joint mentoring programs/opportunities

8. A commitment is shared by partners to establish infrastructures to collect and analyze data on the current and future needs of the RN workforce via

 - Identification of useful workforce data
 - Joint collection and analysis of workforce and education data
 - Joint business case development
 - Assurance of transparency of data

AACN-AONE Task Force on Academic-Practice Partnerships (2012). Reprinted by permission of American Association of Colleges of Nursing, 2013.

The ability to establish and sustain effective partnerships is based on shared mission, values, and trust. Relationships are built through effective, clear communication, and commitment to addressing conflicts collaboratively. Opportunities for moving from contractual affiliations to meaningful partnerships exist from carefully planning initial discussions to evaluating outcomes. However, the efforts involved in developing and sustaining strong collaborative relationships are complex and time-consuming, and they are often influenced by personal commitments or by changes to individual representation within the organization. An interactive toolkit was developed by AACN-AONE (2012) to guide nursing leaders in the development, growth, and evaluation of academic-practice partnerships. Specific questions (Exhibit 9.2) identify activities relevant to development and sustenance of the partnership. Exemplars of strong academic-practice partnerships are provided within the toolkit, focusing on creating a welcoming learning environment and transition into practice, and accessing non-traditional clinical experiences to enhance the home care nursing workforce and improvement in patient care outcomes (AACN-AONE, 2012).

EXHIBIT 9.2 AACN-AONE Interactive Tool Kit for Developing and Sustaining Partnerships

1. Players
    A. Selecting partners
        - How do you identify your partners?
        - Why is this partner a good fit?
    B. Preparing for your first meeting
        - Where do you meet?
        - What do you need to know about your potential partner and the organization?
        - What does your partner need to know about you and your organization?
2. Partnership activities
    A. Conducting initial meeting
        - What is the right partnership activity?
        - What do you have to offer?
        - What is the mutual benefit?
        - What is your vision and do potential partners share the vision?
        - What is the potential initiative/activity and who else needs to be involved?
        - Who from top leadership is involved?
        - What is the business case for the partnership?
    B. Conducting subsequent meetings
        - Do you have clarity on goals and vision?
        - What are the details and the timeline for the initiative?
        - What resources are needed?
        - Will there be an official memo of understanding?
        - What are the expected outcomes?
3. Environmental factors
    A. Time
        - Is this the right time for the partnership?
        - What are the impeding or facilitating issues to partnership development?
        - What is the time commitment?
    B. Space
        - What space, equipment, or supplies are needed?
        - What financial resources are needed?

(continued)

EXHIBIT 9.2 AACN-AONE Interactive Tool Kit for Developing and Sustaining Partnerships (*continued*)

C. Regulation
  • What are the impeding or facilitating policies or regulatory issues?
D. Context
  • How will the partnership be funded?
  • What are the constraints of both partners?

Adapted from American Association of Colleges of Nursing and American Association of Nurse Executives (2012).

Teel, MacIntyre, Murray, and Rock (2011) identified four themes contributing to successful implementation of an innovative academic-practice partnership to increase educational capacity using the coach/preceptor models. Supportive relationships, goodness of fit, flexibility, and communication are examined in Table 9.1. Although additional programmatic research is needed on education innovations, it is helpful for the educator to apply strategies associated with the four themes evidenced in successful partnerships.

TABLE 9.1 Four Themes Contributing to Successful Implementation

Theme	Application Strategy
Supportive relationships	Students, faculty, and preceptors (clinical staff) form a core triad. Elements of supportive relationships • Pairing of student and preceptor • Orientation of preceptors by faculty • Faculty role as advocate between student and preceptor • Continuity of clinical rotations in a single clinical agency
Goodness of fit	Planning for and assessing the innovation for an appropriate "fit." This includes • Presence of an organizational culture that values and supports innovation (academic program and clinical agency) • Recognition of vital roles of faculty and preceptors, including various forms of financial support • Assessment and identification of potential participants (students, preceptors, faculty) and program components for the best "fit"
Flexibility	The partnership stakeholders recognize • Organizational culture, structure, rules, and needs will influence adaptation of innovation • Willingness to change • The value of feedback from students, faculty, and preceptors to be able to adapt and change as needed

(continued)

Theme	Application Strategy
Communication	Multiple modalities of communication are needed to foster effective use of resources and information to meet the needs of students, faculty, and clinical partners and increased flexibility in the partnerships: • Printed literature • Interviews of students, faculty, and preceptors • Websites or portals • E-mail and telephone communication • Regularly scheduled face-to-face meetings with all stakeholders

Adapted from Teel et al. (2011).

In a systematic review of the evidence, Nabavi, Vanaki, and Mohammadi (2012) identified four stages related to the formation and implementation processes of academic and service partnerships. The stages, outlined in Table 9.2, are applicable to a variety of partnerships and create a framework for identifying structures, processes, procedures, and outcomes.

TABLE 9.2 Four Stages of Formation and Implementation of Academic-Service Partnerships

Four Stages	Examples
Mutual Potential Benefits Discovery of interests or issues that could be served by the resources of a partnership	• Nursing workforce shortage • Insufficient number of clinical placements to support increasing enrollments • Insufficient number of qualified/clinically competent faculty • Development of evidence-based nursing practice, including nursing research and translation of nursing research into practice
Moving From Competitor to Collaborator Planning and development of cooperative structural framework that includes 1. Identification and coalition of stakeholders 2. Shared decision or policy making 3. Structure that facilitates interaction between partners	Senior leadership from each partner (academic, service, legislative, regulatory agencies) or other stakeholders identify mutual interests or issues and set mission, goals/purpose, plans, timelines, and deadlines: • Executive/management committee or advisory council • Task force or working groups are formed to promote interaction in a partnership. The focus and activities are to implement the mission of the partnership and develop the methods and means of

(continued)

TABLE 9.2 Four Stages of Formation and Implementation of Academic-Service Partnerships (*continued*)

Four Stages	Examples
	the partnership, including supervision or oversight, identification of roles and responsibilities, framework for decision making, and training needs across organizations in the partnership
	• Development of job descriptions
	• Affiliation agreement and contract auditing
	• Regulatory education and compliance monitoring
	• Preceptor development
	• Continuing education/staff development programs
Joint Practice Process of cooperation between the academic and service organizations to meet mutual goals	New structures and procedures in a partnership bring change to roles and responsibilities for employees in each organization and students:
	• Joint, adjunct, affiliate faculty appointment
	• Preceptorship model
	• Dedicated education unit
	• Clinical scholar model
	• Service learning
	• Interprofessional education
Mutually Beneficial Outcomes There are three realms of benefits to an effective academic-service partnership: 1. Service/practice benefits, 2. Education benefits, and 3. Profession benefits	• Career progression path for clinical nurses into education
	• Clinical nurse job satisfaction
	• Increase in number of clinical faculty
	• Increased educational capacity and admissions
	• Supportive learning environments
	• Improved employment and recruitment opportunities

Adapted from Nabavi et al. (2012).

STRUCTURAL FOUNDATIONS OF ACADEMIC-SERVICE PARTNERSHIPS

CAPACITY MANAGEMENT

In 2009, the National League for Nursing (NLN) commissioned a national survey to examine clinical education in prelicensure registered nursing programs (Ironside & McNelis, 2010). Respondents identified organizational and structural barriers and pedagogical challenges faced in optimizing students' clinical learning (McNelis, Fonachier, McDonald, & Ironside, 2011). The most frequently identified barrier was the lack of high-quality clinical education sites to accommodate student groups and/or lack of learning experiences that supported learning outcomes. Nursing programs are increasingly under pressure to admit and educate more students quickly, given the demand to ease the nursing shortage and to meet the health care needs of 32 million people in the United States who will have health insurance coverage under the Patient Protection and Affordable Care Act. Yet, baccalaureate and graduate nursing programs in the United States turned away more than 75,000 qualified applicants in 2011 due to an insufficient number of faculty, clinical sites, classroom space, clinical preceptors, and budget constraints (AACN, 2012).

Although limited fiscal capital and human resources are constraints, nursing leaders recognize mutual goals and expertise across education and practice required to address complex challenges for improving patient safety, high-quality care, and cost-effective outcomes. When determining capacity relevant to preparing nurses, nursing administrators consider the organization's mission and values, as well as the impact on patient care delivery and nursing staff resources. For example, hiring policies related to educational preparation required for nursing positions and accreditation such as Magnet™ can provide the framework for the type of academic degree programs the agency will host. Many decisions to host students in the service agency also consider the time; resources needed, including personnel, equipment, and space; costs associated with those resources; and the overall number of placement requests from nursing programs. Examples of service agency variables in determining clinical capacity are depicted in Table 9.3.

Service agencies can also examine clinical placement requests in terms of their experience and familiarity with the academic curriculum, model of student supervision used for clinical education, and previous experiences with student performance.

TABLE 9.3 Examples of Service Agency Variables in Determining Clinical Capacity

Operational systems	Determination and monitoring of affiliation agreements/contracts and associated policies that determine roles and responsibilities of the partnership
	Providing The Joint Commission standards required for orientation of nonemployees, which includes students, related to basic life safety and agency operations/resources
	Electronic medical record access and medication-dispensing systems for student use, which include training, surveillance of proper use, and troubleshooting resources
Clinical services	Hours of agency operation
	Types of patient services offered and location of services
	Opening or closing and expansion of patient care units or services
	Changing staffing, skill mix, patient acuity, and census levels that reflect productivity metrics and patient outcome indicators
	Existing and anticipated competency-based education, training, and orientation needs of experienced and newly hired staff

Requests for preceptorships are also carefully considered by agencies in terms of availability of staff with appropriate credentials and educational background, availability, and costs associated with preceptor development courses, and preceptor incentives. The distribution of workload and impact on productivity when clinical staff assume a heavy responsibility for clinical education during a preceptorship is an important factor in determining capacity. Assessment and identification of healthy clinical work environments, as discussed by Schmalenberg and Kramer (2008), is another critical consideration. Nurse educators should consider the systems, framework, and practices that support nurses in developing competence to deliver safe and high-quality patient care as a first step prior to determining whether the clinical unit is appropriate and ready for development of clinical learning experiences and student placements. Nursing schools continue to establish partnerships within nontraditional practice settings and community-based sites to augment acute care experiences. Best practices, noted in the definition of Clinical Practice Environments for Students, include working and learning together with clinical nurse experts from a wide variety of settings, who serve as preceptors and role models (AACN, 2008).

Academic and service partnerships related to capacity are often managed through the use of centralized computer or web-based programs to standardize student placement processes. Additional purposes and functions are to monitor student placement numbers at clinical sites and on units, identify untapped sites and clinical units and the potential for their development to support clinical learning and course objectives, and improved information sharing between nursing programs and service agencies for decision making about current and future needs for clinical placements. Burns and colleagues (2011) describe academic partnership strategies to address the faculty shortage through used of a centralized system by providing job postings, creation of a centralized faculty candidate pool, and clarification of nursing faculty requirements and resources. Use of data derived from placement platforms, including efficacy and quality measurement to drive innovations in clinical education, provides an opportunity for further research. Financial models for sustainability of centralized clinical placement platforms are also evolving from grant-funded sources, to costs shared between academic/service partners, to student use fees.

CLINICAL AFFILIATION AGREEMENTS

The clinical practice environment for students is defined through written agreements, jointly designed to benefit both academic and practice partners with ongoing evaluation and continuous improvement (AACN, 2008). The clinical affiliation agreement is a tool used by a health care agency and an academic program for provision of clinical learning experiences for students. Table 9.4 provides an example of content outlined in a clinical affiliation agreement.

Clinical affiliation agreements typically have multiple clauses that serve to protect the health care agency and the academic program. It is common for the affiliation agreement to be reviewed by legal counsel, risk management, human resources, and agency and nursing program administration to ensure that all interests are represented. The health care agency and academic program both have mandates to provide structure to the affiliation agreement. However, the intent of the partnership is to provide a supportive learning environment and associated clinical experiences for students. The signature authority to establish an affiliation agreement is determined by the leadership structure of each organization. A sample of specific health care agency and nursing program responsibilities are outlined in Table 9.5.

TABLE 9.4 Content Outline of a Clinical Affiliation Agreement

Agreement Component	Description
Shared purpose of health care agency and nursing program	To promote a planned and supervised program of clinical experience for nursing students.
Term period and renewal	Commencement and termination date of affiliation, including reference to early termination terms specified in the agreement.
	Termination without cause: language includes termination without cause or penalty by either the health care agency or nursing program by giving the other party a written notice within a timeframe, such as 30 or 60 days to termination.
Payment terms	Payment for educational services might be stipulated, dependent on the type of service provided, and health care agencies typically exclude payment for wages, worker's compensation, professional liability insurance, health insurance, transportation, meals, room, or uniforms for students.
Employment status	Students are not deemed employees of the health care agency for any purpose; they are present in the agency solely as a part of clinical course curriculum experience.
Responsibilities of the health care agency	The health care agency retains primary responsibility for patient care and treatment.
Responsibilities of the academic program	The academic program affirms that a student is fully matriculated into the program.
Insurance provisions	Language includes reference to policies from both the health care agency and the academic program regarding general liability and professional liability insurance as necessary to insure itself, agents, employees, and students against any claim or claims for damages arising either directly or indirectly in connection with the performance of activities under the agreement of providing clinical experiences.
	Limitations and state government acts might also be described in this section.
Modification and waiver, assignments and compliance with laws and regulations	Affiliation agreements have language reflecting compliance with federal, state, and local laws and regulations.

From University of Colorado Hospital, Anschutz Medical Campus, Aurora, Colorado. Adapted with permission, 2013.

TABLE 9.5 Sample of Specific Health Care Agency and Nursing Program Responsibilities

Health Care Agency	Nursing Program
Provide appropriate supervision of students	Students adhere to health care agency rules, regulations, policies, and procedures, including policies related to patient confidentiality, patient rights, and ethical conduct
Provide students access to rules, regulations, policies, and procedures of the agency	
Provide orientation to the clinical environment that meets regulatory body standards and requirements	Students meet health and immunization status of the health care agency
Provide appropriate emergency care for students incurring sudden onset illness or injury during the clinical experience, including accidental exposure to patient blood or body fluids	Verification of a criminal background check
	Verification of a negative drug screen
	Student proficiency in written and verbal skills
	Student citizenship or visa status

From University of Colorado Hospital, Anschutz Medical Campus, Aurora, Colorado. Adapted with permission, 2013.

Although the affiliation agreement provides the framework for clinical learning experiences, it is important to recognize the collaboration required among academic program faculty and representatives from the health care agency to select appropriate learning environments and experiences that facilitate achievement of specific learning outcomes. The collaborative effort extends to the determination of the type of student supervision required in the clinical environment or model of clinical instruction utilized.

Affiliation agreements and student placements can also be supported by associated internal policies within the health care agency. Policies describe the circumstances under which students can receive clinical experiences as part of an academic program. Accountability of agency personnel and students are identified in policies, which include the process steps for clinical placement of students, orientation of students to the agency, and the process for determination and evaluation of clinical placements in the agency. Recordkeeping of placements and audits of compliance with aspects of the affiliation agreement are also components of an agency's policy. Sample policies from the University of Colorado Hospital, Anschutz Medical Campus (Aurora, Colorado), are illustrated in Table 9.6.

ALLIANCE FOR CLINICAL EDUCATION

The Alliance for Clinical Education (ACE) is an example of an academic-practice partnership with representation of over 60 nursing schools, health care organizations, and professional and regulatory entities in the Denver metropolitan and surrounding region. The purpose of ACE is to promote collaboration between practice and education in preparing a nursing workforce for the future. The ACE group meets quarterly as a forum to share ideas and information and to make recommendations surrounding best practices, community standards, and regulatory compliance, in an effort to provide the optimum clinical student learning experiences (Article I of the Alliance for Clinical Education, 2006).

This alliance between education and health care organizations not only addresses clinical nursing education issues as primary focus, but it also serves as a forum to connect and inform members of initiatives and changes affecting nursing workforce development occurring within individual organizations, the State of Colorado

TABLE 9.6 Sample Policies

Health Care Agency Internal Policy	Description Relevant to Clinical Placements
Student affiliation experiences	Circumstances for the provision of clinical experiences as part of academic programs
Preceptor policy	Processes by which employees and students are precepted, as well as the process by which preceptors are selected, trained, and evaluated
Background screening policy	Processes and procedures related to reasonable inquiry into the background of employees, vendors, and prospective employees and vendors
Drug- and alcohol-free workplace	Processes and procedures to maintain a drug- and alcohol-free workplace
Urine drug screen multidrug point-of-care testing	Process used for performing CLIA-waived, multidrug screening tests on urine
Employee/volunteer health screens	Procedures for preplacement physicals, fitness-for-duty evaluations, and return-to-work procedures

CLIA, Clinical Laboratory Improvement Amendments.

From University of Colorado Hospital, Anschutz Medical Campus, Aurora, Colorado. Adapted with permission, 2013.

Board of Nursing, Colorado Area Health Education Councils, the Colorado Center for Nursing Excellence, and the Colorado Nurses' Association. ACE bylaws, scope of work, meeting minutes, and documents are open-source materials and can be found at www.coloradonursingcenter.org/alliance-for-clinical-education-ace.

EXPLORATION OF MODELS OF CLINICAL EDUCATION AND SUPERVISION

The IOM (2010) calls for nursing faculty to examine the structures and processes associated with clinical education and to determine the extent to which current clinical experiences are preparing students for the future demands of practice. The determination of high-quality clinical education and associated clinical sites or learning environments is an ongoing dialogue between academic and service leadership (McNelis et al., 2011). High-quality clinical experiences are intended to provide students' time and opportunity to synthesize professional values and roles, and cognitive and psychomotor skills into emerging practice competencies. Support of practice outcome competencies, along the education continuum that includes transition into professional practice, should be a shared priority for academic and service partnerships.

Traditionally, the nursing education model in the United States consists of an academic faculty in a clinical setting providing direct supervision of a number of students in the application of knowledge and skills acquired in the classroom, lab, or simulation setting to assigned patients (Rhodes, Meyers, & Underhill, 2012). The model includes scheduling students into a patient care setting 1 to 3 days per week; scheduling and rotating students into different health care agencies to be exposed to different patient populations (Sullivan, 2010); and requiring students to complete preclinical preparation work on assigned patient(s), developing a nursing care plan or concept map for each assigned patient, and completing other activities such as journaling or process recordings. As student enrollments increase and faculty pools decrease, nursing programs need to use innovation to determine and provide high-quality clinical experiences (Rhodes et al., 2012). Alternatives of clinical education and supervision are emerging. Five types of academic-practice partnerships reflecting collaboration and innovation are described.

INTERPROFESSIONAL EDUCATION

In 2003, the IOM report, *Health Professions Education: A Bridge to Quality*, recommended "all health professionals should be educated to deliver patient-centered care as members of an interdisciplinary team, emphasizing evidence-based practice, quality improvement approaches and informatics" (p. 3). The Joint Commission National Patient Safety goals identify the need for improved communication and collaboration between physicians and nurses to prevent harmful outcomes to patients/clients. With the implementation of the Patient Protection and Affordable Care Act, along with the call from many organizations to improve patient safety, quality, and access to care, the United States Health Resources and Services Administration (HRSA) has created the Center for Interprofessional Education and Collaborative Practice. The aim of the center is to accelerate teamwork and collaboration among health professionals and patients and to break down the traditional silo approach to health professions education.

Among the center's goals are to

- Develop, manage, and evaluate programs to enhance interprofessional collaboration in education and practice
- Actively engage leaders in education, practice, and policy communities
- Develop successful funding streams to ensure sustainability
- Contribute to the development and dissemination of metrics/evaluation parameters for IPE
- Develop a strategy to proactively identify innovations in IPEs, connect innovators, and disseminate lessons learned

Additional work is being done to promote a set of core competencies for IPEs developed by the Interprofessional Education Collaborative (IPEC), a group of six health professions associations (AACN, American Association of College of Osteopathic Medicine, American Association of Colleges of Pharmacy, American Dental Education Association, Association of American Medical Colleges, Association of Schools of Public Health; Interprofessional Education Collaborative Expert Panel, 2011). The core competencies for interprofessional collaborative practice are organized in four domains:

- Domain 1: Values/Ethics for Interprofessional Practice
- Domain 2: Roles/Responsibilities
- Domain 3: Interprofessional Communication
- Domain 4: Teams and Teamwork

In reporting results on the Retooling for Quality and Safety Initiative of the Josiah Macy, Jr. Foundation and the Institute for Healthcare Improvement, Hedrick et al. (2012) discuss the creation of student learning activities and experiences in quality and safety by integrating content into existing medical and nursing program curricula. Specific descriptions and examples of teaching quality and safety innovations in an interprofessional curricula, including challenges to curricula development and student learning, and evaluation strategies are adapted from this article (Table 9.7).

TABLE 9.7 Challenges and Strategies for Integrating Interprofessional Education in Learning Experiences

Challenge	Scope of Challenge	Strategies
Scheduling student participation in interprofessional education (IPE) activities	Health professions students often have different academic and clinical schedules, including time on and off campus and distance learning sites.	Commitment of leadership to IPE Advance planning of IPE prior to other academic program schedules Seeking commonalities in program calendars when students are in the same clinical site or on campus Extending IPE participation beyond formal semester date limits Empowering students to self-schedule meeting time for IPE project work Using information technology for student access to resources and networking with IPE faculty and within their work groups
Learner level and experience	There is variability between health professions students' education level (undergraduate vs. graduate program of study), clinical experiences, age, and lack of general familiarity of backgrounds.	Creating time for students to socialize and start teamwork relationships Deliberate planning to match student groups of similar academic achievement to a learning experience Incorporate student diversity as a strength to create and/or support learning experiences Include students in education planning processes Incorporate feedback or touch base with students throughout project work Provide expectations for accountability and grading
Faculty experience and development of meaningful IPE clinical experiences	Building content of quality improvement and safety into a course or across the curriculum, including application to the clinical setting might be unfamiliar to faculty.	Use of existing academic-service partnerships is valuable in the identification of relevant clinical experiences, access to practice experts, and systems management issues

(continued)

TABLE 9.7 Challenges and Strategies for Integrating Interprofessional Education in Learning Experiences (*continued*)

Challenge	Scope of Challenge	Strategies
	Creating and securing clinical experiences for large numbers of health professions students is difficult.	Identification of activities/projects that contribute to safety or quality of care that meet curricular outcomes and are attainable and manageable for students enhances student engagement and sense of accomplishment

Adapted from Hedrick et al. (2012).

Developing well-functioning teams is a priority because of the complexity in care delivery and need for care coordination among the many providers encountered by a single patient. Interprofessional collaboration focuses on activities that promote integrated models of education and practice among health professions students, including the value of each discipline as a full partner in the delivery and determination of quality and safe patient care. Students learn the professional role and scopes of practice of their discipline, and through IPE an increased awareness of other health professional roles and convergence of roles to work toward the common goal of optimal patient outcomes.

IPE can occur in the classroom, through simulation, activities in the clinical setting, or a combination of these throughout health professions programs. Teaching strategies and learning opportunities to reframe relationships and use collaboration, negotiation, and communication skills are foundational in developing interprofessional partnerships as a standard in professional practice. The differing attitude among professions toward interprofessional collaboration is important to acknowledge (Rees & Johnson, 2007). During the implementation of IPE initiatives or associated activities, the clinical teacher might be in a position to renegotiate traditional roles and responsibilities among staff and establish new ways of working that promote interprofessional competencies.

Example of IPE at the University of Colorado, Anschutz Medical Campus

The Anschutz Medical Campus (AMC) of the University of Colorado was intentionally designed to facilitate collaborative IPE among the health science programs of Dental Medicine, Pharmacy, Nursing, Physical Therapy, and Nursing and Medicine students. The planning of campus design was purposeful in the desire to bring health professions students closer together in classroom, laboratories, and simulation spaces and to create common space and facilities to promote student interaction and socialization. Realizing Education Advancement in Collaborative Health (REACH) is the endeavor of the long-term vision of transforming the delivery of health care through IPE at the University of Colorado Denver.

The University of Colorado AMC health science programs interprofessional faculty are developing a longitudinal curriculum that integrates preclinical and clinical training for all of the health profession students. The focus of the REACH curriculum is in developing competencies in teamwork, communication, collaborative interprofessional practice, quality, and safety, with an additional focus on vulnerable and underserved populations. In large part, the IPEC core competencies are the foundation for the curriculum and build on the existing interprofessional ethics course as a starting point.

The REACH goal is to create a curricular thread that is shared across all professional health programs and spans a timeframe adapted to the 2 to 4 years' length of health professions programs. Health professions students start the REACH curriculum with an orientation to the IPE program on the first day of class, which includes a social mixer for approximately 600 students.

Three core elements of REACH are:

1. *Fundamentals*: Fundamentals of Quality and Collaborative Care is the first step in the REACH curriculum. Students are placed into interprofessional teams of four to eight students, and they complete a series of specific tasks that are designed to explore roles and responsibilities of different professions and to building teamwork and communication skills. Specific skills developed during the use of scenarios include: information sharing, assertion and advocacy, mutual support, inquiry, and situation monitoring. The teams meet every 6 weeks for approximately 2 years.

2. *Clinical Transformations*: Clinical Transformations in Quality and Collaborative Care is the second step in the REACH curriculum. This is a simulation experience for students, and it takes place in the Center for Advancing Professional Excellence, which includes a high-fidelity simulation center. During the simulation experience, students undergo training in the TeamSTEPPS (Strategies and Tools to Enhance Performance and Patient Safety) curriculum for clinical communications developed by the Agency for Healthcare Research and Quality (AHRQ) and the Department of Defense (AHRQ, 2007). The simulation experience mimics real-life scenarios found in health care. The goal of the simulation is to expose students to complex patient situations, in which collaborative care is needed to optimize patient outcomes. Communication is the focus of the simulation. Students also learn how to react to situations when they do not know what actions to take, and they then use reflection to examine individual and team behaviors to establish safety and quality of care provided.

3. *Clinical Integrations*: Clinical Integrations is the third step in the REACH curriculum. Building on content and experiences in Fundamentals and Clinical Transformations, the curricula in this step allow students to achieve the competencies of the program through authentic clinical experiences, which also meet education outcomes for each health profession program and comply with accreditation requirements for each program. The clinical experiences are varied and scheduled within students' existing programs, and they are close in alignment with students' education development level. Although structured learning activities form the foundation for Clinical Integrations, flexibility to where and when the activities can be completed has been paramount to success. One example is the Team Structure and Function Project. The goal is to compare and contrast the structure and function of interprofessional clinical care teams with different goals of care. Students attend team meetings in a health care setting to evaluate the team's function using predetermined rubrics and resources, noting areas of strength and areas for improvement. Findings of team structure and function are presented to other student teams and faculty with a facilitated discussion.

PEER TEACHING AND LEARNING

Peer-assisted learning is a collaborative and cooperative teaching and learning strategy, whereby students are active and equal partners. Peers facilitate learning by providing emotional support, feedback through discussions, and assisting with physical skills/tasks (Secomb, 2007). Typically, peer-assisted learning is done in small groups. Small group size can foster interaction and support for learning among members, including ability to provide instant feedback. Although further research is required to support findings in cognitive, psychomotor, and affective development through the use of peer-assisted learning, studies report finding student satisfaction and increased self-confidence with peer teaching and learning (Secomb, 2007).

Peer teaching and learning can also increase student access and involvement in planned learning activities. Other important considerations include determining the types of subjects or content that could be accomplished by peer-assisted learning and measurement of learning results that include cognitive and psychomotor development, determining the level of involvement and collaboration with faculty or staff in health care agencies, and addressing incompatibility of students. An example of peer-assisted Teaching Learning Model (Stables, 2012) is outlined in Exhibit 9.3.

EXHIBIT 9.3 Example of Peer-Assisted Teaching Learning Model

Third-year undergraduate nursing students teach first-year students clinical skills during the first trimester of the program. The clinical skills taught by student peers include:

- Hand-washing
- Temperature measurement
- Pulse measurement
- Blood pressure measurement
- Blood oxygenation saturation measurement
- Urinalysis

Preparation for peer-assisted teaching

- First-year student: Learning resources related to the clinical skills placed on an e-learning platform. Students access the content before the teaching session.
- Third-year student peer: Provide a clinical skills lesson plan, notes, session schedule, and outline of how to teach the skill. Faculty-led drop-in sessions to practice clinical skills in simulation laboratory are scheduled.

Content delivery

- Faculty provide student expectations and learning outcomes to first-year students and oversight to all student groups.
- First-year to third-year student-to-teacher ratio is 5–1
- Location: Skills laboratory

Evaluation of peer-assisted teaching session

- First-year student: Testing of peer-taught clinical skills by faculty prior to progression to clinical site. Questionnaire regarding quality of the peer-assisted teaching session.
- Third-year student peer: Verbal feedback from faculty about teaching skills during session. Questionnaire regarding quality of the peer-assisted teaching session.

Adapted from Stables (2012).

SERVICE LEARNING

Service learning is an "education experience in which students participate in an activity that meets the needs of a specific community and reflect on the service in such a way as to further understand the course content, the broader role of the discipline and their sense of civic responsibility" (Otterness, Gehrke, & Sener, 2007, p. 40). Service learning requires a relationship between the academic and a community-based agency. Both partners establish a need for an identified activity or service that can be provided by students (Reising et al., 2008), which is also connected to structured academic course-work. Use of reflective process is also a component of service learning, and it serves to differentiate service learning from a volunteer experience (Vogt, Chavez, & Schaffner, 2011). Reflective practices include journaling or participation in structured groups for debriefing. In the literature, service learning is linked to increases in student knowledge related to social activism and justice, health care equity (Knight, Mooer, & Groh, 2007; Reising et al., 2008), and cultural diversity (Worrell-Carlisle, 2005).

For application of the service learning model as a short-term immersion experience for baccalaureate nursing students, Vogt et al. (2011) describe the use of camp nursing as providing opportunities for practice of physical assessment, relationship building, and chronic disease management skills. In response to students' needs to connect community health nursing theory to practice and address a decrease in clinical sites and resources, Broussard (2011) describes the integration of a service learning framework that has identified potential activities that are linked to a community assigned to students to promote student interaction with community leaders, and residents alongside public health and social work professionals (pp. 41–42). Other types of clinical experiences that could be reframed as a service learning model directed toward meeting community needs include health screening programs, flu vaccine clinics, development of wellness programs for underserved populations or the elderly, food delivery programs, friendly visitor programs, attending local legislative sessions pertaining to health policy, and faith-based outreach programs serving specific congregations.

CLINICAL SCHOLAR MODEL

The Clinical Scholar Model (CSM) originated in 1984 as a joint initiative between the University of Colorado College of Nursing and University of Colorado Hospital in Denver. The model has expanded in the past three decades to include 12 service agencies and 30 clinical scholars. The service agencies include acute care hospitals as well as county public health, mental health, and rehabilitation facilities. Preheim (2008) identifies the hallmarks of the CSM with sustaining power to be: (a) value-added academic-practice partnership, (b) competency-based and outcomes-focused performance in practice, (c) valuing the clinical nurse expertise, and (d) relationship-centered and caring curriculum.

Qualifications and attributes of the clinical scholar include the following:

1. Expert nurse who exemplifies professionalism and relationship-centered care in practice and conveys a passion for teaching and learning, particularly in the clinical setting
2. Employee of the health care agency, with time dedicated to planning, coordinating, teaching, and evaluating student clinical experiences
3. Master's prepared in nursing
4. Minimum of 5 years' experience in a nursing specialty practice and 2 years of employment within the health care agency
5. Recruited within the health care agency based on experience in practice and as a preceptor
6. Jointly interviewed and selected for hire by the College of Nursing and the health care agency

Clinical nurse experts are a valued and integral part of clinical education. They coordinate placements and learning experiences, provide consistent instruction and supervision, and contribute to evaluation of clinical competencies. Benefits include streamlined communication, liaison to staff for a smoother integration of students into the clinical setting, consistency of involvement, increased relevance of the clinical experience, and curricular modifications (Preheim, Casey, & Krugman, 2006). Exhibit 9.4 summarizes the roles and responsibilities of the clinical scholar.

EXHIBIT 9.4 Roles and Responsibilities of the Clinical Scholar

1. Coordination
   - Confirms scheduled dates, hours, and clinical units preclinical
   - Identifies and negotiates precepted assignments with qualified and available staff nurses
   - Arranges computer training and hospital orientation
   - Assures that staff and preceptors are prepared for arrival and engagement of students in learning activities appropriate for the level of student and course outcomes
2. Clinical education
   - Role models professional behaviors to facilitate socialization as a member of the health care team and nursing profession
   - Clarifies expectations and roles using effective communication and conflict management skills to guide the learning experience
   - Assesses critical thinking and clinical skills, and determines knowledge and application of the nursing process specific to the patient assignment
   - Interacts with individual students to model, dialogue, and provide feedback on performance
   - Provides oversight education to ensure clinical course outcomes are met
   - Conducts clinical conferences to provide an opportunity to reflect on care provided and aspects of professional nursing roles and responsibilities
   - Fosters a trusting and caring relationship, key in developing the student's skills, confidence in performance, and socialization into professional nursing roles
3. Evaluation of student performance
   - Assesses readiness for engagement in clinical practice
   - Serves as a liaison to preceptor and faculty to ensure practice opportunities and skill development according to critical elements for competent practice
   - Consistently evaluates students' clinical performance using standardized clinical evaluation tools and procedures
   - Prepares recommendations for further development and/or revisions of the clinical experience and teaching/learning tools
   - Facilitates development and implementation of joint research and scholarly activities

From Preheim (2008).

DEDICATED EDUCATION UNITS

Emerging in clinical education innovations, developed through academic-service partnerships, is the idea of a triad: students, clinical nursing staff, and faculty members, each with changing roles and responsibilities. As one of the newest innovations in clinical education, Dedicated Education Units (DEUs) have demonstrated outcomes of increased clinical capacity, allowing for increased student enrollments and high student and staff satisfaction with the clinical teaching and learning experience (Moscato, Miller, Logsdon, Weinberg, & Chorpenning, 2007). Central to the DEU concept is that staff nurses have a key educational role in students' knowledge and skill acquisition (Edgecombe, Wotton, Gonda, & Mason, 1999; Moscato et al., 2007). The model also facilitates relationship-building between academic settings and service that use existing resources, support professional nursing development, and are designed to enhance student engagement in and create meaning from practice (Ranse & Grealish, 2007; Warner & Burton, 2009; Wotton & Gonda, 2004). The DEU clinical education model reportedly facilitates teaching and learning of quality improvement and safety competencies (Mulready-Shick, Kafel, Banister, & Mylott, 2009). The development of a DEU for new graduate nurse orientation and role socialization demonstrated improvement in new graduate retention rates and associated quality improvement indicators via increased medication errors reporting and improvement in fall rates (Pappas, 2007).

Rhodes and associates (2012) report the impact of the DEU model on the clinical learning environment. The outcomes included high student satisfaction with their clinical experience, building relationships with DEU nurses that resulted in their feeling a part of the team, and witnessing patient-centered care with identification of patient needs as a priority through immersion of time in the clinical environment. Moscato et al. (2007) describe the key features of the DEU as follows:

1. Clinical unit is an optimal teaching/learning environment.
2. Primary goal is student achievement of learning outcomes.
3. DEU is used solely by one nursing program.
4. Commitment to attain an optimal practice environment for students and staff is shared through collaborative work efforts and communication.
5. Staff nurses, who indicate a desire to teach, are prepared for the clinical teaching role, and nursing faculty members from the academic program support the staff nurse in the instructor role.
6. Students are paired with the staff nurse, who is in the role as clinical teacher throughout the length of the clinical rotation.

The use of registered nurses as preceptors or mentors to nursing students in the clinical setting is well-known and has been employed in the clinical setting for numerous years. Udlis (2008) reports in an integrative review that preceptorships in undergraduate nursing education are as effective as the traditional model of clinical education. Other clinical partnerships that are designed to increase capacity and intentional use of the staff nurse in clinical education, on which the DEU model is based, build on the relationship between staff nurse and student, and include purposeful development of the expert staff nurse in clinical teaching (DeLunas & Rooda, 2009; Kowalski et al., 2007; Kruger, Roush, Olinzock, & Bloom, 2010). The goal in the clinical learning environment is to promote critical thinking in response to actual evolving patient situations during immersion experiences.

TRANSITION INTO PRACTICE

The successful transition of newly graduated, prelicensure nurses into the practice setting has been a focus of interest for nurse educators and employers for decades. Kramer (1974) described the role and values conflict experienced by new nurses as reality shock. Perceived lack of preparation for entry into fast-paced, acute care settings leaves nurses questioning their career choice and impacts safe, high-quality care delivery. In 2002, a National Council of State Boards of Nursing study confirmed the perception that newly licensed nurses are not prepared to safely perform upon entry into practice. Casey et al. (2011) describe the difficulty new graduate nurses have transitioning to acute care practice settings and the lack of perceived support from the organization. Challenges, including managing multiple patient care assignments, communicating with physicians, and caring for dying patients, were identified by students. Students reported needing greater assistance in clinical competencies, role development, and career planning. Nursing faculty awareness and ability to prepare new graduates for entry into practice through competency development is critical to their transition.

Nursing schools seek to increase relevancy of clinical education by involving clinical partners in curriculum development and collaborating in teaching and assessment of learning across classroom and clinical settings. Employers recognize the need for structured and specialized orientation, as well as preceptored experiences to coach and advocate for the new graduate nurse. However, the potential impact on quality and safe patient care, nursing turnover of the new graduate nurse, and impact on the health care team suggest that routine efforts to support entry into practice are inadequate. Benner, Sutphen, Leonard, and Day (2010) emphasize that improvements in prelicensure nursing education are necessary and are the responsibility of schools of nursing. The IOM *Future of Nursing* report (2010) calls for the implementation of nurse residency programs, specifically charging state boards of nursing, accrediting bodies, the federal government, and health care organizations to support transition-to-practice programs.

The emergence of transition-to-practice models and nurse residency programs with a focus on a clinical specialty area demonstrate response in collaborative efforts to promote high-quality and safe care and professional identity. A review of the literature reveals a wide range of definitions, purpose, length, content, and structure of transition-to-practice models, nursing orientation, and nurse residency programs. Common barriers to the design and implementation of a transition program are limited resources and evidence of effectiveness. Despite variations of approaches and fragmentation of effort, the significance of the transition to practice issue and the need for innovative and comprehensive models are evident. Highlights of several transition model exemplars include:

- The National Council of State Boards of Nursing Transition to Practice Program is a regulatory model applicable to both registered nurse and licensed practice nurse post licensure level of practice in all settings (Spector & Echternacht, 2010).
- The University Health System Consortium/American Association of Colleges of Nursing (UHC/AACN) Post-baccalaureate Nurse Residency Program is a national model expanded to 87 sites in 34 states. The Nurse Residency Program is designed in partnership with a College of Nursing and fosters reflection and exploration of nursing professional practice (UHC/AACN, 2008).
- A variety of state models exist to address the specific state needs of education and practice reflected by the nursing shortage and imperative for quality, safe, and cost-effective care. Examples include:
  - Idaho Rural Connection (2006)
  - Massachusetts Initiative (Sroczynsk, Gravlin, Route, Hoffart, & Creelman, 2011)
  - Vermont Nurse Residency Program (Boyer, 2011)
  - Versant RN Residency (Ulrich et al., 2010; Versant RN Residency)
  - Wisconsin's Nurse Residency Program (Bratt, 2009)

ROLES OF PARTICIPANTS

The value of the education mission must be nurtured and demonstrated first and most fundamentally by the chief nurse officer and nursing school dean or director. The challenge is to establish working relationships through awareness of each other's needs and goals, development of trust and effective communication patterns, and engagement to assure that affiliations turn into meaningful partnerships. After the partnership is established, its value must be continuously embraced and cultivated by nurse leaders, faculty, and staff responsible for its planning, implementation, and evaluation. Nursing faculty and agency staff activities influence the relationship and contribute to meeting needs and achieving goals. Roles and responsibilities at each level are important determinants of the effectiveness of the partnership.

The nurse educator role is multidimensional, with clear expectations and opportunities relevant to academic-practice partnership development and sustenance. Nurse educator competencies include the ability to facilitate learning, promote development and socialization, use assessment and evaluation strategies, participate in curriculum design and evaluation of program outcomes, function as a change agent and leader, pursue continuous quality improvement in the nurse educator role, engage in scholarship, and function within the educational environment (NLN, 2005, 2012). Within each of these competencies, task statements delineate specific responsibilities aligning with coordination, education, and evaluation of student learning in the clinical setting. Nursing faculty and clinical instructors are responsible in their roles to facilitate readiness for transition into practice. Nurse educators' understandings of the factors that facilitate or are barriers to effective partnerships are relevant to role development. Similarly, understanding strategies for articulating goals within the formal partnership and developing action plans to attain are key responsibilities of the nurse educator.

A vast range of opportunities for effective partnerships and collaboration await faculty from the academic program and nurses at the staff or unit leader level at the clinical agency. Mutual respect, valuing, and investment are demonstrated through presence, engagement, and effective communication among faculty and unit staff. Nurse educators and clinical faculty influence the quality of the partnership through planning and preparation for the student learning experiences with unit managers and staff. Students who demonstrate readiness and professionalism contribute to the development of a meaningful and valued role to the team and delivery of high-quality and safe care. The appropriate level of student engagement, including expectations for patient assessment, nursing interventions, documentation, and supervision, should be clarified to the team members. Team member roles and responsibilities should be explained to the student. Staff nurses who are prepared for the student's presence and learning needs and who are recognized for their expertise feel valued for their contributions to clinical education. Viewing students as unwanted guests or placements as a commodity become barriers to realizing benefits of the partnership. The relationship of faculty and clinical teachers with the nursing staff and nurse leaders at the patient care unit or service level is vital to an effective partnership. Additional evidence of the partnership might be in the form of joint appointments, preceptor training, student scholarships, and participation in unit-based or nursing education committees relevant to quality, safety, and competency development.

Cronenwett and Redman (2003) describe four types of clinical agency affiliations with nursing schools. The least effective type of affiliation is perceived to be a negative drain on the organization. For example, conflict and concern for safe patient care can occur if students are inadequately prepared for integration into the clinical unit or are accompanied by an unqualified clinical instructor. A second type of affiliation is described as meaningless, with no perceived value or negative impact to the clinical agency. Clinical placements might be viewed as a commodity and routinely requested by the nursing program without consideration of needs or potential benefit to the clinical agency. In the third level of affiliation, value to the partnership is identified. For example, the clinical agency might benefit from a potential source of new graduate nurse employees, and the school of nursing might recognize the relevance of appropriately leveled learning experiences. Significant value of an active partnership is realized only at the fourth level. A clear sense of shared mission and trust are evident with interdependence to achieve goals that could not be accomplished without the partnership. Staff nurses engage in coaching and precepting students, increasing nurse satisfaction and contributing to retention. Nursing faculty interact with clinical experts who inform modifications in curricular design or clinical evaluation tools to assess student performance.

Nursing deans and administrators weigh the impact, benefits, and challenges associated with collaboration in the education of the nursing workforce. Seifer (2000) identified eight principles for developing and sustaining community-based partnerships. Cronenwett and Redman (2003) recommended assessing how each principle was evident in practice, providing an indication of the value of clinical nursing education to the mission and goals of the clinical agency. The eight principles for developing and sustaining community-based partnerships are:

1. Agree on mission, values, goals, and measurable outcomes
2. Demonstrate mutual trust, respect, genuineness, and commitment
3. Build on strengths and assets; address need for improvement
4. Balance power and enable sharing of resources
5. Communicate with clarity, openness, and accessibility; listen, clarify, and validate
6. Establish roles, norms, and processes with input and agreement
7. Provide multidirectional feedback to continuously improve partnership outcomes
8. Share credit for accomplishments

THE FUTURE OF ACADEMIC-PRACTICE PARTNERHSIPS

The NLN in 2003 issued the Position Statement on Innovation in Nursing Education: A Call to Reform, indicating the need for collaboration between educators and health care leadership to prepare the future workforce to function in a complex and rapidly changing health care environment. In 2008, The NLN Think Tank on Transforming Clinical Nursing Education recommended inclusion of quality and safety content in all courses and learning links among classroom, laboratory, and clinical settings.

Incorporating innovation as a strategic plan in the academic environment requires effective leadership to address barriers to innovation, support culture change, and build strong health care and interdisciplinary partnerships (Melnyk & Davidson, 2009). The barriers to innovation in academic programs are mirrored in the service setting. Melnyk and Davidson identify barriers to health care education innovation:

1. Pressure to meet essential regulatory requirements for education and competencies established for nursing practice by national organizations, accrediting agencies, and state boards of nursing are minimal standards.

2. Content-driven curricula not in keeping with the pace of the information explosion. Information management is an application skill. Teaching strategies to access, manage, and evaluate information about health problems across populations require a fundamental change away from a focus on content focus to a focus on health outcomes and on synthesis and application of knowledge and data management.

3. Failure by organization leadership to role-model innovation and support opportunities for innovation, and a lack of clear communication or expectations related to change.

4. Organizational innovation slowed by individuals who subscribe only to established policies and procedures.

5. Individual fear or anxiety with challenging the status quo in organizations and the unknown consequences associated with risk taking related to innovation and change.

Cronenwett (2004) identified the use of academic and service partnerships to enhance patient care and safety in addition to nursing education and research endeavors. To attain the goal of transforming clinical education and addressing the real-world complexities of health care encountered by students, education, and practice innovations should be coupled with teamwork and collaboration among health professionals in academic and service organizations. The goal of transforming clinical education is to improve the level of clinical practice in nursing.

SUMMARY

Academic and service partnerships are forging innovations in clinical education and driving changes in roles for students, faculty, and clinical staff. These innovations and changes will require further evaluation by educators and administrators for curriculum development, additional competencies for practice/teaching, value or cost effectiveness of the innovation or model, and readiness for practice of new graduates. Long-term sustainability of academic-service partnerships should also be examined.

REFERENCES

Agency for Healthcare Research and Quality. (2007). *TeamSTEPPS™: Strategies and tools to enhance performance and patient safety*. Retrieved from http://www.ahrq.gov.qual/teamstepps

Alliance for Clinical Education. (2006). *By-laws*. Retrieved from http://www.coloradonursing center.org/alliance-for-clinical-education-ace

American Association of Colleges of Nursing. (2008). *Essentials of baccalaureate education for professional nursing*. Retrieved from http://www.aacn.nche.edu/education-resources/BaccEssentials08.pdf

American Association of Colleges of Nursing. (2012). *Nursing faculty shortage*. Retrieved from http://www.aacn.nche.edu/news/articles/2012/enrollment-data

American Association of Colleges of Nursing and American Organization of Nurse Executives. (2012). *Academic practice partnerships toolkit*. Retrieved from http://www.aacn.nche.edu/leading-initiatives/academic-practice-partnerships/tool-kit

American Association of Colleges of Nursing and American Organization of Nurse Executives. (2010). *Summary of literature related to academic-service partnerships*. Retrieved from http://www.aacn.nche.edu/leading-initiatives/academic-practice-partnerships/SummaryLiteratureAcademic.pdf

American Association of Colleges of Nursing and American Organization of Nurse Executives. (2012). *Task force guiding principles to effective academic-practice partnerships*. Retrieved from http://www.aacn.nche.edu/leading-initiatives/academic-practice-partnerships/Guiding-Principles.pdf

Benner, P., Sutphen, M., Leonard, V., & Day, L. (2010). *Educating nurses: A call for radical transformation*. San Francisco, CA: Jossey-Bass.

Boyer, S. (2011). Vermont nurses in partnership: Developing nurses competence within a complex, high-acuity healthcare environment. In A. Bushy & D. Molinari (Eds.), *The rural nurse: Transition to practice*. New York, NY: Springer Publishing Company.

Bratt, M. (2009). Retaining the next generation of nurses. The Wisconsin Nurse Residency Program provides a continuum of support. *Journal of Continuing Nursing Education, 40*, 416–25. doi:10.3928/00220124-20090824-05.

Broome, M. (2009). Partnerships: A long walk in the wind. *Nursing Outlook, 57*, 119–120. doi:10.1016/j.outlook.2009.03.006

Broussard, B. B. (2011). The bucket list: A service-learning approach to community engagement to enhance community health nursing clinical learning. *Journal of Nursing Education, 50*, 40–43. doi:10.3928/01484834-20

Burns, P., Williams, S. H., Ard, N., Enright, C., Poster, E. & Ransom, S. A. (2011). Academic partnerships to increase nursing education capacity: Centralized faculty resource and clinical placement centers. *Journal of Professional Nursing, 27*(6), e14–e19. doi:10.1016/j.profnurs.2011.07.004

Casey, K., Fink, R., Jaynes, C., Campbell, L., Cook, P., & Wilson, V. (2011). Readiness for practice: The senior practicum experience. *Journal of Nursing Education, 50*, 646–652. doi:10.3928/01484834-20110817-03

Cronenwett, L. R. (2004). A present-day academic perspective on the Caroline nursing experience: Building on the past, shaping the future. *Journal of Professional Nursing, 20*, 300–304. doi:10.1016/j.profnurs.2004.07.005

Cronenwett, L. R., & Redman, R. (2003). Partners in action: Nursing education and nursing practice. *Journal of Nursing Administration, 28*, 153–155.

DeLunas, L. R., & Rooda, L. A. (2009). A new model for the clinical instruction of undergraduate nursing students. *Nursing Education Perspectives, 30*, 377–380.

Edgecombe, K., Wotton, K., Gonda, J. & Mason, P. (1999). Dedicated education units: A new concept for clinical teaching and learning. *Contemporary Nurse, 8*, 166–171.

Hedrick, L. A., Barton, A. J., Ogrinc, G., Strang, C., Aboumatar, H. J. Audm M. A., … Patterson, J. E. (2012). Results of an effort to integrate quality and safety into medical and nursing school curricula and foster joint learning. *Health Affairs, 31*, 2669–2680. doi:10.1377/hlthaff.2011.0121

Idaho Rural Connection.(2006) Retrieved from http://www.ruralconnection.org/Milestones.html

Interprofessional Education Collaborative Expert Panel. (2011). *Core competencies for interprofessional collaborative practice: Report of an expert panel*. Washington, DC: Interprofessional Education Collaborative.

Institute of Medicine. (2003). *Health professions education: A bridge to quality*. Washington, DC: National Academies Press.

Institute of Medicine. (2010). *The future of nursing: Leading change, advancing health*. Washington, DC: National Academies Press.

Ironside, P. M., & McNelis, A. M. (2010). Clinical education in prelicensure nursing programs: Findings from a national survey. *Nursing Education Perspectives, 31*, 264–265.

Joynt, J., & Kimball, B. (2008). *Innovative care delivery models: Identifying new models that effectively leverage nurses*. White paper produced by Health Workforce Solutions and Robert Wood Johnson Foundation. Retrieved from http://innovativecaremodels.com

Knight, D., Mooer, S., & Groh, C. (2007). Service learning as a component of physician assistant education: The development of a compassionate practitioner. *Journal of Physician Assistant Education, 18*(2), 49–52.

Kowalski, K., Horner, M., Carroll. K., Center, D., Foss, K., & Jarrett, S. (2007). Nursing clinical faculty revisited: The benefits of developing staff nurses as clinical scholars. *Journal of Continuing Education in Nursing, 3*, 69–75.

Kramer, M. (1974). *Reality shock: Why nurses leave nursing*. St. Louis, MO: C.V. Mosby.

Kruger, B. J., Roush, C., Olinzock, B. J., & Bloom, K. (2010). Engaging nursing students in long-term relationships with a home base community. *Journal of Nursing Education*, *49*, 10–16. doi:10.3928/01484834-20090828-07

McNelis, A. M., Fonacier, T., McDonald, J., & Ironside, P. M. (2011). Optimizing pre-licensure students' learning in clinical settings. *Nursing Education Perspectives*, *32*, 64–65.

Melnyk, B. M., & Davidson, S. (2009). Creating a culture of innovation in nursing education through shared vision, leadership, interdisciplinary partnerships, and positive deviance. *Nursing Administration Quarterly*, *33*(4), 288–295. doi:10.1097/NAQ.0b013e3181b9dcf8

Moscato, S., Miller, J., Logsdon, K., Weinberg, S., & Chorpenning, L. (2007). Dedicated education unit: An innovative clinical partner education model. *Nursing Outlook*, *55*, 31–37. doi:10.1016/j.outlook.2006.11.001

Mulready-Shick, J., Kafel, K. W., Banister, G., & Mylott, L. (2009). Enhancing quality and safety competency development at the unit level: An initial evaluation of student learning and clinical teaching on dedicated education units. *Journal of Nursing Education*, *48*, 716–719. doi:10.3928/01484834-20091113-11

Nabavi, F. H., Vanaki, Z., & Mohammadi, E. (2012). Systematic review: Process of forming academic service partnership to reform clinical education. *Western Journal of Nursing Research*, *34*, 118–141. doi:10.177/0193945910294380

National League for Nursing. (2003). *Innovation in nursing education: A call to reform*. New York, NY: Author.

National League for Nursing. (2005). *Core competencies of nurse educator with task statements*. Retrieved from http://www.nln.org/profdev/corecompetencies.pdf

National League for Nursing. (2008). *NLN think tank on transforming clinical nursing education*. Retrieved from http://www.nln.org/facultyprograms/pdf/think_tank.pdf

National League for Nursing, (2012). *Scope of practice for academic nursing leaders*. New York, NY: Author.

Otterness, N., Gehrke, P. & Sener, I. (2007). Partnerships between nursing education and faith communities: Benefits and challenges. *Journal of Nursing Education*, *46*, 39–44.

Pappas, S. (2007). Improving patient safety and nurse engagement with a dedicated education unit. *Nurse Leader*, *5*(3), 40–43.

Preheim, G. (2008). The clinical scholar model: Competency development within a caring curriculum. In M. Oermann (Ed.), *Annual review of nursing education: Clinical nursing education* (pp. 3–23). New York, NY: Springer Publishing Company.

Preheim, G., Casey, K., & Krugman, M. (2006). Clinical scholar model: Providing excellence in clinical supervision of nursing students. *Journal for Nurses in Staff Development*, *22*(1), 15–22.

Ranse, K., & Grealish, L. (2007). Nursing students' perceptions of learning in the clinical setting of the dedicated education unit. *Journal of Advanced Nursing*, *58*, 171–179.

Rees, D., & Johnson, R. (2007). All together now? Staff views and experiences of a pre qualifying interprofessional curriculum. *Journal of Interprofessional Care*, *21*(5), 543–555. doi:10.1080/13561820701507878

Reising, D. L., Shea, R. A., Allen, P. N., Laux, M. M., Hensel, D., & Watts, P. A. (2008). Using service-learning to develop health promotion and research skills in nursing students. *International Journal of Nursing Education Scholarship*, *5*(1), Article 29. doi:10.2202/1548-923X.1590

Rhodes, M. T., Meyers, C. C., & Underhill, M. L. (2012). Evaluation outcomes of a dedicated education unit in a baccalaureate nursing program. *Journal of Professional Nursing*, *28*, 223–230. doi:10.1016/j.prof.2011.11.019

Ridenour, N. (2009). Clinical education reform: Re-envisioning the workforce. *Journal of Nursing Education*, *48*, 419–420. doi:10.3928/01484834-20090717-01

Schmalenberg, C., & Kramer, M. (2008). Clinical units with the healthiest work environments. *Critical Care Nurse*, *28*(3), 65–77.

Secomb, J. (2007). A systematic review of peer teaching and learning in clinical education. *Journal of Clinical Nursing*, 703–716. doi:10.1111/j.1365-2702.2007.01954.x

Seifer, S. (2000). Developing and sustaining community-campus partnerships: Putting principles into practice. Partnership perspectives. *Community-Campus Partnerships for Health*, *1*(11), 7–11.

Spector, N., & Echternacht, M. (2010). A regulatory model for transitioning newly licensed nurses to practice. *Journal of Nursing Regulation*, *1*(2), 18–25.

Sroczynski, M., Gravlin, G., Route, P., Hoffart, N., & Creelman, P. (2011). Creativity and connections: The future of nursing education and practice: The Massachusetts initiative. *Journal of Professional Nursing, 27*(6), e64–e70. doi:10.1016/j.profnurs.2011.08.007

Stables, I. (2012). Development of clinical skills: The contributions of peer learning. *Learning Disability Practice, 15*(8), 12–17.

Sullivan, D. T. (2010). Connecting nursing education and practice: A focus on shared goals for quality and safety. *Creative Nursing, 16*(1), 37–43. doi:10.1891/1078-4535.16.1.37

Teel, C. S., MacIntyre, R. C., Murray, T. A., & Rock, K. Z. (2011). Common themes in clinical education partnerships. *Journal of Nursing Education, 50,* 365–372. doi:10.3928/01484834-2011-429-01

Udlis, K. A. (2008). Preceptorship in undergraduate nursing education: An integrative review. *Journal of Nursing Education, 47,* 20–29. doi:10.3928/01484834-20080101-09

Ulrich, B., Krozek, C., Early, S., Ashlock, C. H., Africa, L. M., & Carman, M. L. (2010). Improving retention, confidence, and competence of new graduate nurses: Results from a 10-year longitudinal database. *Nursing Economics, 28,* 363–376.

University of Colorado Denver, Anschutz Medical Campus. (n.d.). Retrieved from http://www.ucdenver.edu/academics/degrees/health/REACH

University Health System Consortium/American Association of Colleges of Nursing. (2008). *Executive summary of the post-baccalaureate residency program.* Retrieved from http://www.aacn.nche.edu/leading-initiatives/education-resources/NurseResidencyProgramExecSumm.pdf

Vogt, M. A., Chavez, R., Schaffner, B. (2011). Baccalaureate nursing student experiences at a Camp for children with diabetes: The impact of a service-learning model. *Pediatric Nursing, 37*(2), 69–73.

Warner, J. R., & Burton, D. A. (2009). The policy and politics of emerging academic-service partnerships. *Journal of Professional Nursing, 25*(6), 329–334. doi:10.1016/j.profnurs.2009.10.006

Worrell-Carlisle, P. (2005). Service-learning: A tool for developing cultural awareness. *Nurse Educator, 30*(5), 197–202.

Wotton, K., & Gonda, J. (2004). Clinical and student evaluation of a collaborative clinical teaching model. *Nursing Education and Practice, 4,* 120–127.

10

Assessment Methods

MARILYN H. OERMANN

Through the process of assessment, the teacher collects information about student learning and performance. With this information the teacher can determine further learning needs, plan learning activities to meet those needs, and confirm the outcomes and competencies met by the students. Students also assess their own learning and performance, and identify areas in which they need more practice and review. Assessment also provides information on the quality of the teaching, courses, practice experiences, curriculum, and other aspects of the educational program.

This chapter explains assessment, evaluation, and grading in nursing education. Methods are described for assessing learning, and examples are provided for many of these methods. Tests are a common assessment method used in nursing education, and various types of test items are described in Chapter 11. There is a separate chapter, 12, on clinical evaluation, and methods such as rating scales are presented in that chapter.

ASSESSMENT

Assessment is the collection of information about student learning and performance. Assessment that provides information about the student's progress in the course and further learning needs is diagnostic: this is feedback for the teacher and students to identify gaps in learning and plan relevant instructional strategies. Assessment also is used at designated times in the course such as midterm and final to confirm the outcomes of learning and determine students' grades. The data collected through assessment provide the basis for students' grades.

Assessment also provides information about the quality of teaching in the course. At the end of a course, students typically evaluate the effectiveness of the teacher and quality of the instructional methods, feedback to students, interactions with them, availability, and other areas. Students, graduates, and alumni assess the nursing program as part of program evaluation. Other uses of assessment are to select students for admission to the educational institution and school of nursing, and placement of students in appropriate courses in the nursing program.

There are five principles the teacher should use when assessing student learning:

1. *Identify the outcomes, objectives, or competencies to be assessed.* Another way of thinking about this is: What is being assessed? The goal in assessment is to determine if students are meeting or have met the intended outcomes, objectives, and competencies.

2. *Select appropriate assessment methods.* The methods for assessing learning, for example, a test or written assignment, should provide information about the particular outcome, objective, or competency being assessed.
3. *Meet students' needs.* The assessment should provide feedback to individual students about their progress in meeting the outcomes and further learning needed. The most important role of assessment is identifying where further learning is needed and planning appropriate strategies to help students learn and improve their performance.
4. *Use multiple assessment methods.* Decisions about learning and performance are often high stakes, having serious consequences for students, and should not be based on one test or assignment. Multiple assessment methods are needed to provide data for determining if the outcomes of a course were met.
5. *Recognize the limitations of assessment when making decisions about students.* One teacher-made test, for example, may not be a true measure of the student's learning about that content. The test may have flaws in its design, and other factors may influence the results. (Nitko & Brookhart, 2011)

EVALUATION

Evaluation is the process of making judgments about student learning and performance. The teacher analyzes test scores, collects other assessment data, and then makes a value judgment about the *quality* of learning and performance. There are two types of evaluation: formative and summative. Formative evaluation occurs throughout the instructional process and provides feedback to students (Oermann & Gaberson, 2014). In formative evaluation, the teacher assesses learning, gives prompt and specific feedback to students about gaps in learning and performance and how to improve, and plans further instruction to guide their learning. High-quality formative evaluation has been linked to improved learning and student achievement (Koh, 2008). Giving prompt, specific, and instructional feedback is critical to the learning process and a characteristic of quality teaching. Bourgault, Mundy, and Joshua (2013) compared audio and written feedback on clinical assignments, and students reported that audio feedback was more personal, was easier to understand, included more constructive comments, and was more effective in meeting the course outcomes than traditional written feedback. Data collected through formative evaluation should not be graded.

Summative evaluation "summarizes" what students have learned. This is evaluation at the end of a point in time, for example, at midterm and the end of a course, for determining grades.

GRADING

A grade is a symbol (A through F, pass–fail) that represents the student's achievement in a course. Grades are for summative evaluation, indicating how well the student performed in individual assignments, clinical practice, the laboratory, and the course as a whole.

There are different grading systems that can be used. A common grading system is with letters (A, B, C, D, E or A, B, C, D, F), sometimes combined with + and –. Grades also can be represented by percentages (100, 99, 98, . . .), which, in turn, can be used to assign a letter grade, for example, A = 90% to 100%. There are other grading systems such as Honors (exceptional performance in all areas), High Pass (exceptional performance in most areas), Pass (completely satisfactory performance in all areas), and

Fail (unsatisfactory performance), and two-dimensional systems such as pass–fail and satisfactory–unsatisfactory, which are used frequently for grading in clinical courses.

The grade is based on the data collected through the various assessment methods in the course. Each of these methods should be weighted in the overall course grade based on the emphasis of the outcomes and content evaluated by them in the course. For example, a unit examination in an adult health nursing course should count more in the course grade than a journal assignment completed once in clinical practice.

NORM- AND CRITERION-REFERENCED INTERPRETATION

There are two main ways of interpreting test scores and other assessment data. When tests are scored and papers and other assignments are graded, the result is a number. The number itself, however, has no meaning. For example, if the teacher tells students their scores on a test are 20 or 22, what does that mean? Scores need to be referenced or compared to some standard or to other students' scores. A score of 22 might be the highest score possible on the test or the highest score among the students who took it. To interpret a score, there needs to be a reference to compare the score against.

Test scores and the scores resulting from other types of assessment can be interpreted using norm- or criterion-referenced standards. In norm-referenced interpretation, each student's score is compared to those of a norm group. The norm group is often other students' test scores: students who perform better than their peers receive higher scores (Nitko & Brookhart, 2011). Grading on a curve is an example of norm-referenced interpretation. Students' scores are rank ordered from highest to lowest, with grades based on where a student's score falls in the ranking. For example, the top 10% of students might receive an A and the lowest 10% an F.

In clinical practice, a tool on which student performance is rated on a scale of below to above average is norm-referenced: each student's clinical performance is compared to the group of learners. Norm-referenced interpretation does not indicate what a student can and cannot do; it reflects instead if the student's performance is better or worse than other students in the clinical group (Oermann & Gaberson, 2014).

In criterion-referenced interpretation, students' tests and other scores from an assessment are compared to preset criteria, not to how well they performed in relation to other learners. The grades are based on what the student has learned and can do. With criterion-referenced interpretation, the teacher might indicate the percent of items answered correctly on a test, total score received on a term paper, or competencies met (Miller, Linn, & Gronlund, 2009). In clinical evaluation with criterion-referenced tools, students would be evaluated as to whether they could perform the clinical competencies on the tool or have met the outcomes of the clinical course. The competencies are used as the standards for evaluation rather than how other students in the group performed in clinical practice (Oermann & Gaberson, 2014).

OUTCOMES FOR ASSESSMENT

Students need to know what they are expected to learn and the clinical competencies they should develop. Outcomes are the cognitive processes and practice behaviors students should demonstrate at program completion (Iwasiw, Goldenberg, & Andrusyszyn, 2009, p. 182). Competencies are the knowledge, skills, and values students need to develop to achieve those outcomes. Billings and Halstead (2009) defined outcomes as the characteristics that students should display at a particular point in time and competencies as the behaviors needed to develop those characteristics. Some teachers refer to the outcomes of their courses as objectives—the specific knowledge, skills, and values students should exhibit at the end. Nitko and Brookhart (2011) use the term learning targets, what the student should achieve at the end of the instruction. Regardless of the labels used in a particular nursing program, the outcomes should be clearly stated and measurable, guiding students in their learning and the teacher in developing the instruction and planning the assessment. The teacher selects assessment methods to determine if students have achieved these learning outcomes and developed the competencies.

Outcomes, or objectives, may be written in three domains of learning: they can specify knowledge to be gained (cognitive domain), values to be developed (affective domain), and skills to be performed (psychomotor domain). These domains were introduced in Chapter 3. Each of the domains levels its learning outcomes in a taxonomy. The cognitive domain includes knowledge and higher level cognitive skills. The most widely used cognitive taxonomy has six levels of learning, increasing in complexity: knowledge, comprehension, application, analysis, synthesis, and evaluation (Bloom, Englehart, Furst, Hill, & Krathwohl, 1956). These are defined in Table 10.1 with an example of an objective written at each level. In 2001, Anderson and Krathwohl modified the cognitive taxonomy: the knowledge level was renamed as remember, and evaluation was placed prior to synthesis, which was renamed as create. The taxonomy of the cognitive domain is valuable in planning the assessment because it helps the teacher focus the test item or other assessment method on a particular cognitive level (Oermann & Gaberson, 2014). If the outcome relates to application, the assessment should determine if students can apply what they are learning to a new situation or in a new context. By using the taxonomy, the teacher can avoid assessment methods that focus on recall of facts and memorization when the intended outcomes of learning are at a higher level.

The affective domain taxonomy levels values, attitudes, and beliefs from knowing them to internalizing them as a basis for decisions. The psychomotor domain focuses on the development of motor skills. Learners progress through three phases of learning: cognitive (understanding what needs to be done), associative (gradually refining performance until movements are consistent), and autonomous or automatic performance of the skill (Schmidt & Lee, 2005). There are different taxonomies for psychomotor skill learning. Of the three domains, the cognitive taxonomy is used most frequently for planning assessment.

TABLE 10.1 Cognitive Domain Taxonomy

1. *Knowledge*: Recall of facts and specific information
   List two symptoms of heart failure.

2. *Comprehension*: Understanding and ability to explain material
   Describe classes of heart failure based on functional capacity.

3. *Application*: Use of information in a new situation
   Apply clinical practice guidelines to care of patients with heart failure.

4. *Analysis*: Ability to break down material into its parts and identify the relationships among them
   Compare psychometric properties of instruments for measuring the quality of life of patients with heart failure.

5. *Synthesis*: Ability to combine elements to develop a new product
   Develop plan for managing patients with acute decompensated heart failure.

6. *Evaluation*: Ability to make value judgments based on internal and external criteria
   Evaluate the strength of the evidence related to follow-up care of patients with heart failure.

ASSESSMENT METHODS

Tests are a common assessment method for determining students' learning in a course and certifying nurses' knowledge in the clinical setting, for example, competency tests during orientation. While tests are used frequently for assessing students' learning and determining grades, they are not the only assessment method to be used. In a study by Oermann, Saewert, Charasika, and Yarbrough (2009), nurse educators reported using papers, group projects, and case study analyses more frequently than tests for grading in their courses, although the tests counted more in the students' grades. Other assessment methods are: papers and other written assignments (formal papers, reflective journals, short papers, concept maps, writing-to-learn activities, and others); cases; multimedia; portfolios; discussions and conferences; group projects; simulations; standardized patients; Objective Structured Clinical Examination (OSCE); and self-evaluation. Some of these are used predominantly for assessment in the classroom or online environment, such as formal papers and multimedia, and others are designed for assessing learning and performance in a simulated or laboratory setting, such as simulation and OSCE.

TESTS

A test is a set of items to which students respond in written or sometimes oral format. Tests are typically scored based on the number of correct answers, are administered in the same way to all students, and are usually timed.

Tests are used for admission to a college or university and to the nursing program. Once admitted students may take tests to place out of courses in the program. For example, they may have had a genetics course and may not need to take a similar course in the nursing program. Tests also can be used to determine the appropriate level of a course, for example, which research methods course would be best for the student in a graduate nursing program. In many prelicensure nursing programs students take tests as they progress through each level and at the end of the program to identify gaps in learning and assess their risk for not passing the National Council Licensure Examination for Registered Nurses (NCLEX-RN®). These tests provide feedback to students and faculty for developing a learning plan for students to be successful as they continue through the nursing program, improve their test-taking strategies, and prepare for the NCLEX-RN (Harding, 2012; Heroff, 2009). Another use of tests is for evaluating student learning and performance at the end of a nursing program. Tests used in this way are for program evaluation and accreditation rather than indicating what students have learned in a particular course.

The NCLEX-RN and National Council Licensure Examination for Practical Nurses are tests used to validate nurses' knowledge and competencies to engage in safe and effective practice at the entry level. Certification examinations verify nurses' knowledge and competencies in a specialized area of practice.

There are many types of test items that can be used for assessment of learning in nursing courses. Chapter 11 describes different types of test items and principles for writing each of those items on a test.

PAPERS AND OTHER WRITTEN ASSIGNMENTS

Papers and other types of written assignments enable students to search for literature and resources, analyze theories and their application to practice, build their higher level thinking skills, analyze issues and situations in health care, and improve writing skills (Oermann & Gaberson, 2014). When written assignments are used for summative evaluation and are graded, they should provide assessment data for specific outcomes of the course. All too often students complete assignments that are not geared to any particular objective or goal of the course; these assignments may have been in a course for years but are no longer relevant for the aims of the current course. Papers and other types of writing assignments should be carefully selected based on the outcomes of the course. If an objective of a course is to identify resources for evidence-based practice, students could prepare a short paper on reputable websites such as the Agency for Healthcare Research and Quality and The Joanna Briggs Institute, journals such as *Evidence-Based Nursing* and *Worldviews on Evidence-Based Nursing*, and other sources of information they could use in the practice setting. In this way the paper is designed to assess if students can identify relevant resources for evidence-based practice in nursing.

Faculty members should review periodically the papers and other written assignments in courses to confirm they are still relevant, meet specific outcomes of the course, are not "busywork," and are not too repetitive. While some repetition is important to develop knowledge and cognitive and writing skills, once students have mastered writing certain types of papers, the teacher might transition to a new assignment. Faculty in a school of nursing should periodically review assignments across courses to ensure they build on one another.

Formal Papers

Students at all levels of nursing education need to write effectively (American Association of Colleges of Nursing, 2006, 2008, 2011). Term papers and other types of formal papers in a course, which include drafts and feedback from the teacher on the substance of the paper and the writing style and quality, enable students to develop their writing as a skill (Oermann, 2013). To improve writing ability, it is critical for students to prepare drafts of papers, get prompt and specific feedback on the content and writing, and rewrite the papers based on that feedback. Through this process students learn how to write "in the discipline" and communicate their ideas effectively to a professional audience (The Writing across the Curriculum [WAC] Clearinghouse, 2011a).

Because formal papers are difficult for students to write, Luthy, Peterson, Lassetter, and Callister (2009) suggest dividing them into smaller assignments that build on one another and are more manageable for students. For example, one of the assignments might be a quality improvement paper related to the focus of the course. Students might first prepare a paper on a problem they identified in the clinical setting related to patient safety or quality care and data they examined to support that problem. The next assignment might be a literature review on the problem and related interventions that have been used to improve quality of care. The third assignment might be a proposal for a quality improvement project and how it would be implemented on the unit. This strategy of dividing term papers into smaller writing assignments is also valuable for the teacher because feedback can be given to students as they are thinking through the content of the paper and writing individual sections. Students can use the feedback in revising their drafts and writing the subsequent paper.

There are many types of formal papers students can write in a course, such as, term papers, research proposals, integrative literature reviews, and papers analyzing theories and their application to patient care, among others. Exhibit 10.1 lists examples of formal papers for assessment in a nursing course.

EXHIBIT 10.1 Examples of Formal Papers for Assessment

- Term paper
- Research paper and development of research proposal
- Literature review and systematic review
- Evidence review (paper in which students critique and synthesize evidence and report on its application to clinical practice)
- Paper analyzing theories and their use in patient care
- Paper comparing different interventions and evidence base
- Concept analysis paper
- Critical analysis paper in which students analyze issues, compare options, and develop arguments for a position
- Case study analysis with written rationale

Adapted from Oermann and Gaberson (2014), pp. 170–171. Copyright 2014. Reproduced with the permission of Springer Publishing Company, LLC.

Reflective Journals

Reflective journals encourage students to reflect on their experiences and think critically about them. Chan (2013) found that writing narratives and journaling had a positive effect on students' critical thinking and allowed teachers to assess difficulties students were experiencing. With reflective journals students gain an awareness of their environment and ability to self-assess (Schuessler, Wilder, & Byrd, 2012). Journals also provide an opportunity for faculty to give feedback to students (Langley & Brown, 2010; Lasater, 2011; Lasater & Nielsen, 2009). In assessing journals for higher level thinking, the Lasater Clinical Judgment Rubric can be used to provide feedback to students and for them to assess their own thinking (Lasater, 2011).

Davies and colleagues (2013) used reflective journals to assess student learning in an undergraduate gerontological nursing course. As part of the course, students visit older adults who share their life experiences with them. Students then write reflective journals based on these visits, which are evaluated in the course. Reflective journals also have been used effectively for assessment in service learning and study abroad experiences as a way of encouraging them to think about the meaning of their experiences and for faculty members to provide feedback (Adamshick & August-Brady, 2012; Carpenter & Garcia, 2012; Vogt, Chavez, & Schaffner, 2011). While some teachers assess journals for summative evaluation and grading, when the aim of the journal is to reflect on experiences and gain meaning from them, journals should be used for feedback purposes only.

Short Papers

Another type of written assignment for assessment is a short paper that focuses on a specific content area or outcome (Oermann, 2006). For example, students might write a one-page paper that compares two similar patient problems and how to differentiate them in an assessment; a paragraph that describes the ISHAPED (I = Introduce, S = Story, H = History, A = Assessment, P = Plan, E = Error Prevention, and D = Dialogue) bedside handoff process; and a two-page paper that examines nursing interventions and supporting evidence for a patient with a particular health problem. Short assignments provide an opportunity for teachers to give quick feedback on students' knowledge, higher level thinking skills, and sometimes also writing skills. Short assignments can be completed by students individually or as a small group activity, and can be used for formative and summative evaluation.

Concept Maps

In a concept map students illustrate how concepts relate to one another. In clinical practice concept maps can help students plan their care for a patient, organize information, and visualize how the assessment data, problems, treatments, medications, and other information are interrelated. Students can develop a concept map as part of their planning for clinical practice and then revise the map after caring for the patient. Concept maps also enable students to apply theory to practice, demonstrate their synthesis skills, and enhance critical thinking (Kirkpatrick & DeWitt, 2009; Lee et al., 2013). Hunter Revell (2012) used concept maps to teach graduate nursing students how to link theoretical and clinical knowledge. The weekly concept maps promoted theoretical thinking and engagement. An example of a concept map is in Figure 10.1.

Daley and Torre (2010) reviewed 35 studies on the use of concept maps in medical education and found that they promoted meaningful learning, were an additional resource for learning, provided feedback to students, and could be used for assessment of learning. With concept maps teachers can identify knowledge gaps and provide additional instruction (Torre, Durning, & Daley, 2013). While concept maps are assessed typically for formative purposes, they also can be graded, especially if students explain the relationships among concepts in the map.

Writing-to-Learn Activities

Writing activities in which students think about course content, reflect on their learning, and raise questions about the content are often referred to as writing-to-learn activities. These are short, informal, and frequently impromptu (Oermann, 2013; WAC Clearinghouse, 2011b). They can be used for assessment but should not be graded. For example, at the end of an online session or in-class presentation, the teacher may ask students to list content about which they have questions, summarize a key learning from the class or their readings, define a term they learned in class, or write a few sentences about how the class compared to their readings. With these short writing activities students can self-assess where further learning is needed, and teachers can provide feedback to individual students and the class as a whole.

Other Written Assignments

There are many other written assignments that can be developed to assess student learning and writing ability. Students can prepare summaries of readings and their implications, analyze scenarios with a rationale supporting their analysis, prepare nursing care and teaching plans, develop discharge and follow-up plans, write up assessments, analyze quality and safety issues in the health care setting, and evaluate interactions, among others. Depending on the type of assignment, they can be assessed formatively or graded.

Assessment of Papers and Other Written Assignments

For any written assignment, the teacher needs to have specific criteria for assessment, which should be shared with students prior to beginning the paper. The criteria depend on the type of assignment. For formal papers the quality and comprehensiveness of the content, use of relevant and current literature, organization of the paper, writing style, and reference style would be considered. For other types of written assignments, some of these criteria would not be appropriate.

FIGURE 10.1 Example of a concept map.

Condition: Testicular Cancer

Physiology: Testicular cancer is a rare tumor that arises from the germinal cells (cells that produce sperm) of the embryonal tissues and causes less than 1% of all cancer deaths in men. Testicular tumors are classified as seminomas or nonseminomas. Seminomas are composed of uniform, undifferentiated cells that resemble primitive gonadal cells. This type of tumor represents 40% of all testicular cancer and is usually confined to the testes and retroperitoneal nodes. There are two types of seminomas: classical (occur between the late 30s and early 50s) and spermatocytic seminomas (occur around age 55, grow slowly, and do not metastasize). Nonseminomas show varying degrees of cell differentiation and include embryonal carcinoma (occur most often in 20- to 30-year-olds, grows rapidly, and metastasizes), teratoma (can occur in children and adults), choriocarcinoma (rare and highly malignant), and yolk cell carcinoma derivatives (most common in children up to 3 years of age and have a very good prognosis). Sometimes, testicular tumors are "mixed," containing elements distinctive to both groups. Staging is categorized typically as: Stage I (confined to testes); Stage II (regional lymph node spread); and Stage III (spread beyond the retroperitneal lymph nodes). The initial treatment for testicular cancer is surgical resection of the involved testicle (orchiectomy; Taber's, 2009).

Handoff Communication

S (Situation)	Assess what is currently happening in a short statement	Patient presents with_____ Stage and classification_____
B (Background)	Summarize important past assessment data for your patient here. Place lab results and medications on the concept map.	**Age:** **Allergies:** **Social Alerts:** **Mental Status:** **Safety Risk:**
A (Assessment)	Use the assessment data to complete your concept map. Make your nursing diagnosis and plan.	**Nursing Diagnosis:** Place the Nursing Diagnoses in prioritized order on the concept map **Plan:** Place the Nursing Interventions Classification (NIC) on the concept map

IMPLEMENT YOUR PLAN OF CARE

R (Recommendation)	Evaluate your nursing care and make recommendations related to the achievement of your desired outcomes. Were they met, or do new goals need to be established?	Evaluate Your Care		
		Diagnosis	**Nursing Outcomes Classification (NOC)**	**Outcomes Met?**
		1	Patient verbalizes understanding of disease process, diagnostic procedures and treatment options, and available resources	☐ Yes ☐ No
		2	Patient appears relaxed and verbalizes decreased/absent pain	☐ Yes ☐ No

(continued)

FIGURE 10.1 Example of a concept map. (*continued*)

Evaluate Your Care		
Diagnosis	Nursing Outcomes Classification (NOC)	Outcomes Met?
3	Patient demonstrates ability to cope with bodily changes through open discussion and participation in care	☐ Yes ☐ No
4	Patient shares feelings/concerns related to sexual activity and reports satisfaction with physical intimacy	☐ Yes ☐ No

Nursing Diagnosis: Deficient Knowledge of disease process, diagnostic/treatment regimen, and prognosis as evidenced by questions.
NIC: (1) Provide information on disease process; encourage questions related to diagnosis and treatment options, and prognosis; (2) Explain lab tests/procedures; (3) Provide pre-op/post-op teaching; (4) Provide referrals to reputable informational resources and support groups.

Nursing Diagnosis: (Risk for) Sexual dysfunction related to disease process, pain, hormonal changes. infertility.
NIC: (1) Provide private time for the patient and his partner to ask questions, express concerns, and clarify information; (2) Offer the opportunity for sexuality and fertility counseling after discussing the impact of the surgery on anatomy and function.

Nursing Diagnosis: Pain (acute) related to inflammation, tissue damage, tissue compression, or nerve irritation from tumor metastasis in the perineum, groin, or abdomen, as evidenced by complaint of pain.
NIC: (1) Assess pain level systematically and often; (2) Analgesic administration; (3) Relaxation techniques/medication; (4) Trans-cutaneous electric nerve stimulation (TENS); Hypnosis, Heat/cold application.

Patient Initials:
Condition: *Testicular Cancer*
Age:

Link and Explain:
• Nursing Interventions Classification (NIC)
• Laboratory and Diagnostic Procedures
• Medications

Nursing Diagnosis: Disturbed body image related to orchiectomy as evidenced by verbalizations.
NIC: (1) Assess feelings and perceived impact on personal relationships; (2) Acknowledge client feelings, fears, and frustrations/ assess prior coping strategies; (3) Include patient in self-care activities and treatments; (4) Provide information/referral to resources/support groups for testicular cancer

(Use the nursing diagnosis list for any others that are specific to your patient/family)
P _____
E _____
S _____
NIC:

Medications:
a. Chemotherapy
b. NSAIDs/ acetaminophen
c. Opiods/ opiod-NSAID combination drugs
d. Hormone replacement

☐ **Medication sheet used for additional medications**

Laboratory and Diagnostic Procedures:
a. Testicular self-exam
b. Diagnostic ultrasound. CAT scan, MRI, Chest x-ray, Bone Scan
c. Laboratory tumor markers (Alpha feto-protein, human chorionic gonadopropin) t-op laboratory studies
d. Sperm banking

☐ **Lab sheet used for additional laboratory results**

From Wittmann-Price, Reap Thompson, Sutton, and Eskew (2013), pp. 176–177. Reprinted with permission.

The teacher should develop a rubric for evaluating the paper. A rubric is a scoring guide, specifying the criteria to be assessed and points allotted to each criterion. Students should have the rubric ahead of time so they can prepare the paper accordingly. Nitko and Brookhart (2011) view a rubric as useful for both instructional purposes and assessment because it guides students in writing the paper and teachers in assessing it. In a study of how faculty teach writing in a baccalaureate nursing program, teachers reported that they explain the rubric to students and also provide examples of well-written papers (Troxler, Vann, & Oermann, 2011). Table 10.2 provides an example of a rubric for scoring a written assignment in a nursing course.

TABLE 10.2 Rubric for Scoring Written Assignment

Content		
Content relevant to purpose of paper, comprehensive	Content relevant to purpose of paper	Content not relevant to purpose of paper, no depth
5	3	1
No errors in content	Few errors in content	Many errors
3	2	1
Current evidence synthesized and integrated in paper	Relevant evidence in paper but not synthesized	Limited evidence in paper
7	4	1
Organization		
Content well organized	Organization understood but could be improved	Poorly organized
3	2	1
Multiple perspectives explored in paper	Some alternate perspectives explored	No alternate perspectives explored
3	2	1
Writing Style and Format		
Sentence structure clear, correct grammar and punctuation, no spelling errors	Sentence structure adequate; some grammar, punctuation, and spelling errors	Poor sentence structure; many errors in grammar, punctuation, and spelling
3	2	1
Format consistent with requirements	Parts of paper missing or not consistent with requirements	Missing sections, does not meet requirements
3	2	1
References current, no errors in APA	References limited but current, some errors in APA style	Few and old references, errors in APA style
3	2	1

Total Points _____ (sum points for total score)

Adapted from Oermann and Gaberson (2014), pp. 175–176. Copyright 2014. Reproduced with the permission of Springer Publishing Company, LLC.

Following are principles for assessing papers and other written assignments:

1. Written assignments should be planned to guide students in meeting specific outcomes of the course, and the criteria for assessment should address those outcomes.
2. The number of required papers in a course should be reasonable, based on the outcomes to be met, and consider the number of drafts to be submitted with teacher feedback.
3. Written assignments should foster students' higher level thinking about the content rather than summarizing what they have read.
4. The directions about the purpose and format of the paper should be clear, students should know the dates when drafts and the final paper are due, and they should have the rubric ahead of time.
5. In evaluating papers in which students analyze issues, the criteria should focus on the rationale for the position, not the specific position.

6. The teacher should read papers anonymously (to avoid potential bias); read each paper twice before scoring (to gain an overview of how students approached the topic as the rubric may need to be modified if no students addressed a particular content area); and grade papers in random order (to avoid bias, as papers read first may be scored higher than those at the end).

7. If unsure about a grade on a paper or other assignment, the teacher should have a colleague read the paper, also anonymously. (Oermann & Gaberson, 2014)

CASES

Integrative cases, unfolding cases, and case studies are strategies for teaching clinical judgment, problem solving, and decision making and helping students engage in higher level learning (Harrison, 2012; Popil, 2011). They also are appropriate for assessing those outcomes. Cases typically present a clinical scenario that integrates various concepts followed by questions about that scenario. Often the scenarios are short to avoid directing students' thinking in advance (Oermann, 2008). Students analyze the case and might identify patient problems and possible interventions, apply theories and other knowledge to the case, and discuss it from different points of view. Questions can ask students what they noticed in the situation, to analyze the scenario and decide on actions that are appropriate or if no actions are needed, and to reflect on how patients might respond to those actions. In this way the case and questions foster clinical judgment in nursing (Tanner, 2006).

Unfolding cases simulate a changing scenario similar to what might occur in actual clinical practice. With this method the case unfolds to reveal new information about the situation. With unfolding cases students can identify the most salient aspects of a case, develop their clinical imagination, and learn to think like a nurse (Benner, Sutphen, Leonard, & Day, 2010; Day, 2011). Case studies are longer and provide background information about the patient, family, community, or other context. In their analysis of a case study, students can describe the theories that guided their analysis, cite related literature, and provide a rationale for their analysis and any decisions they made.

Cases can be analyzed by students individually or in small groups in class, online, or in postclinical conferences. Discussions about the case expose students to other possible approaches and perspectives that they may not have identified themselves. With this method, the teacher can provide feedback on the content and thought process used by students to arrive at their answers. When grading cases, the teacher first establishes criteria for grading, develops a rubric, and scores answers to the questions using the rubric (Oermann & Gaberson, 2014). Cases are also useful in preparing students for thinking through higher level test items such as on the licensure examinations. Exhibit 10.2 provides an example of an integrative case, unfolding case, and a case study.

MULTIMEDIA FOR ASSESSMENT

Short segments of a digital recording, a video from YouTube, and other media clips can also be used for assessment. Rather than describing a case in print form, the scenario can be visualized in a media clip. These can be used in class to explore if students can apply their learning to the scenario in the multimedia, placed online for student analysis individually or in groups, and used in place of a written case or case study. Media clips allow students to visualize the clinical situation and get a sense of what the experience is like for patients, families, and providers. They can also be used to encourage discussion about different sides of an argument and points of view (Clifton & Mann, 2011).

Questions can be developed by the teacher related to the multimedia for students to answer, either for formative or summative purposes.

EXHIBIT 10.2 Examples of Cases for Assessment

Case

Your patient fell at home and was admitted yesterday with a hip fracture. She is scheduled for surgery today. At shift report the nurse says the patient had lab work done on admission, but she does not know the results. Later you find that the patient's hemoglobin is 5.0 g/dL and hematocrit is 16%.

1. What were unsafe practices in this situation?
2. Which 2013 *National Patient Safety Goals* were not met? What are the implications of these to nursing practice?
3. What should have been done?

Unfolding Case

Your 93-year-old patient in a long-term care facility has a Stage I pressure ulcer at her sacrum. The patient is also coughing and tells you she is too weak to get out of bed for lunch.

1. Describe what the pressure ulcer should look like. What other data should you collect? Why?
2. Develop a plan of action for this patient, with a rationale.

   The following day the patient is coughing more, has shortness of breath, and is more fatigued. A nurse tells you in report it looks like the patient has a blister on her sacrum.

1. What does this new information mean?
2. What are possible problems of this patient? List them in priority and provide a rationale for your prioritization.
3. What will you report to the nurse at handoff?

   The patient's daughter comes to find you on the unit and tells you how angry she is that a nurse moved her mother to a chair.

1. What would you say to her? Why?
2. How can you provide patient-centered care in this situation?
3. Develop a new plan for this patient and family with a rationale for your approaches.

Case Study

A patient comes to the emergency department with severe abdominal pain and diarrhea. The patient has lost 12 pounds in the past 2 weeks and has no appetite. The nurse does not detect any masses, but there is abdominal tenderness and pain. The patient's wife indicates the patient has been healthy except for this "flu," which has lasted for 2 weeks. She says the patient travels frequently and was recently in Portugal and Canada. The patient does not smoke or drink alcohol. The wife explains that last year the patient was treated for depression but is fine now and has no prior health problems. They have two children, and the grandparents are currently watching them.

1. What are possible problems that the patient might have?
2. What assessment data would you collect from the medical record? Why is this information important to deciding what is wrong with the patient? List the two questions you would ask the wife next.
3. What laboratory tests would you expect to be ordered? Why?
4. Add laboratory values to the case and discuss with a peer how that information would influence decisions about the patient's problems.

PORTFOLIO

In a portfolio students collect materials they have developed in the course that provide documentation that they have met the course outcomes. For clinical courses the materials and projects in the portfolio demonstrate their clinical knowledge and competencies. Portfolios are valuable for assessment because they contain the evidence for judging if students have met the outcomes of the course. Portfolios developed for a course can be used later for job applications and career development. Nurses can continue to add materials and documentation of their accomplishments to their portfolios. In this way the portfolio represents the continued development of the nurse's expertise over the years.

There are two types of portfolios: best work and growth (Nitko & Brookhart, 2011). Best-work portfolios contain examples of students' "best" products of learning; when used for assessment these products provide evidence that students have met the outcomes of the course. Growth portfolios are designed for formative evaluation. With a growth portfolio students collect evidence of their work with narrative reflections about each item in the portfolio (Holmboe, Davis, & Carraccio, 2008).

The contents of the portfolio depend on the course outcomes to be assessed. Students can select papers and projects they completed in the course, group projects, self-reflections on clinical and other experiences, and other products they developed that demonstrate their learning and achievement. Holmboe et al. (2008) suggested that when portfolios are used for summative evaluation and grading, the portfolio content should be standardized across students but also provide an opportunity for students to include products they believe reflect their professional development. The evaluation should be based on specific, measurable criteria, which are known to students. In some programs portfolios are presented at an oral defense; in those situations teachers can confirm their assessment of the content and the grade they assigned for the portfolio assignment (Holmboe et al., 2008). The time commitment to develop a portfolio is one of the main issues with its use (Buckley et al., 2009).

Although portfolios can be prepared and submitted as hard copies, electronic portfolios can be updated, stored, and shared more easily with others. With electronic portfolios students can also include multimedia and links to show relationships among materials.

DISCUSSIONS AND CONFERENCES

Discussions are an exchange of ideas between two or more people (Gaberson & Oermann, 2010). These are often informal but may also be planned discussions about a particular topic. In a discussion the teacher can assess students' knowledge of a topic, explore decisions made and the reasoning underlying those decisions, and provide feedback to learners. Open-ended questions rather than ones answered with a "yes–no" response encourage students' higher level thinking and promote discussion about alternate perspectives and approaches. Chan's (2013) systematic review of studies on critical thinking revealed that asking higher level questions, a sequence of questions from low to high level, and multiple questions rather than only one promoted critical thinking among nursing students. These questions are an effective method for assessing students' critical thinking because the teacher can ask students about other perspectives of the situation, possible options and implications of each, and a rationale for their thinking. Nickitas (2012) suggested that in a discussion students can argue their thoughts and decisions, which improves their critical thinking and problem solving.

Conferences are planned discussions on a topic. These include pre- and postclinical conferences, interprofessional conferences, and other types of seminars in which the student participates. In a conference students can develop their oral communication skills and ability to lead and engage others in discussing an issue or a problem and deciding on actions to take. Although most clinical conferences are face-to-face with the teacher or preceptor, Cooper, Taft, and Thelen (2004) evaluated the use of online conferences. Students identified the opportunity for equal participation as one of the benefits of holding clinical conferences in an online format following the clinical experience. Students also preferred the flexibility of this method. In a project by Terry (2012), a patient created a digital story about his health care experience and then engaged in online discussions with students. These discussions enabled students to reflect more deeply on how nursing care is delivered and patients' perceptions than in a traditional clinical conference.

Assessment of student participation in a conference is typically best for formative evaluation because the teacher can provide feedback to students as a group and individually during the discussion. This feedback can encourage students to consider other points of views and think more broadly about a topic. The teacher also can clarify any misunderstandings and share how the teacher would analyze a situation and arrive at a decision. However, conferences can be evaluated for summative purposes, including how well a student led a conference and the quality of students' participation in it. If conferences are assessed for grading purposes, specific criteria need to be established and shared with students prior to their leading or participating in the conference. These criteria include how well the student led the group discussion, presented ideas to the group, encouraged critical thinking about the topic and consideration of alternate perspectives, and encouraged peers to participate in the discussion. The criteria should also address the leader's knowledge of the topic and preparation for the conference.

GROUP PROJECTS

Group projects encourage cooperative and active learning, and the development of problem solving, teamwork, and communication skills (Gagnon & Roberge, 2012; Noonan, 2013). These outcomes are important to students' future practice where they will work in teams and need to collaborate with others. Some group projects are short term with students meeting in class, online, or out of class for the time it takes to develop the product, such as a poster or group presentation. Other groups, however, are long term, for example the length of the course, for cooperative learning purposes. With either type of group, the group products and individual student participation in the group efforts can be assessed.

Group projects can be assessed in three ways. A group grade can be determined, and each student in the group receives that grade. The main issue with this approach is it does not account for individual student participation in the group work. A second method is for students to specify their contributions to the group product or complete a self-assessment of their participation in the group. The teacher can then evaluate and grade each student's contribution and provide a grade for the group or grade only the individual student's contributions. Students can also evaluate each other's participation, reducing the chance of some people not participating in the group work (Shiu, Chan, Lam, Lee, & Kwong, 2012). A third way of grading group projects is for students to prepare a group and an individual product, with both of these evaluated and graded.

When group projects are assessed, the teacher needs a rubric developed specifically for evaluating that project (Nitko & Brookhart, 2011). The rubric should include criteria related to the substance of the group project and also to the process of working as a team. Two examples are provided of rubrics for assessing group projects. The rubric in Exhibit 10.3 was designed to evaluate a group presentation of an assignment in which students explored the literature to answer a selected clinical question. The rubric includes criteria on the substance of the project, for example, the literature review and synthesis of the findings, the quality of the presentation, and how well the students actively engaged the audience in the discussion. The rubric in Exhibit 10.4 is a peer evaluation for a group project in which students critiqued research studies.

SIMULATIONS

Chapter 5 presents types of clinical simulations in nursing, how to integrate and implement them in a nursing curriculum, evaluation using simulations, and debriefing. With simulations students can analyze scenarios, make decisions about problems and actions to take, carry out interventions, demonstrate techniques and skills, and evaluate the effects of their decisions. In simulations students can engage in the deliberate practice of skills, improving their performance (Oermann et al., 2011).

Simulations are valuable not only for instructional purposes but also can be developed for assessment of competencies. They can be used for both formative and summative evaluation. For formative evaluation, in the debriefing session, teachers can provide feedback to students to further develop their clinical judgment and reflective thinking skills (Dreifuerst, 2012; Lasater, 2011). The debriefing provides an opportunity to explore different perceptions of what occurred in the simulation, link theory to the experience, examine actions taken or not taken and other possible approaches, and analyze each student's role. Debriefing is also an oppportunity for the teacher to provide feedback to students for their continued learning.

When simulations are used for summative evaluation, there needs to be standardization across students so that there is consistency with the evaluation, and the tools must be valid and reliable. Scalese and Issenberg (2008) indicated that for assessment the simulation needs to present the same clinical findings, task, or scenario repeatedly to each student, and the teacher or other evaluator needs to be trained in the process, use of the tools, and scoring.

Principles for implementing simulation-based assessment for summative evaluation include:

- The simulation should be developed to assess particular course outcomes or competencies. The teacher begins with the outcomes or competencies and then determines the optional assessment method using simulation.
- The teacher should match the features and fidelity of the simulator to the competencies to be assessed. For example, a task trainer might be more appropriate for evaluation of a specific skill than use of a human patient simulator.
- For some competencies a combination of simulation modalities (e.g., task trainer and standardized patient) are needed to best represent a real patient encounter. This decision should be based on the outcomes and competencies to be assessed.
- The testing situation needs to be the same for each student, that is, it needs to be reproducible. The use of simulators and standardized patients are well suited for assessment where high-stakes decisions will be made (Scalese & Issenberg, 2008).
- The tool for rating performance in the simulation must be valid and reliable. Nursing faculty and educators in clinical settings should not use simulation for high-stakes decisions without assurance that the rating tool and process are valid and reliable based on carefully done studies.

EXHIBIT 10.3 Rubric for Evaluating a Group Presentation of an Assignment

Criteria	Failure (0)	Poor	Fair	Excellent	Score
Organization	Presentation is highly disorganized. Some members lack contribution. Presentation is lacking in smooth transition and logical progression.	Poor (10–15) Presentation is disorganized. Presenters contribute at varying lengths and levels. Most members demonstrate lack of preparedness. Presentation is lacking in smooth transition or logical progression.	Fair (16–17) Presentation is fairly well organized. Presenters contribute at varying lengths or levels. Most members demonstrate preparedness. Presentation is mostly smooth and logical in progression.	Excellent (18–20) Presentation is highly organized. Presenters contribute equitably and demonstrate preparedness. Presentation exhibits flow, and material is presented in a logical progression. Smooth transitions take place between presenters.	Score
Content: synthesis of literature review	Failure (0) Content is inaccurate or unclear. Literature review is weak or incomplete.	Poor (25–39) Presents a poor review of the literature. Content is inaccurate at times. Conclusions are inaccurate at times. The area of exploration lacks clarity.	Fair (40–44) Presents a fair review of the literature. Lists findings. Content is mostly accurate. Conclusions are mostly accurate. A basic exploration of the area is presented.	Excellent (45–50) Presents a thorough review of the literature. Synthesizes findings. Content is accurate. Conclusions are accurate. In-depth exploration of the area is presented with supportive evidence.	Score
Creativity and engagement	Failure (0) Gives a lecture only. Audience is not engaged. No evidence of creativity. Provides no activities, handouts, or supportive materials to educate peers.	Poor (10–15) Gives a lecture-type presentation using PowerPoint with supportive images. Audience is minimally engaged. Provides a handout to educate peers.	Fair (16–17) Engages audience at times. Demonstrates elements of creativity in the presentation. Provides an activity or handout to educate peers.	Excellent (18–20) Actively engages audience through multiple means and creatively throughout the presentation. Provides appealing activities, handouts, or other relevant and supportive means to educate peers.	Score
References and APA format	Failure (0) References are not mentioned or listed.	Poor (5–7) Reference list presented with many errors in APA 6th edition format. In-text citation missing. Uses fewer than five references, or references are outdated or lack credibility.	Fair (8) Reference list presented with few errors in APA 6th edition format or in-text citation missing. Uses fewer than 10 references that are current (<5 years old) and reputable.	Excellent (9–10) Reference list accurately presented in APA 6th edition format. In-text references cited appropriately. Uses 10 or more reputable references < 5 years old.	Score

Total Score out of 100 points

EXHIBIT 10.4 Rubric for Peer Evaluation of Group Project

Instructions: Rate each member, excluding yourself, on whether the member of your group met the criterion of a substantive and meaningful contribution to each of the areas indicated. After completing the rating, compare the score to the descriptions at the bottom of the document to see if your rating matched the description of the member's performance.

Use the following rate scale: 0 = No and 1 = Yes

	Member's Name	Member's Name	Member's Name	Member's Name	Member's Name	Member's Name
Participated in group discussions						
Contributed ideas during group meetings or by written means						
Participated according to agreed upon group role						
Assisted in problem resolution						
Positively challenged others in the group to deepen understanding of critique or apply research concepts correctly						
Supported other group members to encourage a sense of group cohesion						
Organized and influenced the logical flow of the group's writing						
Carried his or her share of the workload						
Met deadlines established by the group						
Submitted individual contributions of sufficient quality to be used by the group, including results of turnitin reports						
Total Points: Add down each column for maximum score						

Comments:

Note: Your individual ratings of each group member will be kept confidential by the instructor.

10—Full Participation. This individual was a true team player, committed to the totality of the project and who made significant content and process contributions. He or she may have contributed in one primary area, but he or she was clearly committed to making the whole project a success.

8—Strong Selective Participation. This individual made a significant contribution to the project, but within a clearly defined scope; he or she limited participation to a particular content or process role—and showed initiative in that area—but did not view the overall project as his or her responsibility.

6—Weak Participation. This individual did not cause any problems, but made little substantive contribution to content or process. He or she showed little initiative and contributed only what was specifically requested.

3—Virtually Absent. This individual was frequently not involved with the project; he or she often missed meetings or other important communications, was consistently unprepared, and/or contributed substandard work that required correction by fellow team members; this individual exhibited little effort and made minimal contribution to the project.

0—Totally Absent. This individual was totally absent from this project, and the end product in no way reflects a contribution on his or her part.

- Evaluators need to be trained on the process and use of the tool. Parsons and colleagues (2012) developed a formal training program for faculty members to use their tool in assessing performance in simulation. As part of the training, the evaluators come to consensus on the minimum expectations of student performance in the simulation to indicate passing each competency on the tool. Findings suggested that training and dialogue about the use of the tool in assessing a particular scenario improve reliability.

STANDARDIZED PATIENTS

Standardized patients are actors trained to portray the role of a patient with a specific condition. With standardized patients, students can be assessed on interpersonal and communication skills, history and physical examination techniques, and other competencies. Standardized patients are often used for formative evaluation, as they are prepared to provide both written and oral feedback to students about their performance (McWilliam & Botwinski, 2010). However, because standardized patients recreate the same patient condition and clinical situation each time they are with a student, providing for consistency in the assessment, they can be used for summative evaluation and high-stakes decisions. Performance-based assessments with standardized patients are widespread in medicine (Hawkins & Boulet, 2008). They are being used increasingly for assessment in nursing programs. Rutherford-Hemming and Jennrich (2013) indicated that standardized patients allow students to practice in a safe environment and receive feedback on their performance, preparing them for clinical practice.

OBJECTIVE STRUCTURED CLINICAL EXAMINATION

Another assessment method is an OSCE. With OSCEs students rotate through stations where they perform a skill or activity, analyze cases or are tested on their knowledge and ability to apply that in scenarios, and interact with standardized patients. Because OSCEs have a high degree of standardization, they are effective for assessing skills in nursing (Mårtensson & Löfmark, 2013). At each station in the OSCE, students are evaluated on their performance often with rating scales or checklists. If standardized patients are incorporated in the OSCE, they also can rate the performance. OSCEs are often used for assessment at the end of a semester or program (Kardong-Edgren, 2013).

Following are principles for setting up an OSCE for formative or summative evaluation:

- An examination blueprint should be developed that specifies the skills and other competencies to be assessed and types of scenarios to be used. Case scenarios should be written based on this blueprint and by faculty members who have expertise in the content and competencies.
- Multiple OSCE scenarios can be developed to provide more than one assessment of students' knowledge and performance. McWilliam and Botwinski (2010) reported that in their school of nursing, faculty members write 10 case scenarios, and students are randomly assigned to 5 of those. They believe this process avoids assessment errors due to the specificity of the content of the scenario and provides a better measure of the students' actual performance.
- The content validity of the scenarios should be established prior to using them for an OSCE. The OSCE scenarios should be updated as needed.

- Standardized patients should be trained to portray the patient role and skilled in assessing students' competencies and providing feedback to them (McWilliam & Botwinski, 2010).
- Rating scales, checklists, and other tools used for evaluation must be valid and reliable, including interrater reliability. The validity and reliability of the tools should be established prior to using them for summative evaluation. Nulty, Mitchell, Jeffrey, Henderson, and Groves (2011) suggested using a holistic scoring tool to allow judgments of performance as a whole rather than discrete skills.
- Evaluators, and standardized patients if their role includes giving feedback to students and rating their performance, need to be trained on the expected performance and proper use of the tools.
- If OSCEs are used for summative purposes, a standard needs to be set as to the score that differentiates students who pass from those who do not.

SELF-EVALUATION

An important outcome of a nursing education program at all levels is the ability of students to evaluate their own learning and performance. With this self-reflection students can identify areas in which continued learning and development need to occur. Self-evaluation is a developmental process. With a positive teacher–student environment, students will be more likely to share reflections and own assessment with their teachers than in an environment that is punitive and viewed as not facilitating their learning. Self-evaluation is for formative evaluation only and not graded.

SUMMARY

Assessment is the collection of information about student learning and performance. It is critical to determining the student's grade in a course because assessment provides the data on which the grade is based. Assessment also reveals gaps in learning and performance and the need for further instruction. When the teacher adds a value judgment about the quality of learning and performance, the process is evaluation. Formative evaluation occurs throughout the instructional process and provides feedback to students. Summative evaluation "summarizes" what students have learned. This is evaluation at the end of a point in time, for example, midterm and the end of a course, for determining a course or clinical grade.

A grade is a symbol (A through F, pass–fail) that represents the student's achievement in a course and clinical practice. Grades are for summative evaluation, indicating how well the student performed in individual assignments, practice settings, and the course as a whole. Test scores and the scores resulting from other types of assessment can be interpreted using norm- or criterion-referenced standards. In norm-referenced interpretation, each student's score is compared to those of a norm group. In contrast, in criterion-referenced interpretation, students' tests and other scores from an assessment are compared to preset criteria, not to how well they performed in relation to other learners. Clinical courses can be graded with letter grades, such as A through F, or as pass–fail and other two-dimensional systems.

There are many methods teachers can use to assess students' learning in a course and performance skills. Tests are a common method in nursing education. Another assessment method used frequently in courses is written assignments. Students can prepare formal papers such as term papers. These types of papers enable students to search for literature and resources, analyze theories and their application to practice, build their higher level thinking skills, reflect on issues and situations in practice, and improve writing. When assignments are used for summative evaluation and are graded, they should be selected to provide assessment data for specific outcomes of a course. The teacher should use a scoring rubric for evaluating the paper. A rubric specifies the criteria to be used for assessing the paper and points allotted to each criterion.

Another type of written assignment is a reflective journal. A journal can be used to encourage students to think critically about clinical practice and decisions they have made in the practice setting, evaluate decisions, and become more self-aware. Short papers provide an opportunity for teachers to give quick feedback on students' thinking and judgments and sometimes also writing skill. For example, students might write a short paper that analyzes a safety issue they identified in clinical practice. Another type of written assignment is a concept map. In a concept map, students think about how concepts relate to one another and illustrate these relationships. Concept maps help students organize information about patients and other data and visualize how the assessment data, problems, treatments, medications, and other information relate to one another. There are many other written assignments that can be developed to assess student learning and writing ability.

Writing activities in which students think about course content, reflect on their learning, and raise questions about the content are often referred to as writing-to-learn activities. These are short, informal, and frequently impromptu. They can be used for giving feedback to learners but should not be graded.

With integrative cases, unfolding cases, and case studies, students can apply theory and other knowledge to practice situations and develop their higher level thinking skills. These are also appropriate for assessment. Cases typically present a clinical scenario that integrates various concepts followed by questions about that scenario. Students analyze the scenario and might identify patient problems, possible interventions, and alternate ways of approaching the situation; apply theories and other knowledge to the case; and discuss it from different points of view. Rather than describing the scenario in print form, short segments of a digital recording, a video from YouTube, and other media clips can also be used to present the scenario.

In a portfolio students collect materials they have developed in the course that provide documentation that they have met the course outcomes. Portfolios are valuable for assessment because they contain the evidence for judging if students have met the outcomes of the course.

Conferences are planned discussions about a topic. These include pre- and post-clinical conferences, interprofessional conferences, and other types of seminars in which the student participates. In a conference students can develop their oral communication skills and ability to lead and engage others in discussing an issue or a problem and deciding on actions to take.

Group projects encourage cooperative and active learning, teamwork, and communication, among other outcomes. Some group projects are short term, with students meeting in class, online, or out of class for the time it takes to develop the product such as a poster or group presentation. Other groups are long term, for example, the length of the course, for cooperative learning purposes. Group projects can be assessed in three ways: (1) a group grade can be determined, and each student in the group receives that grade; (2) students can specify their contributions to the final group product, complete a self-assessment of their participation, or evaluate each other's contributions, and the teacher can incorporate those contributions into the grade; or (3) students can prepare a group and an individual product, with both of these graded.

With simulations students can analyze scenarios and make decisions about actions to take, demonstrate techniques and skills, and implement care. These activities and others completed in a simulation can be assessed for feedback to students and for summative grading. Standardized patients are actors trained to portray the role of a patient with a specific condition. With standardized patients, students can be assessed on interpersonal and communication skills, history and physical examination techniques, and other competencies. Another assessment method is an OSCE. With OSCEs students rotate through stations where they perform a skill or activity, analyze cases or are tested on their knowledge and ability to apply it in scenarios, and interact with standardized patients.

An important outcome of a nursing education program at all levels is the ability of students to evaluate their own learning and performance. With this self-reflection students can identify areas in which further learning and development need to occur.

REFERENCES

Adamshick, P., & August-Brady, M. (2012). Reclaiming the essence of nursing: The meaning of an immersion experience in Honduras for RN to bachelor of science students. *Journal of Professional Nursing, 28,* 190–198. doi:10.1016/j.profnurs.2011.11.011

American Association of Colleges of Nursing. (2006). *The essentials of doctoral education for advanced nursing practice.* Washington, DC: Author.

American Association of Colleges of Nursing. (2008). *The essentials of baccalaureate education for professional nursing practice.* Washington, DC: Author.

American Association of Colleges of Nursing. (2011). *The essentials of master's education in nursing.* Washington, DC: Author.

Anderson, L. W. (Ed.), Krathwohl, D. R. (Ed.), Airasian, P. W., Cruikshank, K. A., Mayer, R. E., Pintrich, P. R., . . . Wittrock, M. C. (2001). *A taxonomy for learning, teaching, and assessing: A revision of Bloom's Taxonomy of Educational Objectives* (Complete edition). New York, NY: Longman.

Benner, P. E., Sutphen, M., Leonard, V., & Day, L. (2010). *Educating nurses: A call for radical transformation.* San Francisco, CA: Jossey-Bass.

Billings, D. M., & Halstead, J. A. (2009). *Teaching in nursing: A guide for faculty* (3rd ed.). St. Louis, MO: Saunders.

Bloom, B. S., Englehart, M. D., Furst, E. J., Hill, W. H., & Krathwohl, D. R. (1956). *Taxonomy of educational objectives: The classification of educational goals. Handbook I: Cognitive domain.* White Plains, NY: Longman.

Bourgault, A. M., Mundy, C., & Joshua, T. (2013). Comparison of audio vs. written feedback on clinical assignments of nursing students. *Nursing Education Perspectives, 34,* 43–46.

Buckley, S., Coleman, J., Davison, I., Khan, K. S., Zamora, J., Malick, S., . . . Sayers, J. (2009). The educational effects of portfolios on undergraduate student learning: A Best Evidence Medical Education (BEME) systematic review. BEME Guide No. 11. *Medical Teacher, 31,* 282–298. doi:10.1080/01421590902889897

Carpenter, L. J., & Garcia, A. A. (2012). Assessing outcomes of a study abroad course for nursing students. *Nursing Education Perspectives, 33,* 85–89. Retrieved from http://dx.doi .org/10.5480/1536-5026-33.2.85

Chan, Z. C. Y. (2013). A systematic review of critical thinking in nursing education. *Nurse Education Today, 33,* 236–240. doi:10.1016/j.nedt.2013.01.007

Clifton, A., & Mann, C. (2011). Can YouTube enhance student nurse learning? *Nurse Education Today, 31,* 311–313. doi:10.1016/j.nedt.2010.10.004

Cooper, C., Taft, L. B., & Thelen, M. (2004). Examining the role of technology in learning: An evaluation of online clinical conferencing. *Journal of Professional Nursing, 20,* 160–166.

Daley, B. J., & Torre, D. M. (2010). Concept maps in medical education: An analytical literature review. *Medical Education, 44*, 440–448. doi:10.1111/j.1365-2923.2010.03628.x

Davies, S. M., Reitmaier, A. B., Smith, L. R., & Mangan-Danckwart, D. (2013). Capturing intergenerativity: The use of student reflective journals to identify learning within an undergraduate course in gerontological nursing. *Journal of Nursing Education, 52*, 139–149. doi:10.3928/01484834-20120213-01

Day, L. (2011). Using unfolding case studies in a subject-centered classroom. *Journal of Nursing Education, 50*, 447–452. doi:10.3928/01484834-20110517-03

Dreifuerst, K. T. (2012). Using debriefing for meaningful learning to foster development of clinical reasoning in simulation. *Journal of Nursing Education, 51*, 326–333. doi:10.3928/01484834-20120409-02

Gaberson, K. B., & Oermann, M. H. (2010). *Clinical teaching strategies in nursing* (3rd ed.). New York, NY: Springer Publishing Company.

Gagnon, J. J., & Roberge, G. D. (2012). Dissecting the journey: Nursing student experiences with collaboration during the group work process. *Nurse Education Today, 32*, 945–950. doi:10.1016/j.nedt.2011.10.019

Harding, M. M. (2012). Efficacy of progression testing in predicting nursing student academic success. *Journal of Nursing Education and Practice, 2*(2). doi:10.5430/jnep.v2n2p137

Harrison, E. (2012). How to develop well-written case studies. *Nurse Educator, 37*, 67–70. doi:10.1097/NNE.0b013e3182461ba2

Hawkins, R. E., & Boulet, J. R. (2008). Direct observation: Standardized patients. In E. S. Holmboe & R. E. Hawkins, *Practical guide to the evaluation of clinical competence* (pp. 102–118). Philadelphia, PA: Mosby Elsevier.

Heroff, K. (2009). Guidelines for a progression and remediation policy using standardized tests to prepare associate degree nursing students for the NCLEX-RN at a rural community college. *Teaching and Learning in Nursing, 4*(3), 79–86. doi:10.1016/j.teln.2008.12.002

Holmboe, E. S., Davis, M. H., & Carraccio, C. (2008). Portfolios. In E. S. Holmboe & R. E. Hawkins, *Practical guide to the evaluation of clinical competence* (pp. 86–101). Philadelphia, PA: Mosby Elsevier.

Hunter Revell, S. M. (2012). Concept maps and nursing theory: A pedagogical approach. *Nurse Educator, 37*, 131–135. doi:10.1097/NNE.0b013e31825041ba

Iwasiw, C. L., Goldenberg, D., & Andrusyszyn, M-A. (2009). *Curriculum development in nursing education* (2nd ed.). Boston, MA: Jones and Bartlett.

Kardong-Edgren, S. (2013). A wake up call with an Objective Structured Clinical Examination. *Clinical Simulation in Nursing, 9*, e3–e4. Retrieved from http://dx.doi.org/10.1016/j.ecns.2012.11.002

Kirkpatrick, J. M., & DeWitt, D. A. (2009). Strategies for assessing/evaluating learning outcomes. In D. M. Billings & J. A. Halstead. *Teaching in nursing: A guide for faculty* (3rd ed., pp. 409–428). St. Louis, MO: Saunders.

Koh, L. C. (2008). Refocusing formative feedback to enhance learning in pre-registration nurse education. *Nurse Education in Practice, 8*, 223–230. doi:10.1016/j.nepr.2007.08.002

Langley, M., & Brown, S. (2010). Perceptions of the use of reflective learning journals in online graduate nursing education. *Nursing Education Perspectives, 31*, 12–17. doi:10.1043/1536-5026-31.1.12

Lasater, K. (2011). Clinical judgment: The last frontier for evaluation. *Nurse Education in Practice, 11*, 86–92. doi:10.1016/j.nepr.2010.11.013

Lasater, K., & Nielsen, A. (2009). Reflective journaling for development of clinical judgment. *Journal of Nursing Education, 48*, 40–44.

Lee, W., Chiang, C. H., Liao, I. C., Lee, M. L., Chen, S. L., & Liang, T. (2013). The longitudinal effect of concept map teaching on critical thinking of nursing students. *Nurse Education Today, 33*, 1219–1223. doi:10.1016/j.nedt.2012.06.010

Luthy, K. E., Peterson, N. E., Lassetter, J. H., & Callister, L. C. (2009). Successfully incorporating writing across the curriculum with advanced writing in nursing. *Journal of Nursing Education, 48*, 54–59.

Mårtensson, G., & Löfmark, A. (2013, February 7). Implementation and student evaluation of clinical final examination in nursing education. *Nurse Education Today*. [Epub ahead of print]. doi:10.1016/j.nedt.2013.01.003

McWilliam, P., & Botwinski, C. (2010). Developing a successful nursing objective structured clinical examination. *Journal of Nursing Education, 49,* 36–41. doi:10.3928/01484834-20090915-01

Miller, M. D., Linn, R. L., & Gronlund, N. E. (2009). *Measurement and assessment in teaching* (10th ed.). Upper Saddle River, NJ: Prentice Hall.

Nickitas, D. M. (2012). Asking questions and appreciating inquiry: A winning strategy for the nurse educator and professional nurse learner. *Journal of Continuing Education in Nursing, 43,* 106–110. doi:10.3928/00220124-20111201-01

Nitko, A. J., & Brookhart, S. M. (2011). *Educational assessment of students* (6th ed.). Upper Saddle River, NJ: Pearson.

Noonan, M. (2013). The ethical considerations associated with group work assessments. *Nurse Education Today, 33,* 1422–1427. doi:10.1016/j.nedt.2012.11.006

Nulty, D. D., Mitchell, M. L., Jeffrey, C. A., Henderson, A., & Groves, M. (2011). Best Practice Guidelines for use of OSCEs: Maximising value for student learning. *Nurse Education Today, 31,* 145–151. doi:10.1016/j.nedt.2010.05.006

Oermann, M. H. (2006). Short written assignments for clinical nursing courses. *Nurse Educator, 31,* 228–231.

Oermann, M. H. (2008). Using short cases for teaching "thinking" in a nursing course. In N. Facione & P. Facione (Eds.), *Critical thinking and clinical reasoning in the health sciences: An international multidisciplinary teaching anthology* (pp. 123–129). Millbrae, CA: California Academic Press.

Oermann, M. H. (2013). Enhancing writing in online education. In K. H. Frith & D. J. Clark (Eds.), *Distance education in nursing* (3rd ed., pp. 145–162). New York, NY: Springer Publishing Company.

Oermann, M. H., & Gaberson, K. B. (2014). *Evaluation and testing in nursing education* (4th ed.). New York, NY: Springer Publishing Company.

Oermann, M. H., Kardong-Edgren, S., Odom-Maryon, T. Hallmark, B., Hurd, D., Rogers, N., . . . Smart, D. (2011). Deliberate practice of motor skills in nursing education: CPR as exemplar. *Nursing Education Perspectives, 32,* 311–315.

Oermann, M. H., Saewert, K. J., Charasika, M., & Yarbrough, S. S. (2009). Assessment and grading practices in schools of nursing: National survey findings Part I. *Nursing Education Perspectives, 30,* 274–278.

Parsons, M. E., Hawkins, K. S., Hercinger, M., Todd, M., Manz, J. A., & Fang, X. (2012). Improvement in scoring consistency for the Creighton Simulation Evaluation Instrument. *Clinical Simulation in Nursing, 8*(6), e233–e238.

Popil, I. (2011). Promotion of critical thinking by using case studies as teaching method. *Nurse Education Today, 31,* 204–207. doi:10.1016/j.nedt.2010.06.002

Rutherford-Hemming, T., & Jennrich, J.A. (2013). Using standardized patients to strengthen nurse practitioner competency in the clinical setting. *Nursing Education Perspectives, 34,* 118–121.

Scalese, R. J., & Issenberg, S. B. (2008). Simulation-based assessment. In E. S. Holmboe & R. E. Hawkins, *Practical guide to the evaluation of clinical competence* (pp. 179–195). Philadelphia, PA: Mosby Elsevier.

Schmidt, R. A., & Lee, T.D. (2005). *Motor control and learning: A behavioral emphasis* (4th ed.). Champaign, IL: Human Kinetics.

Schuessler, J. B., Wilder, S., & Byrd, L. W. (2012). Reflective journaling and development of cultural humility in students. *Nursing Education Perspectives, 33,* 96–99.

Shiu, A. T. Y., Chan, C. W. H., Lam, P., Lee, J., & Kwong, A. N. L. (2012). Baccalaureate nursing students' perceptions of peer assessment of individual contributions to a group project: A case study. *Nurse Education Today, 32,* 214–218. doi:10.1016/j.nedt.2011.03.008

Tanner, C. A. (2006). Thinking like a nurse: A research-based model of clinical judgment in nursing. *Journal of Nursing Education, 45,* 204–211.

Terry, L. M. (2012). Service user involvement in nurse education: A report on using online discussions with a service user to augment his digital story. *Nurse Education Today, 32,* 161–166. doi:10.1016/j.nedt.2011.06.006

Torre, D. M., Durning, S. J., & Daley, B. J. (2013). Twelve tips for teaching with concept maps in medical education. *Medical Teacher, 35,* 201–208. doi:10.3109/0142159X.2013.759644

Troxler, H., Vann, J. J., & Oermann, M. H. (2011). How baccalaureate nursing programs teach writing. *Nursing Forum, 46*, 280–288. doi:10.1111/j.1744-6198.2011.00242.x

Vogt, M. A., Chavez, R., & Schaffner, B. (2011). Baccalaureate nursing student experiences at a camp for children with diabetes: the impact of a service-learning model. *Pediatric Nursing, 2*, 69–73.

Wittmann-Price, R. A., Reap Thompson, B., Sutton, S., & Eskew, S. (2013). *Nursing concept care maps for safe patient care*. Philadelphia, PA: F. A. Davis.

The Writing Across the Curriculum Clearinghouse. (2011a). *What is writing in the disciplines?* Retrieved from http://wac.colostate.edu/intro/pop2e.cfm

The Writing across the Curriculum Clearinghouse. (2011b). *What is writing to learn?* Retrieved from http://wac.colostate.edu/intro/pop2d.cfm

Developing and Using Tests

KATHLEEN B. GABERSON

A test is a measurement instrument, designed to assess learners' knowledge and cognitive abilities. Teachers use test results to make important educational judgments and decisions that affect learners, teachers, patients, future employers, and the educational program. Like every measurement instrument, a test must produce relevant and consistent results to form the basis for sound inferences about what learners know and can do. Good planning, careful test construction, proper administration, accurate scoring, and sound interpretation of scores are essential for producing useful test results. This chapter presents a brief discussion of assessment concepts that influence the quality of test results, and then describes the process of planning, constructing, administering, scoring, and analyzing tests.

ASSESSMENT QUALITY OF TESTS

Like any measurement instrument, a test should produce relevant, accurate results. A teacher who constructs a test or decides to use an existing test must be confident in its assessment quality. Two main considerations of the quality of a test are assessment validity and reliability.

ASSESSMENT VALIDITY

Older definitions of validity characterized it as a quality of the test itself; a test was considered to be valid to the extent that it measured the variable of interest. The current concept of validity focuses on the accuracy or appropriateness of inferences about test results and how those results are used. This understanding of assessment validity therefore focuses on the consequences of testing: Do teachers draw relevant, meaningful conclusions about learners' knowledge and abilities based on their test scores, and what are the intended and unintended consequences of those conclusions (Miller, Linn, & Gronlund, 2009; Nitko & Brookhart, 2011; Oermann & Gaberson, 2014)?

Validity is not an either/or condition; the degree of assessment validity for a test depends on the purpose of the test and how the results will be used in educational decision making. A test can be used for different purposes, and inferences about test results can have greater validity for one purpose than for another. For example, the results of a standardized achievement test in pediatric nursing might be highly valid for the purpose of evaluating the quality of the pediatric nursing course and the effectiveness of the teaching, but have low validity for the purpose of assigning final grades for students who completed the course (Oermann & Gaberson, 2014). Teachers can have greater confidence in the validity of their interpretation and use of test scores when they collect evidence of four major considerations for validation: content, construct, assessment-criterion relationships, and consequences (Miller et al., 2009).

The purpose of *content validation* is to determine the extent to which test items accurately represent a particular content domain. A test contains only a sample of all possible items about a content domain that could be written, but teachers usually want to generalize from that sample to the universe of items. Thus, if a student correctly answers 89% of items on a community health nursing test, the teacher usually infers that the student would answer correctly 89% of all items related to that content domain (Oermann & Gaberson, 2014). However, because desired learning outcomes in nursing education programs involve integration of complex abilities, it usually is not possible to make such specific generalizations (Miller et al., 2009). A process for generating test items that adequately represent the desired content domain, the construction of a test blueprint, will be described later in this chapter.

Construct validation concerns the extent to which it is possible to make inferences from test results to more general abilities and characteristics. A construct is a theoretical construction that can be inferred from an observed behavior (e.g., clinical reasoning). Construct validation involves two fundamental issues: construct representation and construct relevance (Miller et al., 2009). If test items do not adequately represent important elements of the construct, assessment validity is decreased. For instance, a test that requires students to solve problems defined only by the teacher is an inadequate representation of the construct of clinical problem solving, because a student's ability to identify clinical problems is an essential aspect of the construct (Oermann & Gaberson, 2014).

Tests that also measure abilities unrelated to the construct of interest, such as familiarity with cultural colloquialisms, spelling skill, or writing ability, also decrease assessment validity. Evidence of construct representation and relevance should be collected during the test development process by clearly defining the meaning of the construct. Other methods include comparing test results of groups known to possess different levels of the ability being measured, comparing test results before and after instruction, and correlating test results with other measures of the same construct (Miller et al., 2009).

Assessment-criterion relationship considerations focus on the extent to which test results (the assessment) predict performance on another assessment (the criterion measure), either in the future (predictive) or at the same time (concurrent). Nursing faculties often use scores from standardized comprehensive exams at the end of a program to predict performance on high-stakes tests such as NCLEX® and certification exams, but they rarely have use for concurrent validity evidence for teacher-made tests (Oermann & Gaberson, 2014).

Concern about the social consequences of testing leads to the need for *consideration of consequences*. All testing has both intended and unintended consequences. Use of standardized testing programs can have the intended effect of identifying students who are likely to pass licensure or certification exams, but the unintended effect might be to increase student anxiety (Oermann & Gaberson, 2014). Assessment validity must take into account both intended and unintended consequences of testing.

Multiple factors influence test validity. Some characteristics of the test itself, such as clerical errors, unclear directions, too few test items, and a noticeable pattern of correct responses, might decrease the validity of inferences made about the test scores. Student factors such as lack of motivation to perform well, test anxiety, illness, or an emotionally upsetting experience might also affect students' performance on tests and thereby decrease measurement validity. Finally, factors associated with the administration and scoring of tests can lower assessment reliability. Such factors include allowing insufficient time for testing, errors in scoring, variability in the amount of aid to students who ask questions during an exam, and failing to follow the protocol for administering a standardized test (Oermann & Gaberson, 2014).

ASSESSMENT RELIABILITY

Reliability concerns the consistency, stability, or reproducibility of test scores. Measurement reliability boosts the teacher's confidence in assessment results. However, perfect consistency is not possible due to the influence of many extraneous factors:

- Instability of the behavior being assessed (e.g., emotional or health status)
- Varying samples of tasks among different forms of the assessment
- Varying assessment conditions
- Inconsistent scoring procedures (Oermann & Gaberson, 2014)

Inconsistency introduces an unknown amount of error into every assessment result. Reliability estimates therefore gauge the amount of measurement error present under varying conditions. The smaller the measurement error, the greater the assessment reliability (Miller et al., 2009).

Assessment reliability is an essential condition for assessment validity. "Teachers cannot make valid inferences from inconsistent assessment results" (Oermann & Gaberson, 2014, p. 37). However, highly consistent results do not guarantee a high degree of validity, because the assessment might be reliably measuring the wrong construct. Assessment reliability only provides the consistency that makes valid inferences possible (Miller et al., 2009).

Because of different types of consistency, there are different methods of determining assessment reliability:

- Stability: consistency over time
- Equivalence: consistency among different forms of the assessment
- Internal consistency: consistency within the assessment itself
- Interrater reliability: consistency of judgments among different raters (Oermann & Gaberson, 2014)

For teacher-made tests, the most commonly used and appropriate method of estimating reliability is internal consistency, also known as the split-length or half-length method. This method shows the degree to which very similar results are obtained from both halves of the same test. Longer tests tend to yield higher reliability estimates because they sample the content domain more fully, so a split-half reliability estimate usually underestimates the true reliability of the whole test. However, this underestimate can be corrected statistically. It is important to remember that a reliability estimate is not a stable property of the test itself; it will fluctuate each time the test is used with different groups of students.

Various factors can affect assessment reliability, arising from three main sources:

- The test itself: test length, homogeneity, and technical quality of test items
- The test-taker: heterogeneity of student ability, test-taking skill, motivation
- Testing conditions: test security (prevention of cheating), adequacy of time (Oermann & Gaberson, 2014)

The degree of reliability desired depends on factors such as the importance of the decisions made, based on test scores; the consequences of such decisions; and whether it is possible to reverse the decision later. For most teacher-made tests, a reliability estimate of 0.60 to 0.85 is desirable (Miller et al., 2009).

TEST PLANNING

Too often, teachers spend too little time and effort preparing tests, and the result is a test with clerical errors and items that are ambiguous, irrelevant to the content domain, and too easy or too difficult. Adequate planning for test construction and careful critique of the completed test items are essential for tests to produce reliable results that can be used to make valid judgments about how much students know about a content domain. This section of the chapter will describe the steps involved in planning and constructing a test.

PURPOSE OF THE TEST AND STUDENTS TO BE TESTED

Decisions involved in planning a test should be based on the purpose of the test and characteristics of the students to be tested. Purpose relates to why the test is given, what it is supposed to assess, and how the results will be used. If a test is intended to measure the degree to which students have met course learning objectives, and the test score will be used to determine a grade, the purpose is summative. A test designed to provide feedback to staff nurses about how much they learned during a continuing education program has a formative purpose. Understanding the characteristics of the learners to be tested helps a teacher determine which test item formats to use, how many items to include, and how to score the test. Student factors that might influence these decisions include English language literacy, academic program level, and previous testing experience, among others (Oermann & Gaberson, 2014).

TEST LENGTH

The ideal length of a test (i.e., the number of test items or total possible points) depends on a number of variables, including the test's purpose, the ability level of the students, the available testing time, and the desired reliability of test results. As noted earlier, longer tests usually produce more reliable results because they sample the content domain more fully. Test length usually is limited by the length of a classroom period. The number of test items that can be completed in a fixed time period should take into account the nature of the assessment tasks. Items with complex assessment tasks, such as analyzing patient data, take more time to complete; therefore, fewer items of those types can be included on a test with a fixed administration time. The majority of students working at their normal pace should be able to complete a test of the appropriate length within the allotted time (Miller et al., 2009; Nitko & Brookhart, 2011).

DIFFICULTY AND DISCRIMINATION LEVEL

The expected difficulty of a test and its ability to distinguish among different levels of achievement are related to the purpose of the test and the way in which results will be interpreted and used. The difficulty of individual test items depends on the complexity of their assessment tasks, the ability of the students, and the quality of teaching. For tests with results that will be interpreted in a criterion-related way, as are most tests in nursing education programs, the ideal difficulty level correctly classifies students according to whether they met the criterion or not. That is, even if a test item is relatively easy, meaning that the majority of students answered it correctly, if students whose total scores met the criterion tended to answer that item correctly and students who failed to meet the criterion tended to answer incorrectly, the item difficulty is appropriate (Miller et al., 2009; Oermann & Gaberson, 2014).

Item difficulty can only be estimated in advance. Teachers with more experience in assessing the selected content domain and with greater knowledge of their students' abilities usually make more accurate estimates. After the test is administered and scored, a teacher can compute the actual item difficulty levels, compare them with the expected difficulty, and revise them for future use if they are much more or less difficult than anticipated.

The ability of each test item to distinguish between students who have greater knowledge of the content domain and those who have less knowledge is its discrimination power. In general, high discriminating power indicates better-quality test items, although this does not indicate item validity. Discrimination power is related to item difficulty. Items that are answered correctly or incorrectly by all students do not discriminate between knowledgeable and less knowledgeable students; items with moderate difficulty tend to have maximum discriminating power (Oermann & Gaberson, 2014).

ITEM FORMATS

Though some students might prefer multiple-choice items or believe that they do better on essay items, the desired learning outcomes, the specific competency to be assessed, and students' ability level should determine the teacher's choice of item formats. Despite common beliefs, no one item format is better than another for testing nursing students, and academic policies that mandate the use of a specific item format on tests do more harm than good. A test that contains several item formats gives students greater opportunity to demonstrate their competency than tests with only one item format (Nitko & Brookhart, 2011).

Each item format has advantages and disadvantages, as explained later in this chapter. Some desired learning outcomes are better measured with certain item formats. For example, a multiple-choice item would be inappropriate to measure a desired learning outcome such as "discuss the comparative advantages and disadvantages of wet-to-dry and autolytic dressings for Stage III pressure ulcers;" an essay format would be more suitable. Students should have adequate practice with the item format types that a teacher will use on tests; this might be accomplished by using various item formats in classroom exercises.

Another common belief is that certain item types assess more objectively than others. Although true-false, multiple-choice, and matching items are often described as "objective," objectivity refers to the manner of scoring, not the format of the item (Miller et al., 2009). Objectively scored items will yield the same total score as long as the same answer key is used by multiple scorers or by the same scorer on repeated occasions. Subjectively scored items such as essay items require a scorer's judgment to determine the extent of correctness and produce more score variability.

SCORING PROCEDURES

The choice of item format affects the choice of test scoring procedures. Use of essay and short-answer items requires hand-scoring, whether the answers are recorded on the test itself or on a separate answer sheet. Answers to multiple-choice, true-false, and matching items are usually recorded on a separate answer sheet that can be hand-scored or, more frequently, electronically scanned. Electronic scoring has the advantage of speed as well as the ability to allow computer-generated test and item analysis reports. The teacher must decide whether available resources suggest the use of hand- or electronic scoring (Oermann & Gaberson, 2014).

TEST BLUEPRINT

The best way to ensure that a teacher will be able to make valid judgments about the meaning of test scores is to construct a test blueprint before beginning to choose or write test items. A test blueprint, also called a test plan, or table of specifications, guides the teacher to write items at the appropriate level to test the desired content areas. Without a test blueprint, teachers often rely on ease of construction in writing items. This often results in tests with a limited sample of assessment tasks that might omit outcomes that are more important but more difficult to assess (Miller et al., 2009).

Essential elements of a test blueprint include (a) a list of major topics or learning outcomes that the test will assess, (b) the level of complexity of assessment tasks, and (c) the emphasis that each topic or learning outcome will have as indicated by the number or percentage of items or points (Oermann & Gaberson, 2014). Figure 11.1 is an example of a blueprint for a unit test on preoperative nursing care. The row headings along the left margin are the main topic areas to be tested, and, in this case, they comprise a general outline of content. A more detailed content outline, a list of relevant learning outcomes, or both can be used instead. The column headings across the top are selected from an updated taxonomy of cognitive objectives (Anderson & Krathwohl, 2001); the teacher who prepared this blueprint chose not to use all of the cognitive levels, but other teachers might use all levels or a different taxonomy. The body of the blueprint is a grid formed by the intersections of topic areas and cognitive levels. The cells in the grid represent one or more test items to be developed related to that content area and cognitive level, and the

FIGURE 11.1 Example of a test blueprint for a unit test on preoperative nursing care.

Content	Cognitive Level				Total Points
	K	C	Ap	An	
I. Preoperative nursing assessment		4	6	5	15
II. Patient safety	2	3	1	2	8
III. Legal and ethical issues		2	2	2	6
IV. Planning nursing care		3	2	3	8
V. Patient and family teaching		2	4		6
VI. Documentation	2	3	4	4	13
Total points	4	17	19	16	56

An, analysis; Ap, application; C, comprehension; K, knowledge.

numbers represent the number of points allotted to that cell. The teacher should judge the appropriate emphasis and balance of content areas and cognitive levels to determine which cells should be filled and by how many points; some cells can remain blank, as in this example (Oermann & Gaberson, 2014).

A test blueprint is a useful tool for guiding a teacher to select or write test items at the appropriate level to assess important content areas and learning outcomes. It also should be used to inform students about the nature of the test and how to prepare for it. Although they might have a general idea of what content areas will be tested, students often lack awareness of the cognitive levels at which they will be assessed. Although instructional objectives should inform students of the expected level of performance, they might not be able to interpret these objectives accurately. Some teachers worry that sharing the test blueprint with students will encourage them to study only the content areas that will be tested. This is not a harmful outcome: with knowledge of the content areas to be emphasized most heavily, students can focus their time and energy on studying those content areas and preparing for assessment tasks at the appropriate levels.

The beginning of the course or unit of study is the best time to share the test blueprint with students. Teachers might need to explain the blueprint and how students should use it to plan their test preparation. If the teacher must make modifications to the blueprint, for example, because of a class cancellation due to weather emergency at the end of a semester, those changes should also be communicated to students (Nitko & Brookhart, 2011; Oermann & Gaberson, 2014).

WRITING THE TEST ITEMS

The teacher should select or write test items that correspond to each numbered cell in the test blueprint. Regardless of item format, teachers should consider the following general rules that contribute to the quality of test items:

1. *Every item should measure something important.* Some teachers include test items that test trivial or obscure content with the intent of determining which students have read all of the assigned material. However, if this content is important, it will be represented as such on the test blueprint, and all students will be prepared to demonstrate the required competency. Others write filler items to meet a targeted number of items (most frequently, 100). There is no reason to set a fixed number of items or points on all tests, other than for ease of calculating a percentage score. It is better to have a smaller number of test items that assess knowledge of important content than to add meaningless items that serve only to increase test-taking time and that might make valid interpretation of scores more difficult (Oermann & Gaberson, 2014).

2. *Every item should have a correct answer.* "Correct" means that experts would agree on the answer (Miller et al., 2009). The teacher must follow the distinction between fact and belief; in some cases, the correct or best response to an item might be a matter of opinion. Citing a specific authority in the item, such as "according to the AORN Recommended Practices," prevents students' justifiably arguing a response other than the one the teacher expected. Items that ask students to state an opinion on an issue and support that position with evidence should not be scored as correct or incorrect, but with variable credit based on the rationale given and soundness of reasoning (Oermann & Gaberson, 2014).

3. *Use simple, clear, concise, grammatically correct language.* Clear wording of test items is essential for students' understanding of the assessment task required. Using simple words and sentence structure is challenging when writing about complex, highly

technical content. The goal is to include enough detail to communicate the intent of the test item but to avoid extraneous words and complex syntax that only increase reading time and that might confuse nonnative English speakers. Linguistic simplification includes using the active voice and simple, short sentences and avoiding negative forms and conditional and subordinate clauses (Bosher & Bowles, 2008). Because of current concerns that even native English speakers are entering postsecondary programs with low reading proficiency, linguistic simplification is likely to benefit all students.

4. *Avoid jargon, slang, and unnecessary abbreviations.* Although health care professionals frequently use jargon and acronyms informally in the practice environment, informal language in a test item might fail to communicate accurately the meaning of the item. Many students are at least somewhat anxious when taking tests, and they might not interpret an abbreviation correctly in terms of the context in which it is used. For example, does RA mean rheumatoid arthritis, right atrium, or right arm? If the desired learning outcome is to define commonly used health care abbreviations, it is appropriate to use the abbreviation in the item and to ask the student to select or supply the definition. As noted, slang, jargon, acronyms, and abbreviations contribute to linguistic complexity for nonnative English speakers. Also, given growing concern about health care errors attributed to poor communication, nurse educators should use only those abbreviations approved for use in clinical settings (Oermann & Gaberson, 2014).

5. *Use positive wording.* Avoid using words like *no*, *not*, and *except* in test items. Negative wording is particularly difficult for nonnative English speakers to understand, but test-anxious students also might not read such sentences accurately. Negative forms are particularly confusing in true-false items. Teachers should avoid asking students to identify the incorrect alternative as the correct response to the item, as in this example of a multiple-choice stem: "Which of the following is NOT an indication for high-level disinfection of surgical instruments and equipment?" This wording tends to reinforce the incorrect alternative, and it might cause confusion when students try to recall the correct information (Oermann & Gaberson, 2014).

6. *Items should not contain irrelevant cues to correct answers.* Flaws in item construction can allow test-wise students to improve their chances of guessing the correct answer when they do not know it, interfering with valid interpretations of their scores. Irrelevant cues include

- A multiple-choice stem that is grammatically inconsistent with one or more alternatives.
- Repeating important words from the stem in only the correct answer.
- Using qualifiers such as "never" and "always" in incorrect alternatives.
- Having a consistent pattern of correct answers being longer than incorrect alternatives or true statements being longer than false statements.
- Using the same response position consistently for correct answers (Oermann & Gaberson, 2014).

7. *No item should depend on another item for meaning.* Items should not be linked such that students who answer one item incorrectly will likely answer the related item incorrectly. An example of such linking is:

1. Which drug should be available in case of malignant hyperthermia? _____
2. What solvent should be used to mix the drug in Item 1? _____

However, a series of items that relate to a particular context such as a diagram, case study, or graph are called interpretive or context-dependent items. This is not a violation of the rule because the items relate to a common context, not to each other (Oermann & Gaberson, 2014).

8. *Eliminate unnecessary information.* Including fictitious patient names or initials in test items increases reading time unnecessarily, might be a distraction from the items' intent, and might introduce cultural bias. If the purpose of an item is to assess whether students can evaluate the relevance of clinical data and use only relevant information to arrive at the correct answer, extraneous data other than patient names can be included (Oermann & Gaberson, 2014).

9. *Request peer critique of the test item.* Colleagues who teach the same content or who are skilled in the technical aspects of item writing are the best critics of newly written test items. If these colleagues are not available for critique, the teacher should set the items aside and return to them in a few days with a fresh perspective to identify clerical errors or lack of clarity (Oermann & Gaberson, 2014).

10. *Prepare more test items than the test blueprint calls for.* This will permit replacement of items discarded in the critique process. Unused extra test items can be kept in a test item bank for future use (Oermann & Gaberson, 2014).

ITEM-WRITING PRINCIPLES FOR SPECIFIC ITEM FORMATS

In addition to the general item-writing rules described above, there are specific principles for writing test items of each format. The following discussion offers helpful suggestions for writing effective test items of various types. For a more in-depth discussion and specific guidelines for developing items of each type, see Oermann and Gaberson (2014).

TRUE–FALSE

A true–false item comprises a statement that the student must judge as true or false. Variations of this format include requiring students to explain why the statement is true or false, or to correct false statements. True–false items are most effective for testing recall of specific information or for understanding of a principle or concept. They are not useful for testing complex thinking and reasoning (Musial, Nieminen, Thomas, & Burke, 2009). Because these items require relatively little time to read, students can respond to a large number of them in a short period of time, allowing the teacher to sample a broad content area. The main disadvantage of true–false items is the 50% probability of guessing the correct answer. However, this probability pertains to a single test item; on a test with many items, the probability of obtaining an adequate score through guessing alone is small (Nitko & Brookhart, 2011).

Examples of true–false items are in Exhibit 11.1. Important principles to follow when constructing these items are (Oermann & Gaberson, 2014):

- Avoid testing recall of trivial information.
- Each statement should be unconditionally true or false without qualification.
- Avoid words such as *usually* and *often*, which typically occur in true statements, and *never, always, all,* or *none,* which are usually in false statements (Miller et al., 2009).
- Each item should include only one idea to be tested; multiple ideas often result in part of the statement being true and part being false.
- Avoid the use of negative wording, particularly in statements that are intended to be false.

EXHIBIT 11.1 Examples of True–False Items

- T F According to the AORN Recommended Practice for Surgical Attire, the scrub top should be donned before the cap. (F)
- T F The circulating nurse should check the position of the patient's feet before surgical drapes are applied. (T)
- T F The ordered preoperative antibiotic dose should be repeated if the procedure lasts 2 hours or more. (T)

- Attempt to make all true–false items similar in length. True items tend to be longer than false items because they often include more precise language.
- Use approximately the same number of true statements and false statements, or include slightly more false than true items, because false statements tend to have higher discrimination power (Waugh & Gronlund, 2013).
- Avoid ordering true–false items in a noticeable pattern, such as TTFF or TFTF.
- For variations in which students are expected to correct false items or supply an explanation for their judgment, award an additional point for correctly changing the wording or providing a satisfactory rationale.

MATCHING EXERCISES

Matching exercises comprise a series of homogeneous items (premises) with the same set of responses. They are most appropriate for assessing students' ability to classify and categorize information such as definitions of terms, generic and trade names of medications, or pharmacologic classifications (Miller et al., 2009). Important principles to follow when constructing matching exercises are listed below. A sample matching exercise is in Exhibit 11.2.

- Write unequal numbers of premises and responses to avoid giving a clue to the final match. Usually the list of responses is longer, but the use of a scannable answer sheet can limit the number of responses. In that case, the list of premises should be longer.

EXHIBIT 11.2 Sample Matching Exercise

Directions: For each description of a pressure ulcer in Column A, select the appropriate stage from Column B. Responses in Column B can be used once, more than once, or not at all.

Column A	Column B
(e) 1. Base of the ulcer is covered by slough or eschar or both	a. Stage I
(d) 2. Exposed bone or tendons are visible or directly palpable	b. Stage II
(b) 3. Shiny or dry shallow ulcer without sloughing or bruising	c. Stage III
(c) 4. Visible subcutaneous fat without exposure of bone or muscle	d. Stage IV
	e. Unstageable

- Keep the lists of premises and responses short. Miller et al. (2009) recommended four to seven items in each column.

- Place premises on the left and responses on the right. Premises usually are longer; students must read each premise and then search the responses for the correct match. The list of the responses therefore is read repeatedly, so short responses help students to find the correct answer quickly.

- Directions for each matching exercise should state the basis on which premises and responses should be matched, and whether each response can be used once, more than once, or not at all (Oermann & Gaberson, 2014).

MULTIPLE CHOICE AND MULTIPLE RESPONSE

Multiple-choice items can be used to assess many types of desired learning outcomes at various levels of the cognitive taxonomy, especially application and analysis. Well-written multiple-choice items include new information in the stem and require students to apply concepts and principles or use analytical thinking to respond to the item. Nursing students need to have experience with multiple-choice testing because they will encounter many of these items on licensure, certification, and other published tests (Oermann & Gaberson, 2014). However, as stated previously, this is not a good reason to use *only* multiple-choice items on nursing tests.

Each multiple-choice item comprises three parts: stem, correct answer, and distractors. The stem is a question or incomplete sentence that must be completed by one of the alternatives. The alternatives or options include the correct answer and a number of distractors. The correct or best answer is also called the keyed response because it is the alternative marked on the answer key. Distractors are incorrect alternatives that appear plausible to students who are unsure of the correct answer. Specific guidelines for writing each of these components are discussed next.

Whether the stem is a question or incomplete statement, it must communicate clearly the intent of the item. The stem should present a problem or issue that relates to an important learning outcome. The student should be able to read the stem and know what type of response the teacher expects (Nitko & Brookhart, 2011). Guidelines for writing the stem include (Oermann & Gaberson, 2014):

- Clearly present sufficient information for the problem to be solved. As a test of clarity and completeness, the item writer should cover the alternatives and judge whether the stem alone specifies what to look for in the alternatives.

- Avoid including extraneous information unless the purpose of the item is to assess students' ability to differentiate relevant from irrelevant data. Humorous content should be avoided because it can be confusing to nonnative English speakers.

- Do not use the stem to teach. The goal of testing is to assess learning, not to teach or reinforce information.

- Eliminate key words from the stem that would provide a cue to the correct answer, such as a word in the stem that can relate to the same concept as a word used in the answer, for example, *aging* and *elderly*.

- Avoid negative wording; ask for the correct or best answer rather than the only incorrect response, as previously discussed. If there is no acceptable alternative wording, consider revising the stem to a true–false, completion, or multiple-response format.

- Avoid ending a stem in the form of an incomplete sentence with "a" or "an" because these words provide clues as to whether the correct answer begins with a consonant or a vowel. Ending the stem with "a/an" is not a good remedy because students then must read each alternative with "a" and then again with "an."

- If the stem is an incomplete sentence, the alternatives should complete the statement at the end of the sentence. A blank in the middle of the sentence, which the correct answer is supposed to fill, acts as a barrier to reading comprehension (Nitko & Brookhart, 2011).

Alternatives are listed under the stem and can vary in number. The more options, the more discriminating the item, as long as all options are plausible. Most standardized tests use four alternatives, but for teacher-made tests, it is not necessary to have the same number of alternatives for every item. Most scannable answer sheets allow up to five alternatives, which reduces the chance of guessing the correct answer to 20%; however, it is challenging to write four plausible distracters. If the teacher can construct only two plausible distracters for one correct answer, a three-option item is certainly acceptable (Popham, 2012; Rodriguez, 2005; Tarrant & Ware, 2012). Guidelines for writing good alternatives include:

- Make all alternatives similar in length, detail, and complexity. The correct answer frequently is the longest because the teacher tends to include more details, which testwise students might recognize.

- Each alternative should contain the same number of parts. If the correct answer contains two parts (e.g., specific pieces of information), and each distracter contains only one part, this provides a cue to the testwise student.

- Alternatives should be grammatically consistent with each other and with the stem (if it is an incomplete sentence).

- All alternatives should sample the same content domain, such as nursing interventions, diagnostic test results, or assessment findings. Avoid including opposite responses in the alternatives because this often is a clue that the correct answer is one of the opposites.

- If words are repeated in each alternative, move them to the stem to decrease reading time. If alternatives contain several parts, such as clinical manifestations of a postoperative complication, and the same word or phrase appears in each alternative, that word or phrase should be moved to the stem.

- If the stem is a complete sentence or question, end it with the appropriate terminal punctuation and begin each alternative with a capital letter. If the alternatives complete an incomplete sentence in the stem, end the stem with a comma or colon as appropriate, begin each alternative with a lower-case letter, and use terminal punctuation at the end.

- Alternatives with ranges of numerical values should not overlap each other. If a portion of the range of values in one distractor is within the range of the correct answer, students might argue that there is more than one correct answer.

- Place each alternative on a separate line and all lines in one column under the stem. Usually items are numbered, and alternatives are lettered; this format helps students avoid making clerical errors when they use a separate answer sheet.

- Avoid using *none of the above* and *all of the above* as alternatives. If a student knows that at least one of the other options is true, *none of the above* can be eliminated;

likewise, if one option is known to be incorrect, *all of the above* is obviously incorrect. Teachers often use *all of the above* when they have difficulty constructing enough plausible distractors, but it is better to use three options (the correct answer and two plausible distractors) or a multiple-response format, to be described later in this chapter.

- If students are required to choose the best rather than the correct answer, the best answer should be supported by consistency among expert practitioners and in the scientific evidence (Oermann & Gaberson, 2014).

Multiple-response items allow students to select one or more options as the correct or best answer. These items might be in combined-response form (also known as multiple-multiple-choice, or complex multiple-choice), or they might simply allow students to indicate every correct alternative (if that option is provided by the electronic scanning software used). Because this item format is used on licensure, certification, and other types of standardized tests, students should have experience with the format during their educational programs. Guidelines for writing items of this variation include:

- In combined-response items, group the options logically rather than randomly to avoid combinations that are internally contradictory.
- Use options an equal number of times in each combination of alternatives. If one of the options appears in every combination, add this information to the stem. Limited use of one option can be a cue to the correct answer for the testwise student (Oermann & Gaberson, 2014).

Examples of multiple-choice and multiple-response items are in Exhibit 11.3.

EXHIBIT 11.3 Examples of Multiple-Choice and Multiple-Response Items

1. According to the Surgical Care Improvement Project, prophylactic antibiotics other than vancomycin should be administered:
   a. for at least 24 hours preoperatively
   b. for at least 72 hours postoperatively
   c. up to 2 hours before incision
   d. within 1 hour of incision
2. Common adverse medication reactions in elderly surgical patients include:
   1. confusion
   2. dry mouth
   3. headache
   4. nausea and vomiting
   5. respiratory depression
      a. 1, 3
      b. 2, 5
      c. 1, 2, 4
      d. 3, 4, 5
      e. 1, 2, 3, 4, 5

SHORT-ANSWER

Short-answer items require a word, phrase, or number as an answer. These occur in two formats: question and completion (also known as fill-in-the-blank). These items are best used to assess recall of specific information and ability to perform calculations. Short-answer items might ask students to label a diagram, identify specific items, or provide correct abbreviations for medical terms. A variation, ordered-response items, requires students to place a list of responses in the proper order. Completion items consist of a statement with a key word or phrase missing; the student must supply the missing material.

Examples of short-answer items are in Exhibit 11.4. Guidelines for writing these items include:

- Do not use verbatim material from textbooks and other readings; doing so can result in assessing only recall of information without comprehension.
- Construct the item so that only one unique word, phrase, or number will correctly complete it.
- Write items that are specific enough that they can be answered briefly. Think of the correct answer first and then write a question or statement to elicit that response. If more than one response could be correct, list all possible correct answers on the answer key.
- Items requiring mathematical calculations should specify the nature of the desired response and degree of specificity.
- For fill-in-the-blank items, place the blank at or near the end of the statement to make it easier for students to discern the intent of the item after reading it only once. Avoid giving grammatical clues such as "a" or "an" and singular or plural forms just before the blank. If more than one blank is used, blanks should be equal in length to avoid giving a clue to desired length of response. More than two blanks might not leave enough of a context for students to grasp the intent of the item.
- Direct students where to record their answers. Instead of filling in blanks within or at the end of the items, students can be asked to write their answers in blanks arranged in a column to the left or right of the item to facilitate scoring (Oermann & Gaberson, 2014).

EXHIBIT 11.4 Examples of Short-Answer Items

1. A patient weighs 220 lbs. You need to prepare an initial dose of 2.5 mg/kg of Dantrolene sodium. What is the correct dose in milligrams? _____ Show your work:
2. According to Spaulding classification, what level of items should receive a minimum of high-level disinfection? _____

ESSAY

Essay items call for a more lengthy response than short-answer ones. They are useful for assessing complex learning outcomes and higher levels of learning. Essay items are appropriate for assessing students' abilities to analyze (patient data, clinical situations, ethical issues); critique (scientific evidence, approaches to solving a problem); and develop (teaching plans, protocols, arguments for and against a position or decision).

Although responses to essay items require students to compose and write responses, the quality of their writing should not enter into the evaluation of their responses.

Limitations in using essay items include:

- Essay items do not provide a broad sample of a content domain. Because of the amount of time needed for students to organize and write their responses to essay items, teachers usually can include only a few of them on a test.

- Essay responses tend to be scored differently by different teachers (Miller et al., 2009) and by the same teacher at different times. Essay items that are highly structured and focused tend to produce greater reliability in scoring.

- Scoring essay responses might produce a carryover effect in which the teacher develops an impression about the student's knowledge and ability from one answer and tends to expect the same quality of response for the next essay item. For this reason, it is best to evaluate all student responses to one essay item before reading responses to the next one.

- Teachers can have the tendency to be influenced by general impressions of or by feelings about students when evaluating essay responses. These impressions and feelings create a halo effect that might influence the teacher's score. For this reason, the identity of the student who wrote each response should be masked until all responses are scored. Students' essay responses can be identified by assigned or selected numbers that are then matched to their names when scoring is complete.

- The teacher's judgment of essay responses often is affected by students' writing abilities. As previously mentioned, teachers should focus on the substance of essay responses and attempt to ignore writing style, grammar, and spelling (Nitko & Brookhart, 2011; Waugh & Gronlund, 2013).

- The first essay responses read in a scoring session tend to be scored higher than those read near the end, due to teacher fatigue and time constraints. This problem is called "rater drift." To prevent rater drift, teachers should read essay responses in random order, rearrange the order before scoring another item, and read each response twice before computing a score.

- Some teachers allow students to choose a subset of essay items to respond to. For example, from a set of six essay items, students are allowed to choose which four they want to answer. Miller et al. (2009) advised against this practice because, when students choose which items to answer, they actually are taking different tests, which affects measurement validity (Oermann & Gaberson, 2014).

In writing essay items, the teacher should: (a) develop items that require analysis, integration, and synthesis rather than summary of the content; (b) use clear wording to direct students to the intended response; (c) prepare students for an essay test by asking questions in class, clinical practice, and online that require clinical reasoning, synthesis of content from various sources, critique of opposing views, and comparison of approaches; (d) indicate the point value of each essay item, an approximate amount of time students should allot to answering it, or both. Students should spend more time responding to items that carry greater weight; and (e) write an ideal answer to each essay item while drafting it to determine whether it is clearly stated and could be answered in a reasonable timeframe. The teacher can save this ideal response to use when constructing a scoring rubric. Examples of essay items are in Exhibit 11.5.

EXHIBIT 11.5 Examples of Essay Items

1. Give three examples of circumstances in which perioperative personnel should wear personal protective equipment when handling used instruments and equipment. (3 points)
2. Critique arguments for and against the practice of suspending Do Not Resuscitate status when patients undergo surgery. Based on your critique, state which position you believe is the strongest and provide a rationale supporting your choice. (7 points)

Essay items can be scored by two methods, holistic and analytic. *Holistic scoring* involves reading the entire response and judging its overall quality. This can be done by comparing each student's response with those of other students and ranking them by degrees of quality. Answers are read to assess the overall quality of response (sometimes by comparing them to a model answer), and then sorted into piles representing different degrees of quality; each pile then receives a particular score. For *analytic scoring*, the teacher identifies the content that should be included in the answer and assigns a number of possible points for each content area. A scoring rubric can be developed that describes how points should be assigned for various degrees of completeness, logic, organization, and accuracy. Use of an analytic rubric also provides feedback to students about the quality of their essay responses (Oermann & Gaberson, 2014).

CONTEXT-DEPENDENT ITEM SETS

A context-dependent item set (also known as an interpretive exercise) is a group of test items that relate to the same introductory material. The introductory material might be a description of a clinical situation, a set of patient assessment findings or laboratory test results; a diagram; a graph; a table; a photograph; or excerpts from health care records, textbooks, or research reports. Students read, interpret, and analyze the introductory material and then respond to each test item related to it. The test items in the interpretive exercise can be in any item format, but all items in the same set should be the same format.

Context-dependent item sets are most appropriate for assessing higher level learning outcomes such as application of knowledge to novel situations, solving problems, making decisions, synthesizing information, and creating or developing new approaches. Interpretive items are also included on licensure, certification, and other standardized tests, so students should have some experience with this type of test item during their academic programs.

A sample context-dependent item set is provided in Exhibit 11.6. Suggestions for developing these item sets are:

- The introductory material or context should provide enough information for analysis without limiting or directing students' thinking or creativity. One approach is to draft the test items first and then construct introductory material that includes the essential information needed to respond to the items.

- The introductory material can include irrelevant as well as relevant information if the intent of the exercise is to assess the student's ability to select relevant data on which to base judgments. All information included, however, should appear logical and pertinent to the situation.

EXHIBIT 11.6 Sample Context-Dependent Item Set

Items 1 to 4 relate to the following situation:

An 82-year-old woman is scheduled for an open reduction and internal fixation of her right femur. She rates her pain at 4 on a 1 to 10 scale and has not received any preoperative sedation. Three days ago, on admission, an indwelling urinary catheter was inserted and it is now draining clear, light yellow urine. While transferring the patient to the OR bed, the perioperative RN notices a reddened area on her sacrum, approximately the size and shape of a silver dollar; the skin is intact with no blistering apparent, and it feels warm to touch. The patient is positioned supine on the fracture OR bed with the left leg supported in a padded stirrup. Her right arm is positioned over her chest in a sling and the left arm is on a padded arm board.

T F 1. According to the National Pressure Ulcer Advisory Panel definitions of pressure ulcers, the perioperative RN should document the lesion on the patient's sacrum as Stage I.

T F 2. This patient is at an increased risk for inability to give informed consent for the surgical procedure.

T F 3. The patient's position on the OR bed increases her risk of compression and stretch injury to the left sciatic nerve.

T F 4. According to the National Guideline Clearinghouse guideline for prevention of catheter-associated urinary tract infections, this patient has an increased risk of such an infection.

- All items in the set should relate directly to the introductory material; students should not be able to arrive at a correct or best answer without reading and analyzing the context.

- The length of the context should correspond to the number of items that relate to it. It is a waste of students' time to read a lengthy scenario before responding to only two test items related to it.

- Arrange the context-dependent item set so that it is clear to the students which items relate to the introductory material. Use a heading to indicate the item numbers in the set (e.g., "Items 34–38 relate to the following patient assessment findings") and consider centering the introductory material horizontally on the page so that it is more visible. If possible, place the context and all items related to it on the same page (Oermann & Gaberson, 2014).

ASSEMBLING THE TEST

The final appearance of a test and the way in which it is administered can affect measurement validity. Confusing directions, haphazard arrangement of components, and clerical errors all contribute to measurement error. Teachers can avoid such errors by following certain test design rules.

ARRANGE ITEMS IN A LOGICAL SEQUENCE

There are various methods for arranging items on the test: by order of expected difficulty, according to the sequence in which the content was learned, and a combination of the two. If using two or more item types, the teacher should first group items of each type together. This allows students to maintain the mental set required to respond to each type of item and prevents errors caused by frequent task changes (Oermann & Gaberson, 2014). Miller et al. (2009) recommended the following order of item formats on a test, from simplest to most complex:

1. True–false
2. Matching
3. Short-answer or completion
4. Multiple-choice
5. Context-dependent item sets
6. Essay items

Using all item formats on a single test is not necessary nor recommended, but the longer the test, the greater variety of item formats can be included. If the test is to contain complex item formats requiring more reading and processing time, they should be combined with only one or two additional item types.

Within each item format, items can be arranged according to the order in which the content was presented in the course, which can help students recall essential information more easily. Finally, in the combination of item format and content sequencing, items can be arranged in order of expected difficulty, easiest items first. Beginning each section with easier items can help anxious students relax so that they can demonstrate their best performance (Gronlund, 2006; Miller et al., 2009; Oermann & Gaberson, 2014).

WRITE DIRECTIONS

The teacher should write a set of clear general directions for the test, including such information as:

- How and where to record responses
- Whether students may write on the test booklet
- The amount of time permitted
- Whether students may ask questions during the test

Each section (according to item format) should begin with a set of directions that specify the assessment tasks. For example, for multiple-choice items, students need to know whether to select the correct or best response.

USE A COVER PAGE

A cover page serves to keep the test items concealed during the distribution of test materials so that the first students to receive the test will not have more time to complete it than students who receive their copies later. If a separate answer sheet is used, the cover page can be numbered to help maintain test security. Students are asked to record their numbers in a specified location on their answer sheets, and when test materials are returned, teachers can identify any missing test booklets. The general directions for the test can be printed on the cover page, allowing the teacher to review them with the students before anyone begins reading and responding to test items.

AVOID CROWDING

Teachers should allow enough space between and around test elements so that each test item is distinct from the others. Tightly packing words on a page might minimize the amount of paper used, but it can also interfere with students' maximum performance by contributing to reading and clerical errors.

KEEP RELATED MATERIAL TOGETHER

In addition to grouping items of the same format together, the teacher should ensure that all parts of a test item appear on the same page, such as the stem and alternatives of a multiple-choice item and the directions and both columns of a matching exercise. As previously mentioned, the introductory material and all related context-dependent items should appear on the same page, if possible (Gronlund, 2006; Miller et al., 2009).

FACILITATE SCORING

If the teacher will be hand-scoring the test, the test or answer sheet layout should facilitate quick, accurate scoring. If students record their answers on the test booklet itself, items should be formatted with scoring in mind. For example, arrange true-false items with columns of Ts and Fs at the left margin and ask students to circle their responses, as in this example:

T F 1. A clean mastectomy incision primarily closed and with a Jackson-Pratt drain should be categorized as a Class II wound.
T F 2. A 10% bleach solution should be used for environmental cleaning of patient care areas for patients infected with *C difficile*.
T F 3. Contact precautions should be used when caring for patients infected with seasonal influenza.

NUMBER ITEMS CONTINUOUSLY

Although test items should be grouped according to format, the teacher should number them continuously from the beginning to the end of the test instead of starting each item format section with item number 1. This technique helps to prevent clerical errors when students record their answers on a separate answer sheet and helps students to recognize items they have skipped.

PROOFREAD

To ensure optimum measurement reliability and validity, the test should be free of spelling, grammatical, and typing errors. The test designer often does not recognize his or her own errors, so a colleague who is familiar with the content should be asked to proofread a copy of the test before it is duplicated. Spell-check and grammar-check features of computer software are insufficient because they do not always recognize words that are spelled correctly but used in the wrong context, or structural errors such as giving two test items the same number.

PREPARE AN ANSWER KEY

For both hand scoring and electronic scoring, the teacher should prepare an accurate scoring key to provide a final check on the accuracy of the test items. This answer key should also be proofread by someone who did not prepare it, verifying that it is accurate. The teacher should also prepare ideal responses to short-answer items and prepare scoring rubrics for essay items.

REPRODUCING THE TEST

Obviously, the teacher must provide a copy of the test for each student, but it is wise to make extra copies for proctors or to replace defective copies that might have been distributed to students. The original copy of the test should be produced on a laser or other high-quality printer, and the copies should be made on a machine that has sufficient toner to produce crisp, dark print without artifacts.

The test should be printed on only one side of each sheet of paper to prevent students from inadvertently skipping items by failing to notice the printing on the back of a page. If students are to record their answers on the test itself, printing on only one side makes hand-scoring easier.

Teachers are responsible for maintaining the security of tests by protecting them from unauthorized access. Dishonest students who gain access to test materials can use them to obtain higher scores than they deserve, contributing to measurement error. Printed tests should be stored in locked areas, and computer files should be password protected or encrypted. Printed drafts and old copies of used tests should be shredded.

PREPARING STUDENTS TO TAKE TESTS

Teachers should create conditions under which students will be able to demonstrate their best performance on tests. One of these conditions involves adequate preparation of students to take tests (Miller et al., 2009; Nitko & Brookhart, 2011).

INFORMATION NEEDS

Students need information about the test to prepare effectively for it. They should have sufficient time to prepare, so the date and time of the test should be announced well in advance. Although many teachers believe that unannounced or pop tests motivate students to study, no credible evidence supports this belief. Students also need to know about the testing conditions, including how much time will be provided, whether they will be able to use resources such as a calculator, number and type of test items, and whether any items, such as cell phones, books, and papers, will not be permitted in the testing room.

Students need to know which content domain will be assessed, the cognitive level at which they will be expected to perform, and the relative weights assigned to each content area. As previously discussed, teachers can communicate this information by sharing and discussing the test blueprint with students.

TEST-TAKING SKILLS

Students need adequate test-taking skills for the type of test to be administered. Skill in test-taking is often called testwiseness, but this term more appropriately refers to the ability to use test-taking skills and experience along with clues from poorly constructed test items to achieve a score higher than a student's true knowledge would predict. All students need adequate test-taking skills so that they are not at a disadvantage when their scores are compared with those of testwise students. Some of these skills are:

- Following test directions
- Reading and understanding test items
- Recording responses accurately
- Using testing time wisely
- Checking answers for clerical errors
- Distributing test preparation and getting adequate rest before a test (Oermann & Gaberson, 2014)

A common misconception is that students should not change their answers to test items because their first response is usually correct. Students should be encouraged to change answers any time they have a good reason for the change, such as later recalling necessary information or getting a cue from another item.

TEST ANXIETY

Teachers should prepare students to approach a test with helpful attitudes. Anxiety is a common response in testing situations, but excessive anxiety is likely to interfere with a student's performance (Miller et al., 2009). Test anxiety is a trait with physical, emotional, and cognitive components. Research evidence demonstrates an interaction among these components: negative thoughts about testing can produce negative feelings that interfere with performance (Poorman, Mastorovich, & Molcan, 2007). Physical feelings and reactions associated with test anxiety relate to autonomic reactivity, producing symptoms of perspiration, increased heart rate, and gastrointestinal upset, although not all test-anxious students have these reactions.

Students whose text anxiety interferes with their test performance can benefit from treatment that addresses the negative emotions (e.g., worry) and thoughts (e.g., distractibility, difficulty concentrating) as well as improvement of test-taking skills. Teachers who identify students who are affected by test anxiety should refer those students for treatment.

TEST ADMINISTRATION

Administering the test is usually the easiest step in the testing process. However, common problems associated with test administration can affect the reliability of test scores and the validity of inferences made about the scores. Careful planning can help teachers prevent or minimize those problems by using such strategies as scheduling the test in a classroom that minimizes potential distractions such as noise and interruptions.

Teachers should distribute test materials efficiently; with large groups of students, several proctors can assist with this process. If a cover page is used, as previously recommended, students should be instructed not to turn to the first page of test items until they are told to start. If there is no cover page, distribute the tests face down and instruct students not to turn them over until told to do so. General instructions about the testing procedures should be given before students are permitted to begin taking the test.

How to respond to student questions during a test is a challenge for most teachers. Some teachers do not answer any questions related to the content of the test items, even to clarify their meaning. In this case, the teacher should provide students with an opportunity to record their questions and concerns on a separate piece of paper to be reviewed later. Teachers who do answer questions during the test should do so quietly and briefly, avoid giving cues to the correct answer, and should ensure careful proctoring of the group while answering one student's question.

Cheating during tests is a common concern. No matter how widespread the practice might be, teachers should protect the security of test materials throughout the testing process so that honest students are not at a disadvantage when their scores are compared with those of students who cheat. A number of methods have been proposed to deter cheating during a test, but the single most effective method is careful proctoring. There should be enough proctors to allow one to respond to student questions or a student emergency during the test. Proctors should devote their full attention to proctoring and not use this time to grade papers, read, or check e-mail. Because of the variety of creative ways in which students can access unauthorized information during a test, it is wise to also prohibit students from bringing certain items into the testing room, including backpacks, caps with bills, facial tissues, water bottles, cell phones, earbuds, and the like (Oermann & Gaberson, 2014).

TEST AND ITEM ANALYSIS

Computer software for scoring scannable answer sheets and analyzing test results is widely available. These applications provide useful information about how well the test as a whole functioned as a measurement instrument and about the effectiveness of each test item.

Test statistics usually include the range and distribution of scores, measures of central tendency (i.e., the average or typical score), measures of variability (e.g., standard deviation) and reliability estimates. These test characteristics help teachers to interpret the test results and make appropriate inferences about them.

To determine the effectiveness of each test item, teachers should review their difficulty and discrimination indexes. Item difficulty (or p-value) is calculated as the percentage of students who responded correctly to that item; values range from 0 to 1.00. The difficulty level is commonly understood to mean that the higher the percentage, the easier the item. However, difficulty is not an intrinsic characteristic of a test item; different p-values can be obtained on the same item by students with more or less ability or by students who were taught by more- or less-effective teachers. Difficulty level is also related to the probability of students' guessing the correct response. Thus, the probability of guessing the correct response to a true–false item is .50, whereas the probability of correctly guessing the answer to a five-option multiple-choice item is .20. Moderately difficult test items have p-values approximately halfway between the chance of blind-guessing and 1.00.

The discrimination index, D, indicates how effectively each test item measures what the entire test measures (Miller et al., 2009). D-values range from –1.00 to + 1.00. Negative values indicate that the item was answered correctly more often by students with low total test scores than by high-scoring students. A D-value of 0.00 means that the item has no discriminating power because equal numbers of high- and low-scoring students answered it correctly. Positive D-values mean that high-scoring students tended to answer the item correctly more often than low-scoring students.

Students often argue that if all or most of them answered an item incorrectly, that item should be deleted from the test, or that students who answered incorrectly should receive an extra point. Difficulty index alone is an insufficient basis on which to delete a test item from scoring: the teacher should carefully review the item in question, and if it measures important content, was expected to be difficult for many students, and is not seriously flawed, it should remain. If there is a fatal flaw, such as omission of the correct answer from a multiple-choice item, that item should be eliminated and the test rescored without it. Review of the discrimination index should help teachers determine whether a very difficult item effectively distinguished between high-scoring and low-scoring groups of students and, if so, that item should be retained (Oermann & Gaberson, 2014).

SUMMARY

A test is a measurement instrument for assessing learners' knowledge and cognitive abilities. Test results allow teachers to make important educational decisions that affect learners, teachers, patients, future employers, and the educational program. A test must produce relevant and consistent results to form the basis for sound inferences about what learners know and can do. Good planning, careful test construction, proper administration, accurate scoring, and sound interpretation of scores are essential for producing useful test results. This chapter discussed assessment concepts that influence the quality of test results, and the process of planning, constructing, administering, scoring, and analyzing tests. Guidelines were presented for writing true–false, matching, multiple-choice, multiple-response, short answer, and essay items, and context-dependent item sets.

REFERENCES

Anderson, L. W., & Krathwohl, D. R. (Eds.). (2001). *A taxonomy for learning, teaching, and assessing: A revision of Bloom's taxonomy of educational objectives*. New York, NY: Longman.

Bosher, S., & Bowles, M. (2008). The effects of linguistic modification on ESL students' comprehension of nursing course test items. *Nursing Education Perspectives, 29*, 165–172.

Miller, M. D., Linn, R. L., & Gronlund, N. E. (2009). *Measurement and assessment in teaching* (10th ed.). Upper Saddle River, NJ: Prentice Hall.

Musial, D., Nieminen, G., Thomas, J., & Burke, K. (2009). *Foundations of educational measurement*. Boston, MA: McGraw-Hill Higher Education.

Nitko, A. J., & Brookhart, S. M. (2011). *Educational assessment of students* (6th ed.). Upper Saddle River, NJ: Pearson Education.

Oermann, M. H., & Gaberson, K. B. (2014). *Evaluation and testing in nursing education* (4th ed.). New York, NY: Springer Publishing Company.

Poorman, S. G., Mastorovich, M. L., & Molcan, K. L. (2007). *A good thinking approach to the NCLEX and other nursing exams* (2nd ed.). Pittsburgh, PA: STAT Nursing Consultants.

Popham, W. J. (2012). *Selected-response tests: Building and bettering* (Vol. 12). Boston, MA: Pearson.

Rodriguez, M. C. (2005). Three options are optimal for multiple-choice items: A meta-analysis of 80 years of research. *Educational Measurement: Issues and Practice, 24*(2), 3–13. doi:10.1111/j.1745-3992.2005.00006.x

Tarrant, M., & Ware, J. (2012). A framework for improving the quality of multiple-choice assessment. *Nurse Educator, 37*, 98–104. doi:10.1097/NNE.0b013e31825041d0

Waugh, C. K., & Gronlund, N. E. (2013). *Assessment of student achievement* (10th ed.). Upper Saddle River, NJ: Pearson Education.

12

Clinical Evaluation

MARILYN H. OERMANN

As students learn about nursing, they develop their knowledge base, higher level thinking skills, and a wide range of practice competencies essential for patient care. Learning concepts in a classroom or an online environment is not sufficient: students need to apply those concepts and other knowledge to clinical situations and be proficient in carrying out care. Teachers guide student learning in the clinical setting and evaluate their performance in practice. This chapter describes the clinical evaluation process, the importance of giving prompt and specific feedback to students as they are learning, principles that are important when observing and rating performance, and grading clinical practice.

WHAT OUTCOMES AND COMPETENCIES SHOULD BE EVALUATED?

Each school of nursing establishes its own program and course outcomes, or objectives, consistent with a range of factors that are described in Chapter 13. Some of those course outcomes relate to care of patients, families, and communities and are best met through clinical practice experiences. In these experiences students learn to apply their knowledge to clinical situations, transfer skills acquired in other settings to patient care, gain essential competencies for practice, and develop their clinical reasoning skills. Students use the nursing process to deliver holistic and patient-focused care (American Nurses Association, 2013). They search for and use evidence to guide decisions, enabling them to learn about evidence-based practice and how it is implemented in patient care. They also learn about high-quality care and the nurse's role in improving health care quality and patient safety (Cronenwett et al., 2007; Cronenwett, Sherwood, & Gelmon, 2009; McKown, McKeon, & Webb, 2011; Sherwood, 2012).

Other outcomes of clinical practice are to develop psychomotor skills; gain informatics competencies (Flood, Gasiewicz, & Delpier, 2010; Institute of Medicine, 2011; Tellez, 2012); learn to collaborate with nurses and other health professionals and function on interprofessional teams; become culturally competent (Giddens, North, Carlson-Sabelli, Rogers, & Fogg, 2012; Hawala-Druy & Hill, 2012); and develop professional values and competencies in patient-centered care (McKeon, Norris, Cardell, & Britt, 2009; Sherwood & Barnsteiner, 2012). In clinical courses, students learn to accept responsibility for their own actions and become self-directed learners. Depending on the course, intended learning outcomes for students can also include gaining leadership and management skills.

These outcomes, and others in a nursing program, can be stated as outcomes or objectives to be met in a clinical course or as clinical competencies to be developed by students. Regardless of the format, these outcomes, objectives, or competencies provide the framework for the teacher to plan clinical activities for students and for assessing their performance. These outcomes are listed in Exhibit 12.1. Not all of the outcomes are relevant to each clinical course, but generally as students progress through a curriculum, they will meet these outcomes and develop related competencies.

EXHIBIT 12.1 Areas of Outcomes or Competencies for Clinical Evaluation

1. Apply concepts and other knowledge in patient, family, community, and global health care
2. Develop higher level thinking and clinical judgment skills
3. Deliver holistic and patient-centered care (nursing process)
4. Use evidence in clinical practice
5. Gain knowledge, skills, and values for improving the quality and safety of care
6. Develop psychomotor, technological, and informatics skills
7. Develop communication skills with patients, families, the interprofessional team, and others with whom the nurse interacts
8. Develop values and cultural competencies essential for care of culturally and ethnically diverse patients
9. Accept responsibility and accountability for own actions and decisions
10. Become a self-directed learner
11. Develop leadership and management skills

CLINICAL EVALUATION PROCESS

In clinical evaluation, the teacher makes judgments about the quality of the students' performance in practice. These judgments indicate whether the student is meeting or has met the outcomes or objectives of the clinical course, and can perform the competencies to be developed in it. Clinical evaluation involves observing students' performance; assessing their understanding of the clinical situation through questions, discussions, and assignments completed by students; and collecting other data about student learning and performance. The teacher then uses these data to determine whether the student is progressing in the course, or at the end, has met each of the outcomes or objectives and can perform the competencies.

Clinical evaluation is a judgmental process (Oermann & Gaberson, 2014). The teacher's judgment influences the data collected through observations of students and other sources, and what those data mean, that is, decisions about the quality of the performance. First, in any clinical situation teachers can make varied observations of performance and collect different types of data on which to base the evaluation. For example, if two teachers observe a student in practice, one might collect information on how well the student interacted with the patient during a procedure, whereas the other focuses mainly on procedural skills, resulting in varied observations on which to judge the performance. Second, teachers can have different interpretations of how well the student performed. For this reason it is important to have multiple sources of data and to collect data over a period of time before arriving at a conclusion about the quality of the student's performance.

Another issue is that the teacher's personal values, attitudes, beliefs, and biases can influence the observations made and decisions about the quality of the performance (Oermann & Gaberson, 2014). Teachers need to be aware of these when evaluating students' performance. For example, a teacher who prefers working with students who are outgoing and initiate conversation can be biased when assessing the performance of a beginning student who is quiet and needs guidance in interacting with patients. Issues with interactions can affect the communication competencies on the clinical evaluation tool, but they should not influence the assessment of other unrelated competencies. As students are learning, it is the teacher's responsibility to guide their development. In this situation, the teacher's goal should be to help this student develop skills and confidence in communication. The teacher's main role is teaching students to gain competencies for practice, not only to evaluate their performance.

FORMATIVE AND SUMMATIVE CLINICAL EVALUATION

The teacher can evaluate students' performance to provide feedback for improving it (formative evaluation) or to indicate the outcomes met and competencies achieved in the clinical practicum (summative evaluation). In formative evaluation, the teacher provides feedback to students about their progress in the clinical practicum and how to improve performance. Feedback enables students to reflect on their performance, identify continued learning needs, and decide how to meet them (Bonnel, 2008). This is good teaching: the nurse educator identifies gaps in learning and performance and provides specific and instructional feedback to resolve those gaps. Students, though, need to reflect on the information provided to them and incorporate the feedback into their own learning (Bonnel). Formative evaluation is diagnostic, and it should not be graded (Nitko & Brookhart, 2011).

At periodic intervals, the teacher summarizes the extent of learning achieved in the course. This is done in relation to the outcomes or objectives to be met, or the expected competencies to be learned, answering questions such as: What outcomes have been met by the student? What is the student's current level of performance? Summative clinical evaluation is typically done at midterm and the end of the clinical practicum to decide on the student's grade. Summative evaluation is for grading—it usually comes too late for students to have an opportunity to improve their performance (Oermann & Gaberson, 2014).

FOCUS ON FORMATIVE EVALUATION

The teacher should focus on giving prompt and continuous feedback to students (formative evaluation) because the feedback will enable them to improve their performance. For feedback to guide student learning and improve performance, it should be

1. *Precise, specific, and instructional.* Saying to a student, "Your organization needs to improve," or writing on a paper that the "content lacks depth" does not specify the problem with organization of care and the paper's content or how to improve. Instead, the teacher should indicate the specific skills and knowledge that are lacking and provide suggestions about what to do next to gain those missing skills. By incorporating guidance on how to improve, feedback is instructional and leads to improved performance.
2. *Delivered using varied and relevant modes.* With oral feedback, the teacher describes the observations made of performance, explains what to do differently, and shares other

ways of thinking about the clinical situation. Some of the best learning occurs when students and teachers engage in dialogue about the feedback. For procedures and psychomotor skills, feedback should be oral (explaining the errors in performance and how the skill should be performed) and visual (demonstrating the correct procedure). The student can then practice the skill under the guidance of the teacher or someone else with expertise. Written comments on students' papers and other assignments provide another mode of feedback and should meet the same criteria: be precise, specific, and instructional.

3. *Prompt.* Feedback needs to be given at the time of learning or shortly thereafter. The longer the time between the performance and feedback, the less effective the feedback is, because students cannot recall the specifics of their performance to be modified.

4. *Individualized, based on the needs of the student.* Students need varying degrees of feedback and positive reinforcement as they are learning, especially in the clinical setting. As they become more clinically competent, they are better able to assess their own performance, but with new experiences they still need feedback on their thinking and judgment as well as skills.

5. *Given in private.* No one likes to be told in public and for others to hear about improvements needed in his or her care. The teacher should be sensitive to the setting in which feedback is delivered: it should be private, and the teacher should be respectful of students and their feelings (Clynes & Raftery, 2008).

Gigante, Dell, and Sharkey (2011) outlined a five-step process for giving feedback to students that reflects the important principles of good feedback. First, the teacher should review the outcomes, objectives, or competencies students need to achieve in the course. These specify what is expected of students in the clinical practicum. Second, the teacher should set the stage for students to receive the feedback, for example, by beginning with this statement: "I am giving you feedback." Then it is clear to students that the information from the teacher is intended to guide their learning and performance. Third, the teacher should have students reflect on their performance and assess its quality—what went well, and what needs improvement from their point of view. Fourth, the teacher should share specific observations of performance with examples and areas for improvement. The last step in this process is for the teacher to recommend specific ways to improve performance.

SUPPORT OF STUDENTS IN THE EVALUATION PROCESS

Being evaluated is stressful, especially in the clinical setting, where patients, family members, other nursing students, nurses, and others can be observing the student provide care and teachers assess performance. Clinical practice in and of itself is stressful for students (Li, Wang, Lin, & Lee, 2011; Manning, Cronin, Monaghan, & Rawlings-Anderson, 2009; Melincavage, 2011; Moscaritolo, 2009), and being evaluated adds to that stress. Students need a supportive learning environment where they are comfortable asking for help and seeking feedback from the teacher. Both teachers and nursing staff need to support students in their learning and be cognizant of the stress students experience in clinical practice. To reduce some of this stress, Dearmon et al. (2013) provided a 2-day, simulation-based orientation for students prior to their first clinical experience. In the simulation, students interacted with standardized patients in realistic clinical situations. Findings indicated that students increased their knowledge and confidence and experienced a decrease in anxiety following the simulation.

SELECTION OF CLINICAL EVALUATION METHODS

Clinical evaluation should be based on the outcomes, objectives, or competencies of the clinical course or practicum. These indicate the expectations for performance and areas to be assessed. The learning activities planned for students, including patient assignments, should enable students to meet these outcomes and become proficient in the identified competencies—the teacher's observations and subsequent assessment should focus on whether the desired outcomes were achieved.

There are different clinical evaluation methods that can be used to assess performance. Using multiple methods takes into consideration individual student needs, abilities, and characteristics and avoids relying on one source of information about student learning (Oermann & Gaberson, 2014). Most often the methods provide data for assessing more than one outcome or objective. For example, an observation of the student completing a health history of an elderly patient would provide data related to assessment, interviewing, communication, developmental needs, and others. In deciding on the evaluation methods for a clinical course, the teacher should review the outcomes or competencies and select methods for assessing them. In this way the methods are geared to the learning expected of students.

The clinical evaluation methods planned for a course should be realistic, considering the types of experiences available in the setting or through simulation, and both student and teacher time. Planning for an evaluation method that depends on a certain type of patient in the clinical setting is not realistic and the evaluation would be better done with simulation or standardized patients. Some methods are not feasible because they might not be available for all of the students or take too much time. Weekly writing assignments might provide data on a number of the course outcomes but require too much time for students considering other course and clinical requirements and demand too much of the teacher's time to review them and give prompt feedback. In such cases, an alternate assessment method might be used such as a group project or discussions with students, or the teacher might use fewer papers, but focused on specific outcomes to be assessed. Bourgault, Mundy, and Joshua (2013) examined the use of audio recordings for providing feedback on weekly clinical assignments rather than written feedback. Students reported that the audio feedback was more personal, contained more positive and constructive feedback, and was easier to understand than written feedback. However, it did not save the faculty time.

CLINICAL EVALUATION METHODS

OBSERVATION OF PERFORMANCE

Oermann, Yarbrough, Ard, Saewert, and Charasika (2009) found in a survey of 1,573 faculty members teaching in prelicensure nursing programs that the main strategy they used to evaluate students' clinical performance was by observing them in the clinical setting. Observations of performance provide data about student achievement of the outcomes and their proficiency in the clinical competencies to be demonstrated. These guide the teacher on *what* to observe. Observations over a period of time in different clinical situations provide more reliable data on student performance than a one-time observation. Holmboe (2008) suggested that increasing the number of observations of performance improves recall and provides more opportunities for practice.

Teachers should share their observations with students and be willing to include student perceptions of their performance. The teacher might have had an incorrect impression, for example, deciding that a student lacked knowledge of a patient's problem, when in fact the student did not understand the teacher's question. Teachers should discuss their observations with students and be willing to modify their judgments about performance.

ANECDOTAL NOTES

Observations of performance should be recorded because otherwise the teacher cannot recall details about the performance and the clinical context. Teachers should develop a strategy for documenting their observations in the clinical setting. Some educators use anecdotal notes, which are narrative descriptions of observations, with or without a judgment about how well the student performed (Di Leonardi Case & Oermann, 2010). Hall, Daly, and Madigan (2010) found in a survey of clinical teachers in six schools of nursing that most (97%) used anecdotal notes. In a study by Hall (2013), faculty identified a variety of uses for anecdotal notes: the most common reason was bringing attention to patient safety concerns. Qualitative findings indicated that anecdotal notes were important for providing accurate feedback to students for formative evaluation.

These notes can be handwritten in the clinical setting or recorded using other devices such as an iPad (Apple Inc., Cupertino, CA) or tablet computer. Zurmehly (2010) suggested that using technologies results in more accurate clinical evaluation because the observations can be recorded in real time. In a study by Swan et al. (2013), the use of tablets by teachers in the clinical setting was hampered by the lack of an Internet connection at some of the sites. At other clinical sites, faculty members were not able to use School of Nursing tablets because of privacy concerns.

CHECKLISTS

For assessment of procedures, skills, and implementation of technology, checklists are typically used. A checklist includes a list of specific actions or steps in a procedure to be observed and a place for marking if the student performed them correctly (Nitko & Brookhart, 2011). Checklists also allow learners to self-assess their performance before it is evaluated by the teacher. They are commonly used for assessing skills in learning laboratories and simulation. In using checklists to assess performance of skills, it is important to focus on the ability of students to perform the skill safely; when there are different ways of carrying out the skill, the teacher should give students this flexibility.

CLINICAL EVALUATION TOOLS (RATING SCALES)

Clinical evaluation tools, which are types of rating scales, are more comprehensive than checklists. They typically list the outcomes or objectives to be met, or competencies to be demonstrated, at the end of the clinical practicum, with a scale for rating their performance. Clinical evaluation tools are intended for summative evaluation. At midterm the teacher can rate how well the student is performing at that point in time, and then at the end of the semester can indicate the outcomes or competencies that were achieved. Rating scales also are used to assess the quality of student performance of particular activities in clinical practice, such as leading a conference, in simulation, and in Objective Structured Clinical Examinations, among other uses.

Rating scales used for clinical evaluation can be pass-fail or satisfactory-unsatisfactory, or they can include multiple levels for rating performance, such as 1 to 4, or below average to exceptional. A pass–fail scale requires only two levels of judgment: did the student achieve the outcome or perform the competency at a satisfactory level to indicate a pass? In a survey of nursing faculty, 83% ($n = 1,116$) used pass–fail rating forms for clinical evaluation (Oermann et al., 2009).

With a system that has multiple levels, the teacher needs to judge the quality of the performance and decide which level it represents on the tool. Nitko and Brookhart (2011) suggested that for this type of instrument, a short description should be included with each number or level for each of the outcomes or competencies to improve consistency across teachers. For example, for the competency "Collects relevant data from patients," the descriptions for each level might be:

4: Collects significant data from patients and other sources, differentiates relevant from irrelevant data, analyzes data from multiple sources to identify additional information needed.

3: Collects significant data from patients, uses multiple sources of data

2: Collects data from patients related to main problems

1: Does not collect significant data and misses important cues in data

Holaday and Buckley (2008) developed a clinical evaluation tool with five levels of competence from dependent (0) to self-directed (4). The ratings are used to get a score that can be changed to a grade for the course.

With the goal of preparing students with the knowledge and skills for improving the quality of care, many faculty are incorporating quality and safety competencies into their clinical evaluation instruments. Exhibit 12.2 provides an example of a clinical evaluation tool that incorporates the Quality and Safety Education for Nurses (QSEN) competencies (QSEN, 2013; Walsh, Jairath, Paterson, & Grandjean, 2010). The Clinical Performance Evaluation Tool in Exhibit 12.2 is a generic tool used in all clinical courses for assessing student performance related to the QSEN competencies. In addition to this tool, each clinical course has its own key with competencies specific to that course. An example of the key that accompanies the first adult health nursing course is in Exhibit 12.3. Guidelines for grading clinical performance for all of the clinical courses in the nursing program are provided in Exhibit 12.4.

Another approach to clinical evaluation developed by Caputi (Appendix C) examines student learning outcomes performed in the clinical setting with learning activities tied directly to the behaviors on the clinical evaluation tool. These behaviors reflect the course outcomes and competencies. Caputi's approach is to also include activities students are required to complete during the clinical experience. A description of this approach with examples is provided in Appendix C.

Regardless of the outcomes or competencies on the tool, the areas rated and the rating scale must be understood by all involved in the process. Teachers, students, preceptors, and others should understand what is meant by each competency to be rated and how to use the scale (Oermann & Gaberson, 2014). In addition, teachers should be able to identify examples of performance that reflect a pass or fail or at each level in the scale. For example, what is passing performance for "collects comprehensive data from patients?" If there are multiple levels in the scale, what is the difference in the collection of data at each level? Teachers should discuss as a group the meaning of each outcome or competency on the tool and acceptable performance. These discussions enable educators to come to consensus about behaviors that demonstrate competency for each of the items on the instrument (Parsons et al., 2012). Teachers, adjunct faculty members, and preceptors can practice using the tool to assess the performance of students in digitally recorded simulations or video clips. Discussing their ratings and rationale improves use of the tool and its reliability. In addition, teachers should review the instrument with students, explaining each outcome and competency and expected performance. Other important principles for using a clinical evaluation tool are listed in Exhibit 12.5.

EXHIBIT 12.2 Example of Clinical Evaluation Tool Integrating QSEN Competencies

CUA   The Catholic University of America School of Nursing

Clinical Performance Evaluation Tool

[date]

Student Name_____ Faculty_____ Facility_____

Fill in appropriate fields to the right and below: Date_____ Midterm
Date_____ Final Evaluation

Student must obtain a Satisfactory "S" grade in all competencies at the final evaluation to pass the course.

Core Competencies	Midterm			Final	
	S	NI	U	S	U
Provides Patient-Centered Care					
• Values					
• Caring/Human Dignity					
• Spirituality					
• Ethics					
• Utilizes and Performs Nursing Process					
Exhibits Teamwork and Collaboration					
• Communication					
• Personnel (Faculty, Staff, Patients, Peers, Family)					
• Oral (Nonverbal)					
• Written (Documentation)					
Incorporates Evidence-Based Practice Into Clinical					
• Exhibits Critical Thinking					
Understands and Applies Quality Improvement Methods					
• Promote Healing					
Promotes Safety					
• Technical Skills					
• Safe Medication Administration					
• Timeliness					
Understands and Utilizes Informatics					
• Appropriate decision making based on core competencies above and implemented with informatics support					

Midterm Comments (Address Strengths and Weaknesses)

by Instructor

by Student

Final Comments (Address Strengths and Weaknesses)

by Instructor

By Student

Student Signature_____ **Date**_____

Faculty Signature_____ **Date**_____

QSEN, Quality and Safety Education for Nurses

EXHIBIT 12.3 Key With Clinical Competencies for Adult Health Nursing Course

 The Catholic University of America School of Nursing
Clinical Evaluation Tool—**KEY**
[date]
N275-Performance I[a]

1. Patient Centered
   a. Elicit patient values, preferences, and their expressed needs as part of the clinical interview, while performing within the process of assessment, planning, intervention, and evaluation in the implementation of the plan of care.
   b. Communicate patient values, preferences, and expressed needs to other members of health care team.
   c. Assess presence and extent of pain and suffering.
   d. Assess levels of physical and emotional comfort.

2. Teamwork and Collaboration
   a. Demonstrate awareness of own strengths and limitations as a team member.
   b. Function competently within own scope of practice as a member of the health care team.
   c. Initiate requests for help when appropriate to situation.
   d. Communicate effectively and appropriately in nonverbal, verbal, and written forms with other team members, while adapting one's own style of communication. Adapt communication styles to meet the needs of the client, team, clinical instructor, and situation.

3. Evidence-Based Practice
   a. Demonstrate knowledge of basic scientific methods and processes.
   b. Differentiate clinical opinion from research and evidence summaries.
   c. Base individualized care plan on patient values, clinical expertise, and evidence.
   d. Read original research and evidence reports related to area of practice.

4. Quality Improvement
   a. Describe strategies for learning about the outcomes of care in the setting in which one is engaged in clinical practice.
   b. Recognize that nursing and other health profession students are parts of systems of care and care processes that affect outcomes for patients and families.
   c. Give examples of the tension between professional autonomy and system functioning.
   d. Explain the importance of variation and measurement in assessing quality of care.
   e. Describe approaches for changing processes of care.

5. Safety
   a. Demonstrate effective use of technology and standardized practices that support safety and quality (medication administration).
   b. Demonstrate effective use of strategies to reduce risk of harm to self or others.
   c. Use appropriate strategies to reduce reliance on memory (such as checklists).
   d. Communicate observations or concerns related to hazards and errors to patients, families, and the health care team.

[a] Competencies for N275 Adults in Health and Illness. Each clinical course has its own key with competencies specific to that course based on QSEN outcomes.

(continued)

EXHIBIT 12.3 Key With Clinical Competencies for Adult Health Nursing Course (*continued*)

> 6. Informatics
>   a. Explain why information and technology skills are essential for safe patient care.
>   b. Navigate the electronic health record.
>   c. Document and plan patient care in an electronic health record.
>   d. Recognize the time, effort, and skill required for computers, databases, and other technologies to become reliable and effective tools for patient care.
>   e. Maintain safety and confidentiality in informatics.

From the School of Nursing, The Catholic University of America, Washington, DC. Copyright 2013. Reprinted by permission of the School of Nursing, The Catholic University of America, Washington, DC, 2013.

EXHIBIT 12.4 Guidelines for Grading Performance

> **The Catholic University of America School of Nursing**
> Clinical Evaluation Tool Guidelines
> [date]
>
> ### Tool Guidelines
>
> - Each student will fill out an evaluation at (1) midterm (2) final.
> - Each faculty member will fill out an evaluation at (1) midterm (2) final.
> - Each row item (boxes) must be checked at (1) midterm (2) final.
> - The Clinical Score will be completed by the Clinical Faculty by placing a √ or an x in the appropriate box for each student.
> - The Clinical Score will be completed by the Student by placing a √ or an x in the appropriate box for each student.
> - The score for Clinical Evaluation will be either *Pass* or *Fail*.
> - A passing grade will be assigned only if *all* the items are checked *S* at the time of the final evaluation.
>
> ### Core Competency Key
>
> - Each core competency (as outlined in *BOLD)* has a template or key, which specifies individual guidelines and examples for each.
> - The keys are based on level of matriculation in each clinical course.
>
> ### Grading Guidelines—Entire course
>
> - The score for each student in the course will be the numeric grade received for the course based on all of the didactic work required in the syllabus.
> - Clinical Performance will be evaluated with a Clinical Performance Tool, and will be scored either *PASS* or *FAIL*.
> - Every student must receive a score of *PASS* on the Clinical Performance Tool to pass the course.
> - A student who receives a *FAIL* on the Clinical Performance Tool will receive *FAIL* for the course and receive a grade of *F* for the course.

From the School of Nursing, The Catholic University of America, Washington, DC. Copyright 2013. Reprinted by permission of the School of Nursing, The Catholic University of America, Washington, DC, 2013.

EXHIBIT 12.5 Guidelines for Using Clinical Evaluation Tools (Rating Scales)

1. Be alert to the possible influence of your own values, attitudes, and biases in observing performance and making judgments about its quality.

2. Use the outcomes, objectives, or competencies to focus your observations. Give students feedback on other observations made about their performance.

3. Collect sufficient data on students' performance before arriving at conclusions and judgments about the quality of the performance.

4. Observe students more than one time before rating performance. Rating scales for clinical evaluation should represent a pattern of the student's performance over a period of time.

5. Observe students' performance in different clinical situations or in simulation, or use additional methods for evaluation.

6. Do not rely on first impressions; these might not be accurate.

7. Always discuss observations with students, have students reflect on their performance and obtain their perceptions, and be willing to modify your own judgments and ratings when new data are presented.

8. Collect data on students' performance as it relates to the outcomes or competencies on the tool. These indicate the expectations for learning and performance and *what* should be evaluated in the clinical setting.

9. Avoid using the clinical evaluation tool as the only source of data about a student's performance—use multiple methods for evaluating clinical practice.

10. Rate each outcome or competency on the tool separately based on your observations of performance and other data you have collected. If you have insufficient information to rate a particular outcome or competency, leave it blank.

11. Rate students' performance based on the data. Do not let your general impressions of the student or personal biases influence the ratings.

12. If the clinical evaluation tool is not effective for judging student performance in your clinical course, revise it. Consider these questions: Does use of the tool yield data for making valid decisions about students' competence? Does it yield reliable, stable data? Is it easy to use? Is it realistic for the types of learning activities students complete and that are available in clinical and simulation settings? Is there consistency across faculty members in their use of the tool.

13. Discuss as a group (with other educators and preceptors involved in the evaluation) each competency on the clinical evaluation tool. Come to agreement as to the meaning of the competencies and what a student's performance would look like for a pass or fail and at each rating level in your tool. Share examples of performance, how you would rate them, and your rationale. As a group exercise observe a digital recording or simulation of a student's performance, rate it with the tool, and come to agreement as to the rating. Exercises and discussions such as these should be held before the course begins and periodically to ensure reliability across teachers and settings.

14. Review the clinical evaluation tool at least annually and modify as needed.

Adapted from Oermann and Gaberson (2014), p. 276. Copyright 2014. Reproduced with the permission of Springer Publishing Company, LLC.

OTHER CLINICAL EVALUATION METHODS

Observations of students, summarizing observations in anecdotal notes, using checklists to assess skills, and rating how well students performed the expected clinical competencies are not the only methods for evaluating clinical practice. Other methods are listed in Exhibit 12.6. These methods, which are also described in Chapter 10, provide additional data about student achievement of the outcomes of the clinical course.

EXHIBIT 12.6 Clinical Evaluation Methods

- Observation
- Anecdotal note
- Checklist
- Clinical evaluation tool (rating form)
- Formal (term) paper
- Short paper
- Reflective journal and other types of journals
- Nursing care plan
- Concept map
- Analysis of interactions in clinical setting and simulation
- Case including unfolding case and case study
- Media clip
- Portfolio including electronic portfolio
- Discussion and clinical conference
- Group project
- Game
- Simulation
- Standardized patient
- Objective structured clinical examination
- Self-evaluation

GRADING CLINICAL COURSES

Clinical courses can be graded as pass-fail or satisfactory-unsatisfactory, or with letter grades such as A through F. Based on a survey of nursing programs, pass-fail appears to be the most common method of grading clinical nursing courses (Oermann et al., 2009). When using pass-fail grading, faculty can specify that the student must pass all of the competencies to pass the course or can identify critical behaviors for passing. When letter grades are used, the grade can be determined according to the number of outcomes or competencies achieved by the student. For example, an A might be assigned if all of the competencies were met and a B if the critical ones and half of the others were achieved (Oermann & Gaberson, 2014). The grade can also incorporate other evaluation methods used in the course. For example, the rating on the clinical evaluation tool can count for 50% of the clinical grade, with the other 50% determined by grades on written assignments, a portfolio, and a conference presentation. Or, the grade might be computed based only on the grades on assignments and other clinical evaluation methods used in the course, with the requirement that students receive a pass on the evaluation tool. In some schools, the clinical assignments and other evaluation methods provide data for determining whether students achieved the outcomes and competencies, but they are not evaluated and graded separately.

There are important principles for the teacher to be aware of related to grading clinical practice. First, the teacher should understand the outcomes to be met in the course, expectations of performance, and the specific evaluation methods used in the course. This information should be communicated in writing to students and reviewed with them. Second, students need to understand how the course is graded. For example, if students must pass the clinical course to progress in the program, no matter what grade they have in the course overall, this information should be in the course syllabus and school policies and should also be reviewed with students. Third, it is important to share all of the evaluation data with students and to consider their feedback on performance. Students should sign any evaluation documents and summaries of performance. Signing does not mean they agree with the evaluation, but it confirms they had an opportunity to read what was written about their performance. Fourth, the most important role of the teacher in clinical practice is to provide continuous feedback to students on their performance and to help them improve. If the teacher identifies problems with performance, it is critical to discuss these with students and to prepare a learning plan with strategies mapped out for the student to correct deficiencies and further develop competencies (Oermann & Gaberson, 2014). Fifth, the teacher should document observations of performance as the course proceeds, discussing those with students so they are aware of their progress. All nurse educators need to be aware of the policies of the nursing program on unsafe clinical performance and failing a clinical course and to follow those precisely.

SUMMARY

Clinical evaluation is a process in which the teacher collects data through observations of performance and other assessment methods and based on those data makes judgments about the quality of the students' performance in practice. These judgments indicate whether the student is meeting or has met the outcomes or objectives of the course, or can perform the competencies expected in the course. Through formative evaluation the teacher provides feedback to students about their progress in the clinical practicum and specifically how to improve their performance. Feedback should be prompt, specific, and instructional; continuous during the learning process; and given in private. Formative evaluation is diagnostic and is not graded. At periodic intervals, such as at midterm and at the end of the clinical practicum, the teacher summarizes the extent of learning and performance. This process is referred to as summative evaluation.

Being evaluated is stressful, especially in the clinical setting, where patients and others can be observing the student provides care and teachers assess performance. Both teachers and nursing staff need to provide a supportive and caring environment for students to learn and for the evaluation process to be less stressful.

Clinical evaluation methods should be selected based on the outcomes or competencies of the clinical course. These indicate the expectations for performance and areas to be assessed. Observations of performance provide data about student achievement of the outcomes and their proficiency in the clinical competencies to be demonstrated. Observations over a period of time in different clinical situations provide more reliable data on student performance than a one-time observation. When assessing a skill or procedure, the teacher might use a checklist, which includes the specific steps to perform the skill or carry out the procedure and a place for marking if the student performed each step correctly and in the right order. Clinical evaluation tools, which are rating scales, are more comprehensive than checklists. They typically list the outcomes or competencies to be demonstrated at the end of the clinical practicum with a scale for rating their performance. Clinical evaluation tools are intended for summative evaluation. Based on a survey of nursing programs, pass–fail appears to be the most common method of grading clinical nursing courses.

REFERENCES

American Nurses Association. (2013). *The nursing process.* Retrieved from http://www.nursingworld.org/EspeciallyForYou/What-is-Nursing/Tools-You-Need/Thenursingprocess.html

Bonnel, W. (2008). Improving feedback to students in online courses. *Nursing Education Perspectives*, *29*, 290–294.

Bourgault, A. M., Mundy, C., & Joshua, T. (2013). Comparison of audio vs. written feedback on clinical assignments of nursing students. *Nursing Education Perspectives*, *34*, 43–46.

Clynes, M. P., & Raftery, S. E. (2008). Feedback: An essential element of student learning in clinical practice. *Nurse Education in Practice*, *8*, 405–411. doi:10.1016/j.nepr.2008.02.003

Cronenwett, L., Sherwood, G., Barnsteiner, J., Disch, J., Johnson, J., Mitchell, P., … Warren, J. (2007). Quality and safety education for nurses. *Nursing Outlook*, *55*, 122–131. doi:10.1016/j.outlook.2007.02.006

Cronenwett, L., Sherwood, G., & Gelmon, S. B. (2009). Improving quality and safety education: The QSEN learning collaborative. *Nursing Outlook*, *57*, 304–312. doi:10.1016/j.outlook.2009.09.004

Dearmon, V., Graves, R. J., Hayden, S., Mulekar, M.S., Lawrence, S.M., Jones, L., … Farmer, J. E. (2013). Effectiveness of simulation-based orientation of baccalaureate nursing students preparing for their first clinical experience. *Journal of Nursing Education*, *52*, 29–38. doi:10.3928/01484834-20121212-02

Di Leonardi Case, B., & Oermann, M. H. (2010). Clinical teaching and evaluation. In L. Caputi (Ed.), *Teaching nursing: The art and science* (2nd ed., pp. 82–141). Glen Ellyn, IL: College of DuPage.

Flood, L. S., Gasiewicz, N., & Delpier, T. (2010). Integrating information literacy across a BSN curriculum. *Journal of Nursing Education*, *49*, 101–104. doi:10.3928/01484834-20091023-01

Giddens, J. F., North, S., Carlson-Sabelli, L., Rogers, E., & Fogg, L. (2012). Using a virtual community to enhance cultural awareness. *Journal of Transcultural Nursing*, *23*, 198–204. doi:10.1177/1043659611434061

Gigante, J., Dell, M., & Sharkey, A. (2011). Getting beyond "good job": How to give effective feedback. *Pediatrics*, *127*, 205–207. doi:10.1542/peds.2010-3351

Hall, M. A. (2013). An expanded look at evaluating clinical performance: Faculty use of anecdotal notes in the U.S. and Canada. *Nurse Education in Practice*, *13*, 271–276.

Hall, M., Daly, B., & Madigan, E. (2010). Use of anecdotal notes by clinical nursing faculty: A descriptive study. *Journal of Nursing Education*, *49*, 156–159. doi:10.3928/01484834-20090915-03

Hawala-Druy, S., & Hill, M. H. (2012). Interdisciplinary: Cultural competency and culturally congruent education for millennials in health professions. *Nurse Education Today*, *32*, 772–778. doi:10.1016/j.nedt.2012.05.002

Holaday, S. D., & Buckley, K. M. (2008). A standardized clinical evaluation tool-kit: Improving nursing education and practice. In M. H. Oermann (Ed.), *Annual review of nursing education* (Vol. 6, pp. 123–149). New York, NY: Springer Publishing Company.

Holmboe, E. S. (2008). Direct observation by faculty. In: E. S. Holmboe & R. E. Hawkins (Eds.), *Practical guide to the evaluation of clinical competence* (pp. 119–129). Philadelphia, PA: Mosby Elsevier.

Institute of Medicine. (2011). *The future of nursing: Leading change, advancing health.* Washington, DC: The National Academies Press.

Li, H. C., Wang, L. S., Lin, Y. H., & Lee, I. (2011). The effect of a peer-mentoring strategy on student nurse stress reduction in clinical practice. *International Nursing Review*, *58*, 203–210. doi:10.1111/j.1466-7657.2010.00839.x

Manning, A., Cronin, P., Monaghan, A., & Rawlings-Anderson, K. (2009). Supporting students in practice: An exploration of reflective groups as a means of support. *Nurse Education in Practice*, *9*, 176–183. doi:10.1016/j.nepr.2008.07.001

McKeon, L. M., Norris, T., Cardell, B., & Britt, T. (2009). Developing patient-centered care competencies among prelicensure nursing students using simulation. *Journal of Nursing Education*, *48*, 711–715. doi:10.3928/01484834-20091113-06

McKown, T., McKeon, L., & Webb, S. (2011). Using quality and safety education for nurses to guide clinical teaching on a new dedicated education unit. *Journal of Nursing Education*, *50*, 706–710. doi:10.3928/01484834-20111017-03

Melincavage, S. M. (2011). Student nurses' experiences of anxiety in the clinical setting. *Nurse Education Today, 31*, 785–789. doi:10.1016/j.nedt.2011.05.007

Moscaritolo, L. M. (2009). Interventional strategies to decrease nursing student anxiety in the clinical learning environment. *Journal of Nursing Education, 48*, 17–23.

Nitko, A. J., & Brookhart, S. M. (2011). *Educational assessment of students* (6th ed.). Upper Saddle River, NJ: Pearson Education.

Oermann, M. H., & Gaberson, K. B. (2014). *Evaluation and testing in nursing education* (4th ed.). New York, NY: Springer Publishing Company.

Oermann, M. H., Yarbrough, S. S., Ard, N., Saewert, K. J., & Charasika, M. (2009). Clinical evaluation and grading practices in schools of nursing: National survey findings Part II. *Nursing Education Perspectives, 30*, 352–357.

Parsons, M. E., Hawkins, K. S., Hercinger, M., Todd, M., Manz, J. A., & Fang, X. (2012). Improvement in scoring consistency for the Creighton Simulation Evaluation Instrument. *Clinical Simulation in Nursing, 8*(6), e233–e238.

QSEN Institute. (2013). Pre-licensure KSAs. Retrieved from http://qsen.org/competencies/pre-licensure-ksas

Sherwood, G. (2012). Driving forces for quality and safety: Changing mindsets to improve health care. In G. Sherwood & J. Barnsteiner (Eds.), *Quality and safety in nursing: A competency approach to improving outcomes* (pp. 3–22). Oxford, England: John Wiley & Sons.

Sherwood, G., & Barnsteiner, J. (Eds.). (2012). *Quality and safety in nursing: A competency approach to improving outcomes*. Oxford, UK: John Wiley & Sons.

Swan, B. A., Smith, K. A., Frisby, A., Shaffer, K., Hanson-Zalot M., & Becker, J. (2013). Enhancing tablet technology in an undergraduate nursing program. *Nursing Education Perspectives, 34*, 192–193.

Tellez, M. (2012). Nursing informatics education past, present, and future. *CIN: Computers, Informatics, Nursing, 30*, 229–233. doi:10.1097/NXN.0b013e3182569f42

Walsh, T., Jairath, N., Paterson, M., & Grandjean, C. (2010). Quality and safety education for nurses clinical evaluation tool. *Journal of Nursing Education, 49*, 517–522. doi:10.3928/01484834-20100630-06

Zurmehly, J. (2010). Personal digital assistants (PDAs): Review and evaluation. *Nursing Education Perspectives, 31*, 179–182.

13

The Context in Which Teaching Takes Place: The Curriculum

SARAH B. KEATING

It is vital that nurse educators take into account the context in which teaching takes place. Such recognition ensures the integrity of the mission and purpose of the curriculum or educational program. Often, both new and experienced teachers focus on the specific content of the classes or sessions they teach and lose sight of the objectives and how they relate to the overall program. The temptation is to adjust the objectives and content to the individual teacher's personal interests and expertise. Such changes can result in the loss of the educational program or curriculum's intent and planned student learning outcomes. If the teacher identifies the need to update the content of a class and thus the objectives, it is important to compare the proposed change to the overall curriculum to discover its impact on the total program. Such changes can involve revision of the curriculum and, depending on the setting, involve other members of the educational team. In the case of major changes, approval processes for the revisions might be necessary through the hierarchal structures in the involved academe or health care setting. These processes focus on curriculum revision. However, if a need for a new curriculum or educational program arises, the processes become that of curriculum development.

This chapter describes the processes for curriculum development or revision for schools of nursing or educational programs related to patient education and staff development in health care settings. To determine whether a curriculum needs revision or a new program is proposed, a needs assessment is necessary to document the need. This chapter reviews the factors that influence educational programs and curricula and provides guidelines for collecting and analyzing data in order to make informed decisions about revising or developing curricula.

To gain an appreciation of the connection of teaching/learning sessions to the curriculum or educational program, the components of the curriculum are described. The influence of the components on the teacher, student/learner, courses or classes, and related learning activities are considered. The importance of program and student learning outcomes and how they direct subsequent instructional strategies and ongoing evaluation of the curriculum or educational program are discussed. Though the setting can vary according to the type of educational program (e.g., schools of nursing or health care agencies), the same processes and components of the curriculum apply. Budget considerations are briefly reviewed as they apply to curriculum/program development and revision.

NEEDS ASSESSMENT

Developing a new educational program or revising an existing one calls for a needs assessment; that is, there must be compelling factors to cause the change or to create a new one. For the purposes of this text, a brief review of possible factors that influence change or the development of new programs in academic or health care settings is discussed as they apply to nurse educators who teach in these programs. Keating (2011) discusses in detail the external and internal frame factors that influence curriculum development and offers outlines for collecting and analyzing relevant data for making decisions related to this activity. Figures 13.1 and 13.2 present models of external and internal frame factors.

FIGURE 13.1 External frame factors for a needs assessment for curriculum development in nursing.

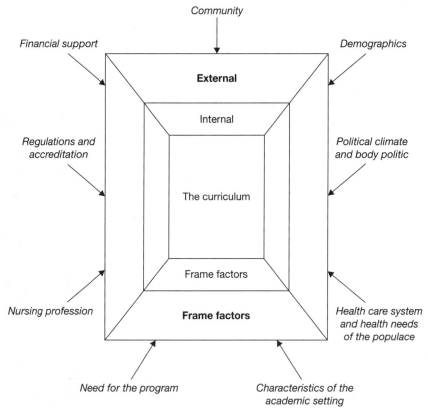

Adapted from Johnson (1977). From Keating (2011), p. 92. Reproduced with the permission of Springer Publishing Company, LLC, 2013.

Faculty members in the academic setting often recognize the need for revision or development of new programs within their schools of nursing. Though the major functions of their role can be that of teaching, research, and scholarly activities, service to the institution and community are also expectations. Service to the institution includes membership on curriculum committees and participation in level and course meetings that concern the need for revision of the program. It is possible that members of committees or level and course coordinators identify the need for change to bring

FIGURE 13.2   Internal frame factors for a needs assessment for curriculum development in nursing.

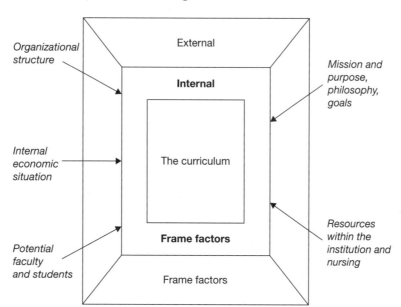

Adapted from Johnson (1977). From Keating (2011), p. 132. Reproduced with the permission of Springer Publishing Company, LLC, 2013.

the curriculum up to date or to adjust learning objectives to improve student learning outcomes. Teachers might be aware of changes in nursing education or the health care system that call for new programs to meet the demands of the profession and needs of the population. In such instances, a new program is indicated.

Nurse educators in health care settings, for example, in staff development and patient education, experience the same indicators for the need to change educational programs or create new ones. Although their central role might be that of teaching staff or patients, at the same time, they often recognize the need for new programs to update staff knowledge and skills or to educate patients on the newest treatment protocols and preventive health care strategies. The organizational structure might be different from that of academe, but nurse educators revise or create new programs and consult with other members of the organization such as nurse administrators, managers, and other members of the multidisciplinary team, including physicians, therapists, pharmacists, and others.

EXTERNAL FRAME FACTORS

No matter what the setting, the need for creation of new programs, or revision of existing ones, the process for change is much the same. There are factors that influence the educational program and curriculum and indicate that a needs assessment in is in order. External frame factors are those outside of the parent institution in which the program is housed, for example, the health care system and its changes, the nursing profession, the community and population served by the institution, competitive schools or agencies, government and political bodies, and accrediting and program approval agencies. Table 13.1 provides examples of external frame factors influencing nursing programs and health care agencies.

TABLE 13.1 Sample External Frame Factors Influencing Educational Programs in Academic and Health Care Settings

External Frame Factor	Academic Settings	Health Care Settings
Health care system and changes in it	New technologies Changes in delivery of care (primary and acute care)	New technologies Health care demands: primary, secondary, tertiary
Nursing profession	Institute of Medicine calls for higher education Certification for advanced practice and leadership roles	Orientation needs Skills updates Continuing education requirements Role of nurse educators in patient education
Community and population served	Role of school of nursing in providing nursing workforce locally, regionally, and nationally Population health care needs, e.g., geriatrics, major causes of morbidity and mortality, etc.	Rural, suburban, urban Type of services (acute, tertiary, extended care, nursing home, rehabilitation, public health, home care, hospice, etc.) Population health care needs, e.g., geriatrics, major causes of morbidity and mortality, etc.
Competitive schools or agencies	Levels of nursing programs in direct competition Possibilities of collaboration Programs articulating with each other (e.g., associate degree leading into baccalaureate or master's programs)	Competitive agencies in the region Specialty units Possibilities for collaboration
Government and political bodies	Involvement in political activities that support higher education Awareness of financial programs that support student financial aid, program development, and research	Regulations governing health care services at state and national levels Medicare and Medicaid reimbursement policies Health insurance and other payers for health care services Regulations affecting professional practice
Accrediting and program approval agencies	Commission on Collegiate Nursing Education or Accreditation Commission for Education in Nursing Regional accreditation Specialty accreditation Board of nursing approval	The Joint Commission Community-based accreditation and by specialty Board approval Government regulations

INTERNAL FRAME FACTORS

Internal frame factors are those that come from within the institution in which the educational program is housed. Similar to external frame factors, these influence the need for change or the creation of new programs. Nurse educators in schools of nursing, as contributing members to the program, participate on curriculum committees and other governance bodies within the school at various levels of the institutional organization, such as division or department curriculum committees, and on university-wide committees. Even faculty senates have influence and approval powers for curricula and their creation, revision, and/or discontinuance. The administrators of the institution also have influence, including the president, vice president(s), provost, dean, associate deans, and chairs or directors of academic programs. All new programs must go through the appropriate echelons of approval bodies from the school or department faculty to the chief administrative officer. Major revisions experience the same approval processes as new programs; however, depending on the extent of the revision, such as minor changes to course objectives, approval at higher levels might not be necessary, and only the curriculum committee in the school and/or faculty approval might be required. Internal frame factors in the academic setting include organizational and administrative structures, physical plant and resources, budget, faculty and staff numbers and qualifications, faculty governance, and the student body and characteristics.

Internal frame factors that influence health care settings are similar to those in schools of nursing and other academic settings. The cost and benefits of educational programs for patients and staff development influence the creation and revision of the curricula. Other factors are the organizational structure (public or private, religion-based or nonsectarian, profit or nonprofit, etc.); administrative echelon; physical plant; budget; nature of the staff, both professional and nonprofessional; governance; and characteristics of the population served. Table 13.2 provides examples of internal frame factors influencing schools of nursing and health care agencies.

TABLE 13.2 Sample Internal Frame Factors Influencing Educational Programs in Academic and Health Care Settings

Internal Frame Factor	Academic Settings	Health Care Settings
Organizational and administrative structures (public or private; religion-based or nonsectarian)	Place of nursing program within the institution (layers of decision making) Sources of funding (e.g., state, tuition, endowments, etc.)	Place of education within agency, power structure, to whom the educator reports? Agency structure (e.g., independent, part of a health care system, governmental agency, etc.) Funding sources
Physical plant and resources	Faculty offices, classroom, labs, conference rooms, media supplies, and services Library and other support	Audiovisual materials, learning labs, classrooms, conference rooms, Internet access and support Supplies and services

(continued)

Table 13.2 Sample Internal Frame Factors Influencing Educational Programs in Academic and Health Care Settings (*continued*)

Internal Frame Factor	Academic Settings	Health Care Settings
Budget	Control for forecasting needs and expenditures	Cost of program and benefit analysis
	External funding resources	Control for forecasting needs and expenditures
	Scholarship and research support	
Governance	Faculty involvement	Place of educational program in the agency
	Student representation	
		Educator involvement in governance
Nature of the staff both professional and nonprofessional	Faculty numbers and qualifications	Qualifications and experience of educators
	Support staff adequacy	Staff support adequacy
Characteristics of the population served	Student body	Patient population
	Community served by the students and faculty	Staff: nursing and other providers of care
Internal program approval	Periodic review by institution: frequency	Administrators
		Advisory Board

Nurse educators should be aware of the environment in which they teach. As educational programs are implemented, and the need for new ones are identified, persons who teach in the programs must be part of the processes for conducting a needs assessment and developing a curriculum. Although teaching dominates their activities, educators' involvement in the needs assessment contributes to dynamic, evolving, and high-quality programs.

COMPONENTS OF THE CURRICULUM

The following discussion describes the components of the curriculum that nurse educators should be familiar with when teaching in an educational program. The components begin with the mission and/or vision of the institution and move through a philosophy statement reviewing the teachers' beliefs about teaching and learning, to an organizational framework to provide a schema for the program. That is followed by an overall goal statement with accompanying end-of-program learning outcomes, usually stated in the form of objectives, and finally to an implementation plan that includes a list of the courses or learning sessions and their objectives. Each component is described briefly as a guide for teachers when they are assessing or orienting themselves to their curricula or educational programs. The importance of involving key stakeholders in the process so that schools and agencies respond to the health care needs of their community cannot be overemphasized.

MISSION AND/OR VISION

The mission of the curriculum or educational program must align itself with the mission of the parent institution. Curran and Totten (2010) provide the rationale for having mission statements in health care agencies with an emphasis on the involvement of key stakeholders, including those populations that the agencies serve.

The Board of Directors of the Association of American Colleges and Universities (AACU) developed a paper on its beliefs about mission statements for higher education in the United States (AACU, 2010). It emphasizes the need for a melding of liberal education and the knowledge and skills desired for the workplace. According to AACU, mission statements and visions should embrace four critical learning outcomes, including "knowledge of human cultures and the physical and natural world, intellectual and practical skills, personal and social responsibility, and integrative learning" (p. 32). Nursing faculty members should look for these major concepts in the parent institution's mission or vision for congruence with those of the school of nursing and seek to identify how they are translated into the curriculum. For example, knowledge of human cultures is identified for the development of cultural competence; knowledge of the natural and physical world applies to the prerequisite knowledge for nursing, including chemistry, biology, anatomy, physiology, and microbiology. Intellectual and practical skills are integral to the development of critical thinking and clinical decisions, as well as the technical skills required to provide nursing care. Personal and social responsibility relate to professional behaviors, and integrative learning applies nursing knowledge to the delivery of nursing care. An awareness of these concepts and their appearance in mission statements help to guide teachers as they carry out their educational activities.

PHILOSOPHY

As with mission and vision statements, a philosophy statement describes the beliefs of the members of the institution and contains additional theories and concepts that help to guide the development of the curriculum or educational program. In schools of nursing, central theories and concepts can include faculty's beliefs about teaching and learning, social justice, diversity, health and illness, professional values, etc. Health care agencies develop philosophy statements that expound on their missions and visions to further explain the rationale and purpose for their services to the community and what is unique about them.

Nurse educators are essential to the development of philosophy statements and their realization. Teachers meet to discuss their personal beliefs about the educational program and come to consensus to produce a philosophical statement that reflects their values and ethics and the critical concepts and theories used in the program to deliver the program or curriculum. Nurses considering positions as teachers or those in current teaching positions should review the philosophy statements of their institutions to assure congruence with their personal beliefs and values. If conflict is discovered, the issues should be discussed with others to possibly review the statements, or if incongruity exits and cannot be changed, the individual should consider finding a position in a nursing program with values and beliefs similar to his or her own.

Ricci (2011) describes change and the leadership process involved when examining the mission and vision, and when planning a curriculum or educational program. He differentiates between the mission and vision, with the mission stating the overall purpose of the institution and the vision expressing the institution's aspirations for the future. Both guide philosophical discussions by the key stakeholders and the subsequent development of the plan for delivering the program and its evaluation. When developing or revising a program, participants in the change process should review the philosophy to ensure that it includes current beliefs and that the major concepts and theories that apply to the program are present. From the statement, an organizational framework serves as the scaffolding or support for the curriculum. The philosophy assists teachers in choosing a framework that encompasses the mission, vision, and beliefs about the program and its services.

ORGANIZATIONAL FRAMEWORK

An organizational framework for an educational program or curriculum is essential to the integration of the theories and concepts identified in the mission, vision, and philosophy and serves as an outline on which to build the goals, objectives, courses or sessions, and content into a plan for delivering the program. Professional and accreditation standards often serve as frameworks. For example, in health care agencies, there are requirements to meet the standards defined by The Joint Commission. Another example is the American Cancer Society's (ACS) Guidelines on Nutrition and Physical Activity for Cancer Prevention (ACS, 2013).

Though not specified in the Accreditation Commission for Education in Nursing (ACEN) Standards and Criteria (ACEN, 2013; http://www.acenursing.net/manuals/SC2013.pdf) or the Commission on Collegiate Nursing Education (2012) standards for accreditation (www.aacn.nche.edu/ccne-accreditation/standards-procedures-resources/overview), many schools of nursing use these standards as organizational frameworks. Many baccalaureate and higher degree programs use the American Association of Colleges of Nursing's (AACN's) Essentials of Baccalaureate Education for Professional Nursing Practice, Essentials of Master's Education in Nursing, and Essentials of Doctoral Education for Advanced Nursing Practice as frameworks (AACN, 2012; www.aacn.nche.edu/education-resources/essential-series).

Although not as common, both agencies and schools of nursing sometimes use nursing and health-related models or theories as a framework on which to organize the program, for example, systems theory, health belief models, stress and adaptation, health-illness continuum, and others. Tables 13.3 and 13.4 provide examples of organizational frameworks in a health care setting and school of nursing. Organizational frameworks, in addition to providing guidelines for the program, also provide schemata for assessment of student learning outcomes and evaluation of the program. For example, teachers can return to the framework to assess certain concepts; identify where they are taught in the nursing program; identify the objectives (or outcomes), content, and learning activities associated with them; and analyze the level of achievement that students reach in meeting the relevant objectives.

TABLE 13.3 Organizational Framework for a Health Care Agency Educational Program for Cancer Prevention: Target Population, Grades Kindergarten to Sixth (K–6) Grade

ACS Guideline	End-of-Program Goal	Patient Education Objectives
Achieve and maintain a healthy weight throughout life	The majority of children (80%) in grades K–6 will achieve and maintain recommended weight for age and height.	Children will: Describe the benefits of healthy weight over a lifetime. Exhibit healthy eating behaviors. Achieve recommended weight for age and height.
Be physically active	Children in grades K–6 will participate in daily physical activities.	Children will: Describe the benefits of daily physical activity. Participate in physical activities in school, at home, and in the community.

(continued)

ACS Guideline	End-of-Program Goal	Patient Education Objectives
Eat a healthy diet with an emphasis on plant foods	At least 80% of children in grades K–6 will consume healthy diets in the home, school, and community environments.	Children will: Describe healthy diets by listing healthy foods with an emphasis on plant foods. Children will be provided with healthy foods at school and during community events. Parents of children K–6 will attend nutrition classes sponsored by the school.
Public, private, and community organizations work together to apply policy and environmental changes that promote cancer prevention behaviors	Schools, parent–teacher organizations, the local health department, and ACS will work together to apply policy and environmental changes that promote cancer prevention behaviors.	A community advisory board will be organized to initiate healthy eating and physical activities for school-aged children. The advisory board will collaborate with the health care agency in implementing multi-pronged educational programs in the community to promote healthy eating and physical activity for school-aged children.

ACS, American Cancer Society.

Source: Adapted from American Cancer Society: *Summary of the ACS guidelines on nutrition and physical activity.* http://www.cancer.org/Healthy/EatHealthyGetActive/ACSGuidelinesonNutrition PhysicalActivity forCancerPrevention/acs-guidelines-on-nutrition-and-physical-activity-for-cancer-prevention-summary

TABLE 13.4 Organizational Framework for an Associate Degree Nursing Program Curriculum Based on ACEN Standard 4 Curriculum

Standard	End-of-Program Objective	Year 1 Objectives	Year 2 Objectives
The curriculum includes cultural, ethnic, and socially diverse concepts and may also include experiences from regional, national, or global perspectives.	The graduate will provide culturally competent nursing care for ethnically and socially diverse populations.	The student will: Analyze ethnically, culturally, and socially characteristics in the patient population served by nursing. Recognize differences in populations served. Adapt nursing care according to the cultural needs of the patients served.	The graduate will provide culturally competent nursing care for ethnically and socially diverse populations.

(continued)

Table 13.4 Organizational Framework for an Associate Degree Nursing Program Curriculum Based on ACEN Standard 4 Curriculum (*continued*)

Standard	End-of-Program Objective	Year 1 Objectives	Year 2 Objectives
The curriculum incorporates established professional standards, guidelines, and competencies, and has clearly articulated student learning and program outcomes.	The graduate will incorporate ethical, professional standards and competencies in the provision of nursing care.	The student will analyze professional nursing standards and their relationship to ethical nursing care.	The graduate will incorporate ethical, professional standards and competencies in the provision of nursing care.
The curriculum and instructional processes reflect educational theory, interdisciplinary collaboration, research, and current standards of practice while allowing for innovation, flexibility, and technological advances.	The graduate will integrate nursing and interdisciplinary knowledge, best practice standards, and technological advances into the delivery of nursing care.	The student will: Analyze interdisciplinary coordination for health care provision. Describe best practice standards. Utilize technology in the delivery of patient care services.	The graduate will integrate nursing and interdisciplinary knowledge, best practice standards, and technological advances into the delivery of nursing care.
Student clinical experiences reflect current best practices and nationally established patient health and safety goals.	The graduate will provide safe, competent, and knowledgeable nursing care that reflects national patient health and safety goals.	The student will: Describe the national patient health and safety goals. Integrate social and scientific knowledge with the liberal arts into nursing care strategies. Provide safe patient care.	The graduate will provide safe, competent, and knowledgeable nursing care that reflects national patient health and safety goals.

ACEN, Accreditation Commission for Education in Nursing.

Source: Adapted from ACEN: Standard 4. Curriculum. Associate (p. 4), http://www.acenursing.net/manuals/SC2013.pdf

OVERALL PROGRAM GOALS AND PURPOSE

Based on the mission and/or vision, philosophy, and organizational framework, a purpose statement or overall goal(s) sets the stage for defining the specific objectives, competencies, or student learning outcomes that the curriculum or educational program purports to achieve. The literature is crowded with terms signifying educational goals or aims, objectives, and the steps for completing them. Most nurse educators express the steps toward achieving desired learning outcomes in terms of objectives to be met. The advantage to this format is the ability to measure the outcomes and, therefore, assess and evaluate the success of the program. For the purposes of this chapter, goals are identified as the overall aims or purpose of the program, and program learning outcomes are a description of the "product" of the program, that is, what the graduate or participant in the program will achieve. Student learning outcomes are the objectives or steps the learner takes to reach the outcomes and goals of the program. Multiple texts and articles in the literature provide educators with recipes for developing behaviorally stated objectives and student learning outcomes. Expressed in behavioral terms, the objectives of specific courses or learning sessions help to define what student learning outcomes are expected from the teaching/learning process (Todd, 2012).

IMPLEMENTATION PLAN

Program, Level, and Student Learning Outcomes

To carry out the educational program or the curriculum, an implementation plan must be organized according to the program goals and learning outcomes. In order to reach these outcomes, a series of steps are necessary to assist the learner to progress through the program and reach the ultimate goal. For a school of nursing, the curriculum can be divided into segments according to the level of progress toward the final year, such as the sophomore, junior, and senior years. For a health care agency, the program can be self-contained and consist of only one session or multiple sessions depending on the target audience. For example, in staff development, an orientation program can consist of instilling in the new employees the organization's mission and philosophy, familiarizing them with policies and procedures, reviewing the necessary skills to assure the employees' competency and patient safety, and assigning them to mentors. In these examples, the program learning outcomes are listed and filter down to the various levels of the program. Table 13.5 provides an example of one program learning outcome in a baccalaureate curriculum as it is tracked from the end of the program, through the senior, junior, and sophomore levels to course objectives at each level.

TABLE 13.5 Sample Tracking of a Program Learning Outcome in a Baccalaureate Nursing Program[a]

Level Student Learning Outcomes (SLOs)	Relevant Course Number and SLOs
Senior-Level SLO	N400 Community Health Nursing:
Provide evidence-based therapeutic nursing interventions for culturally diverse patients and families in a wide variety of health care and community settings.	Demonstrate evidence-based practice in nursing interventions for patients, families, and communities. Apply culturally competent nursing care concepts to the care of patients, families, and communities in the community setting.
Junior-Level SLO	N300 Nursing Care of Adults in Acute Care:
Integrate evidence-based therapeutic nursing interventions into the care of ethnically and culturally diverse patients and families.	Analyze evidence-based concepts into the nursing process and the delivery of therapeutic nursing interventions for patients and families. Implement culturally competent nursing care in the acute care setting.
Sophomore-Level SLO	N200 Introduction to Professional Nursing:
Develop nursing care plans that reflect evidence-based practice and therapeutic interventions in the care of ethnically and culturally diverse patients.	Describe the concept of evidence-based practice. Describe the nursing process and therapeutic nursing interventions. Compare ethnically and culturally diverse patient groups and their health care needs.

[a]Program Learning Outcome (PLO): The graduate will provide evidence-based therapeutic nursing interventions for culturally diverse patients and families in a wide variety of health care and community settings.

A familiarity with educational taxonomies is helpful when assessing or developing objectives to fit the level of learner, as illustrated in the table. Note that the novice learner objectives use terms such as "describes," the intermediate learner "integrates," and the senior learner "provides." Once the level objectives are identified, course or session objectives with their sequencing fall into place. This becomes the "Program of Study." Exhibit 13.1 is an example of a Program of Study for a master's program in a school of nursing and Exhibit 13.2 for a Staff Orientation Program.

EXHIBIT 13.1 Sample Program of Study for a Master of Science in Nursing Administration Program

Year 1 Fall Semester	Spring Semester
• Theoretical and Scientific Foundations of Nursing (3) • Introduction to Quantitative and Qualitative Statistics (3) • Research in Nursing (3)	• Analysis of Health care Organizations (3) • Health care Policy and Political Action (3) Nursing Leadership Strategies (3)
Year 2 Fall Semester	**Spring Semester**
• Informatics and Technology in Health care Systems (3) • Health care Economics (3) • Administration Role Development and Practicum I (2) • Nursing Project or Thesis Proposal (1)	• Human Resources and Budget Management (3) Administration Role Development and Practicum II (2) • Nursing Project or Thesis Defense (4)
Total Credits: 36	

EXHIBIT 13.2 Sample Program of Study for a 6-Month Staff Orientation Program in an Acute Care Hospital With Responsible Parties

Month 1

- *Week 1:* Class: Description of mentoring program and assignment to mentor for observational experiences: educator and mentors
- *Week 2:* Class: Mission, vision, and philosophy of the agency: chief executive officer, chief nursing officer, chief operations officer

Patient care assignments to continue throughout the 6 months with the assigned mentor

- *Week 3:* Class: Agency personnel policies: human resources staff
- *Week 4:* Class: General agency policies and procedure: educator

Month 2

- *Weeks 1 and 2:* Class and lab practice: Skills competencies assessment and updating: educator
- *Weeks 3 and 4:* Class: Policies and procedures specific to assigned unit: educator and mentor

(continued)

Month 3

- *Weeks 1 and 2:* Class and lab practice: Skills competencies assessment and updating: educator
- *Weeks 3 and 4:* Meeting: Performance assessment for probationary period: educator and mentor

Month 4

- *Weeks 1 and 2:* Class and lab practice: Skills remediation and updating: educator
- *Weeks 3 and 4:* Staff governance participation: educator

Month 5

- *Weeks 1 and 2:* Class: Review of agency and unit policies and evaluation of orientation program: educator. (*Weeks 3 and 4:* patient care assignment)

Month 6

- *Weeks 1 and 2:* Meeting: Final performance assessment for probationary period: educator and mentor

---

The final step in curriculum development following the plan and sequencing of courses or sessions of study is to develop outlines for the course or sessions. The following briefly describes the classic components for a course description. In colleges and universities, the course usually has a number with a prefix that indicates its discipline (e.g., NURS100 for a nursing course). Following the identifier, the title of the course appears, which introduces the major concepts taught in the course, for example, NURS100 Introduction to Professional Nursing. A brief description is listed, comprised of usually no more than three sentences and captures the essence of the course. For example, for NURS100: Describes nursing as a profession, its history, and its role in the interdisciplinary health care system. Course objectives follow and should align with level and program student learning outcomes. Using NURS100 as the exemplar, one objective could be: compares the profession of nursing to the definition of a profession.

A content outline follows that contains the topics specific to the objectives and the timeframes related to when they are introduced, discussed, and assessed. The learning activities associated with the objectives and content accompany the topical outline and include such strategies as discussion, lecture, group assignments, role playing, and so forth. The methods for measuring student progress toward meeting the learning outcomes are provided, and their contribution to the course grade are listed. These include quizzes, tests, essays, participation in discussions, and others. Finally, statements on academic dishonesty and provisions for disability are reiterated according to academic polices.

Parallel descriptions for courses and sessions apply to the health care setting. At the very least, the session should include the title for the session, a brief description, the expected learning outcomes/objectives, a topical outline, timeframe, and description of the learning activities such as demonstration-return demonstration, lecture, group work, and so forth. A statement on how the outcomes and effectiveness of the session will be measured should be mentioned, such as a quiz or ratings of the session according to objectives and teaching effectiveness.

CONCEPT OR CONTENT MAPPING

It is helpful for educators to review the curriculum or program as a whole to insure that certain concepts or content critical to delivering the program are covered in the implementation. To accomplish this task, it is useful to create content or concept maps that trace the concept throughout the program. The concept maps are also illustrations for students to identify relationships between concepts and the logic underlying the concept and its application to nursing practice. Several articles discuss the usefulness of concept maps in teaching/learning situations for nursing students and staff in hospitals (All & Huycke, 2007; Conceição & Taylor, 2007; Vacek, 2009; Wilgis & McConnell, 2008). Figure 13.3 is an example of a simplified concept map that traces the concept of social justice in a baccalaureate curriculum. Novak and Cañas (2012) provide an extensive discussion on the purpose of concept maps, the theory underlying them, and how to construct them. Concept maps were also discussed in Chapter 10.

FIGURE 13.3 Sample concept map of social justice content in a baccalaureate nursing curriculum.

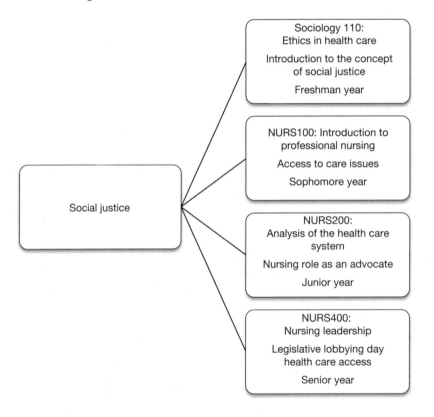

BUDGET CONSIDERATIONS

BUDGETS IN THE ACADEMIC SETTING

Though teachers are not directly involved in the process of budget planning or management, they should have an appreciation for its place in developing and revising educational programs and curricula. In academic settings, the dean or director of the school, college, or department usually has control over budget development and requests for funds to run the program. The dean or director also estimates additional budget items to supplement normal expenditures. The everyday costs to implement a curriculum include faculty and staff salaries and benefits; office equipment and supplies; audiovisual materials; computer hardware and software for faculty, staff, and classroom support; simulation and other skills lab equipment and supplies; faculty development activities including research, scholarly activities, and travel; and the physical facilities such as offices, classrooms, conference rooms, labs, and others. Additional funding beyond the usual includes the costs associated with program development and revision such as released time for faculty members involved in the process and additional office supplies to support the development activities. Periodic program approval and accreditation expenses are part of the budget, including accreditation fees and, similar to program approval, released time for faculty and staff and the additional associated materials. These costs are some examples of the costs for maintaining a nursing program in the academic setting and are not necessarily complete.

Forecasting budget needs for the future as well as decisions about the expenditures and maintenance of the budget is usually within the dean or director's prerogative; however, these functions can differ according to the organizational schema and political climate of the institution within which the program is housed. Size of the program also influences how the budget is administered, for example, in small programs the dean or director might be solely responsible for planning, requesting, expending, maintaining, and reporting on the budget. Larger programs might have an administrative assistant to whom the dean delegates budget responsibilities.

Sources of funding are critical to the life of the program and the assurance of its quality. In large multipurpose colleges and universities, nursing programs are often targeted as expensive, owing to the clinical nature of the program and the low student-to-faculty ratio required for safe clinical supervision of students. Nursing's reply to these challenges usually points out that nursing students and their prerequisites from the sciences and liberal arts provide many full-time equivalents for the other disciplines.

Funding for the program is dependent on the nature of the parent institution, with income from the general funds if state-supported or tuition and endowment funds for private schools. All programs, whether state-funded or private, cannot rely solely on these sources of funds, and thus grants, donations in the form of endowments and scholarships, and some revenue-generating opportunities are sought. Faculty are involved in these activities such as grant writing with released time for research and program development as rewards if the grants are funded. Revenue-generating programs include faculty practice clinics with Medicare, Medicaid, and health care insurance plans reimbursement funding. Charging additional lab fees to cover costs and special tuition rates through continuing education are additional sources of funds to pay for the cost of supplies and services and faculty and staff salaries.

All of these factors point out the need for teachers to be aware of the sources of funding for and the costs to run the educational program. Many deans and directors share budget planning and spending with faculty members to involve them in the process and to seek their input on cost savings and revenue generation. Such activities contribute to an appreciation of the budget and its influence on the implementation and quality of the program.

BUDGETS IN THE HEALTH CARE SETTING

Financial support for staff development and/or patient education varies widely in health care agencies. Depending on the size of the institution, its purpose for service to the community, and the sources of funding, the budget for educational purposes can be set aside separately or as part of another department within the agency. Large academic and non-academic medical centers usually have an educational department staffed by educators (usually nurses) who have expertise in developing programs and teaching. Services include staff development, orientation of new staff, and patient education. One nurse might serve as the educator and acts as coordinator for the programs with staff nurses, physicians, and other health care professionals teaching in the program. The budget for this type of structure is usually within the agency's overall budget or set aside to target specific educational services. In larger institutions, the education department might be composed of several staff members, usually nurses or health educators, and coordinated by a manager who has administrative support staff. Budget responsibilities fall to the manager of the program who accounts for staff salaries and benefits, office supplies and services, media and computer hardware and software, and associated facilities such as conference rooms, classrooms, and laboratories.

To be accredited, The Joint Commission (2012) requires that health care agencies meet its standards. Most standards imply or address educational needs including those related to staff orientation, staff qualifications and continuing education, and patient education. Agencies need to document that these services are present and effective, and, thus, educational services are integral to the functioning of the agency. It should be noted that each time policies and procedures change in the institution or The Joint Commission issues revised standards, it is necessary for staff to receive education to comply with national standards (e.g., safety regulatory requirements).

Several articles in the literature provide examples of these types of services. Gannon (2011) describes an assessment of an academic medical center and its role in establishing a learning organization for the benefit of patients, staff, and health care students. Burfeind (2009) provides an example of the need for staff development when updating professionals on The Joint Commission's National Patient Safety Goals. Bragg et al. (2011) describe the creation of Geriatric Research, Education, and Clinical Centers in the Veterans Administration that focus on geriatrics education for staff and students. Michel (2009) describes a patient safety education program that involves patients, and Hill et al. (2011) studied the need for patient education regarding falls after discharge from the hospital. Stonecypher (2009) describes the development of a patient education tool for post-stroke patients and the involvement of the multidisciplinary team in its development.

The nurse educator's role is to make the case for educational needs in the agency and the associated costs for their delivery. Cost savings realized by the implementation of educational programs for staff and patients provide a significant rationale for the existence of the program. Larger institutions might have several educators on staff with administrative assistant support. Smaller institutions depend on individual staff members' identification of educational needs, development of programs, and their implementation. Costs associated with these activities are absorbed into the time spent in delivering the services as a part of the care provided.

Health departments and other governmental agencies use general funds to pay for educational programs. Again, depending on its size, there might be dedicated nurse educators or health educators to provide staff development/orientation and patient education services as indicated. If it is a large department within the agency, the chief coordinator of the education department is responsible for the budget, whereas smaller agencies might depend on separate requests to the agency administrator for the educational program. Nonprofit agencies in the community also provide patient education services. These agencies often rely on donations, endowments and, to some extent, fees for services. The agencies might employ nurse or health educators or integrate the services into the specific care services that they provide.

As with academic settings, it is necessary for the educator to document the need for education, justify its expense, and manage the funds that are provided. Although educational services in health care settings are vital to maintain a competent staff and provide preventive and health maintenance educational services for patients, the importance of education is often lost. Nurses in these settings have a responsibility to bring the need to the attention of the administrators and the public, and to develop budgets for the services that are reasonable in cost, justify their need, and are sustainable over time.

SUMMARY

Chapter 13 reviewed the role of nurse educators in schools of nursing and health care agencies in the context of the educational programs in which they teach. It compared the differences between curriculum development and revision and pointed out the necessity for examining the external and internal frame factors that influence change or the creation of a new program. The major components of the curriculum were described, and their interrelationships, the implementation of the curriculum, and its evaluation were discussed. Mention of concept and content maps illustrated how educators can track concepts or content throughout the curriculum to assure their presence and levels of understanding in the program. Brief overviews of the budget process for programs in both the academic and practice setting were presented.

REFERENCES

Accreditation Commission for Education in Nursing (ACEN). (2013). Accreditation manual. Section III. Standards and criteria glossary. Atlanta, GA: ACEN.

All, A., & Huycke, L. (2007). Serial concept maps: Tools for concept analysis. *Journal of Nursing Education, 46*, 217–224.

American Association of Colleges of Nursing. (2012). *Essentials series*. Retrieved from http://www.aacn.nche.edu/education-resources/essential-series

American Cancer Society. (2013). *ACS guidelines on nutrition and physical activity for cancer prevention*. Retrieved from http://www.cancer.org/healthy/eathealthygetactive/acsguidelineson nutritionphysicalactivityforcancerprevention/index

Association of American Colleges and Universities. (2010). The quality imperative: Match ambitious goals for college attainment with an ambitious vision for learning. *Liberal Education, 96*(1), 30–35.

Bragg, E., Meganathan, K., Shay, K., Gilman, S. C., Zeiss, R. A., & Hettler, D. L. (2011). The impact of VA's Geriatric research, education, and clinical centers on academic affiliates. *Gerontology & Geriatrics Education, 32*(1), 5–21. doi:10.1080/02701960.2011.550211

Burfeind, D. (2009). Healthcare policy news: The joint commission announces 2009 National Patient Safety Goals. *Dermatology Nursing, 21*(2), 106.

Commission on Collegiate Nursing Education. (2012). *Standards for Accreditation*. Retrieved from http://www.aacn.nche.edu/ccne-accreditation/standards-procedures-resources/overview

Conceição, S., & Taylor, L. (2007). Using a constructivist approach with online concept maps: Relationship between theory and nursing education. *Nursing Education Perspectives, 28*, 268–275.

Curran, C. R., & Totten, M. K. (2010). Mission, strategy, and Stakeholder. *Nursing Economics, 28*, 116–118.

Gannon, S. C. (2011). Assessing the academic medical center as a supportive learning community. *Journal of Research Administration, 42*, 74–87.

Hill, A. M., Hoffmann, T., Beer, C., McPhail, S., Hill, K.D., Oliver, D., … Haines, T. P. (2011). Falls after discharge from hospital: Is there a gap between older peoples' knowledge about falls prevention strategies and the research evidence? *Gerontologist, 51*, 653–662. doi:10.1093/geront/gnr052

Keating, S. B. (2011). *Curriculum development and evaluation in nursing* (2nd ed.). New York, NY: Springer Publishing Company.

Michel, A. (2009). Patient involvement enhanced patient safety. *Texas Board of Nursing Bulletin,* *40*(2), 6.

Novak, J. D., & Cañas, A. J. (2012). *The theory behind concept maps and how to construct them.* Retrieved from http://cmap.ihmc.us/publications/researchpapers/theorycmaps/ theoryunderlyingconceptmaps.htm

Ricci, A. (2011). Managing the organizational vision, mission, and planning: Five steps toward a successful leadership strategy. In *20th Annual International Leadership Conference, Strategic Leadership.* Dallas, Texas: The Chair Academy.

Stonecypher, K. (2009). Creating a patient education tool. *Journal of Continuing Education in Nursing, 40,* 462–467. doi: 10.3928/00220124-20090923-06

The Joint Commission. (2012). *About the joint commission.* Retrieved from http://www.joint commission.org/about_us/about_the_joint_commission_main.aspx

Todd, R. J. (2012). *School librarians as teachers: Learning outcomes and evidence-based practice 2002.* Retrieved from ERIC database (ED472883).

Vacek, J. (2009). Using a conceptual approach with concept mapping to promote critical thinking. *Journal of Nursing Education, 48,* 45–48.

Wilgis, M., & McConnell, J. (2008). Concept mapping: An educational strategy to improve graduate nurses' critical thinking skills during a hospital orientation program. *Journal of Continuing Education in Nursing, 39,* 119–126.

Program Evaluation

DONNA L. BOLAND

In today's world of increasing accountability, evaluation has moved to the forefront of importance, especially in the educational arena. At the most basic level of conceptual interpretation, evaluation is about making judgments regarding the value or worth of something. In this case it is about the value of an institution or educational program based on preconceived expectations and the worth of the institution or educational program to one or more entities. It is an expectation that judgments made about value and worth are based on information collected through a variety of qualitative and quantitative methods deemed appropriate by those charged with the responsibility of making the judgment calls. Evaluation provides decision makers with information about the institution or program's aims, purpose, and goals, and how well it is functioning in relation to these intentions.

This chapter focuses on various theories and theoretical frameworks that underpin evaluation efforts and discusses evaluation models and their use in approaching evaluation systematically. The chapter also examines research methodologies for generating useful evaluative information, especially within the context of nursing programs, connections between accountability and accreditation, and approaches to developing and implementing program evaluation meaningful to nursing programs.

THEORETICAL UNDERPINNINGS

The ability to understand the theory that drives evaluation is critical from a variety of perspectives. Theory provides an explanation as to why we do something: in this case—evaluate. It positions us to examine our practice and revise it as guided by the knowledge gained through the assessment of that practice. Theory also plays a valuable role in shaping our thinking about how to approach and carry out meaningful evaluation. There is continued discourse as to whether evaluation is grounded in science, or is a tool that allows us to implement the scientific method to achieve evaluation purpose and goals. Program evaluation has matured as both theory and method in response to societal needs and requirements for productivity and efficiency. Embedding evaluation into the need for accountability has pushed the science of evaluation into a publicly credible field, seeded by specific theories and nurtured by models.

Alkin and Christie (2004) discuss the roots of evaluation and the various contributions made by those recognized within this scientific field. Some of the most recognized leaders in evaluation research included in Alkin and Christie's discussion are highlighted in the following presentation on theoretical development of the field of evaluation. They conceptualized the evolution of theories into three distinct theoretical branches, based on their review, and they attached conceptual labels to each of these branches, based on their perceptions of theoretical similarities among the works. These labels were *use*, *methods*, and *valuing* (Alkin & Christie, 2004, p. 12). Although Christie and Alkin (2013) continue to refer to these three branches in their recent publication, the theorists and their branch categories are not mutually exclusive, based on characteristics identified. What are important to the development of evaluation science are the theoretical underpinnings evident in some of today's evaluation models. The following discussion highlights some of the notable theorists and their contributions to the evolution of the state of evaluation science.

USE- OR UTILIZATION-ORIENTED EVALUATION THEORISTS

Theorists who fall into this category share the philosophy that evaluation should be used to generate information valuable to decision makers; they include such notables as Daniel Stufflebeam, Michael Patton, David Fetterman, and Marvin Alkin (Christie & Alkin, 2013). These theorists share the point of view that the main emphasis of evaluation efforts is concentrated on the collection of information that facilitates decision making. Using this theoretical orientation, the ultimate goal of evaluation is to facilitate decisions that support changes important to the institution or program.

The value placed on the contribution of evaluation was directly related to decision making. An example of this theoretical orientation was the context, input, process, and product (CIPP) model developed by Daniel Stufflebeam and Egon Guba. CIPP includes the four essential components they believed to be critical in creating a useful evaluation (Stufflebeam, 1971, 2013). Stufflebeam advocated for an evaluation process that was both cyclic and sustainable, in that information should be continually available to support quality improvement efforts. According to Stufflebeam, evaluation designs should attend to such conceptual standards as utility, feasibility, propriety, and accuracy.

- The *utility* standard is intended to ensure that an evaluation will serve the information needs of intended users.
- The *feasibility* standards are intended to ensure that an evaluation will be realistic, prudent, diplomatic, and frugal.
- The *propriety* standards are intended to ensure that an evaluation will be conducted legally, ethically, and with respect for the welfare of those involved in the evaluation, as well as those affected by its results.
- The *accuracy* standards are intended to ensure that an evaluation will reveal and convey technically adequate information about the features that determine worth, or merit, of the program evaluated (Alkin & Christie, 2004, p. 45).

Michael Quinn Patton's utilization-focused evaluation theory was built on the foundation laid by Stufflebeam. Patton, however, argued that it was critical to identify and involve in the evaluation process those stakeholders who would be primarily users of evaluation findings in an effort to increase utility of the evaluation process and resulting outcomes. Patton (2008, 2012) continues to refine his view of utilization-focused evaluation in a reality where we are able to generate more information than we can assimilate and apply to complex and often convoluted decisional issues.

Michael Scriven's early writings argued that evaluators needed to place a value on their findings in an effort to increase the usefulness of evaluation to decision makers. He suggested that the focus of evaluation efforts is to examine how causal associations relate directly to program quality. This thinking continues to be in vogue in today's reality. Scriven was a proponent of *goal-free* evaluation, determining which program outcomes to examine, rather than starting with the objectives of the program. He believed evaluation should determine the real accomplishments (and nonaccomplishments) of the program (Alkin & Christie, 2004, p. 33; Scriven, 1991, 2013). Few evaluation theorists have supported Scriven's sense of assigning a good or bad dichotomous approach in interpreting evaluation results. Egon Guba and Yvonna Lincoln also supported the notion of valuing as critical to evaluation. However, they placed the responsibility for making valuing interpretations on the shoulders of the stakeholders, based on the belief that "there are multiple realities based on the perceptions and interpretations of the individuals in the program to be evaluated" (Alkin & Christie, 2004, p. 42). Their approach to the role of evaluator was to navigate these various perceptions in facilitating stakeholders' ability to reach consensus on the issues and decisions to be made.

METHODS-FOCUSED EVALUATION THEORISTS

Other evaluation theorists directed their attention to methodological issues related to attainment of specified program goals and objectives. Ralph Tyler, known to many in the discipline of nursing, was an early leader in promoting the need to set behavioral objectives, identify situations in which the learners are able to demonstrate those behaviors, and find measures that generated the best information in determining how well the program or institution was meeting its goals. This information was used to support or reject assumptions regarding the effectiveness of a particular program (Madaus, 2013). Other theorists who expanded on Tyler's orientation to evaluation included Donald Campbell, who, joined by Stanley, wrote the 1966 classic text on experimental and quasi-experimental designs for research, which continues to serve as a valued resource for evaluation researchers when exploring methods and their contribution to evaluation efforts.

In the late 1960s, evaluation research gained in popularity as a legitimate science, thanks to the works of Edward Suchman, who argued that scientific methods were important to the legitimization and value of evaluation studies (Christie & Alkin, 2013). Suchman is credited with the creation of five criterion categories that provide a framework for evaluation research. They include:

1. Effort (quantity and quality of activity that takes place)
2. Performance (criteria that measure the results of effort)
3. Adequacy of performance (degree to which performance is adequate to the total amount of needs)
4. Efficiency (examination of alternative paths or methods in terms of human and monetary costs)
5. Process (how and why a program works or does not work) (Christie & Alkin, 2013, p. 21)

These categories are still used today in designing evaluation research activities.

Also included in the methods branch was Thomas Cook, who explored the application of scientific designs for use in evaluation research. Additionally, he advanced the importance of the role of stakeholders within the design structure. He argued that the key to good evaluation was stakeholder involvement into the integration of the evaluation process. Stakeholders make valuable contributions to the identification of the problem to be examined, integral to the generation and interpretation of evaluation information. Cook recognized that, although the identification of appropriate methodologies was critical to evaluation outcomes, there are variables that are difficult to control for, but that have a confounding effect on evaluation findings and interpretation of those findings. The concept growing out of this orientation was that program evaluation had to be studied within each program's unique context, and that study methods needed to match the contextual uniqueness surrounding each program (Christie & Alkin, 2013).

CONTEXTUALLY FOCUSED THEORISTS

Theory-driven evaluation came into vogue in the early 1980s, due to the contributions of Huey-Tsyh Chen and Peter Rossi, who believed that theory-driven evaluation is critical to the generation of meaningful evaluation outcomes (Christie & Alkin, 2013). Context is central in theory-driven evaluation, but Chen drew on social science theories to help inform the context surrounding program evaluation activities. From his perspective, theory informs context and improves the internal and external validity of evaluation outcomes (Chen, 2013).

In keeping with the context theme, Carol Weiss was among the first to reason that politics intrudes on program evaluation in three ways: "(1) programs are created and maintained by political forces; (2) higher echelons of government, which make decisions about programs, are embedded in politics; and (3) the very act of evaluation has political connotations" (Weiss, 1991, p. 213). Guided by her thinking, the scientific approach to evaluation activities is essential but not all-inclusive of factors. Certainly the focus on accountability is politically driven, which continues to support her supposition. Lee J. Cronbach incorporated the concept of policy into his orientation by suggesting that evaluation should inform conversations and decisions of those responsible for setting program policies. He believed that stakeholders were critical, both in shaping the questions that drive evaluation activities and in arriving at judgments based on the issues at hand (Alkin & Christie, 2004).

CURRENT EVALUATION THEORISTS

Evaluation theories continue to emerge from the groundwork laid by these and others devoted to developing the science of evaluation. Over the past 10 years, the theory of empowerment evaluation has gained in popularity. Although empowerment evaluation incorporates the tenets of utilization and decision making, it distinguishes itself from other theories, including utilization evaluation theory, by emphasizing the use of information to drive decisions that enable the decision makers to improve "their lives and the lives of those around them, [which] produces an extraordinary sense of well-being and positive growth" (Wandersman et al., 2012, p. 12). The principles that guide empowerment evaluation have historical roots and are guided by theoretical and philosophical tenets. These principles also resonate with both internal and external expectations to which higher education programs are being held, including, among others, professional accreditation and institutional accounting activities that encourage positive growth.

Wandersman et al. (2012) identified nine principles associated with empowerment that educators should incorporate into their perspectives on evaluation (Exhibit 14.1). In nursing, education processes need to be developed to evaluate the evaluation process as part of being "accountable." It is important that stakeholders understand that evaluation processes and resulting outcomes can be perceived as either good or not so good within the context of the desired aim or purpose of the evaluation process. There are various reasons that affect the perceived value or worth of the process. It is therefore important that cyclic evaluation processes should be evaluated on a periodic basis. Evaluation of evaluation can employ both formative (process-oriented) and summative (outcome-oriented)

EXHIBIT 14.1 Perspectives on Evaluation: Nine Principles Associated With Empowerment

- *Principle one* argues the need to focus on program improvement as the end goal of evaluation activities. Improvement both provides a clear end goal and acts as a purposeful guide to evaluation designs.

- *Principles two and three* focus on the inclusion and engagement of stakeholders in the establishment of goals, design, collection, interpretation, and application of evaluation information. They argue that the more involved the community of interest is, the more meaningful and useful the results.

- *Principle four* highlights the need for democratic participation in the evaluation process. This principle is translated to mean that participation should be authentic, and every attempt should be made to leverage individual talent held among stakeholders in moving the evaluation process forward. Participatory equality leads to transparency of the evaluation process and a valued sense of control over the process.

- *Principle five* addresses the need for a social justice orientation. Although the concept of social justice grew out of a social-political theoretical framework, it can be easily applied to nurse educators, assuming that as a collective, program improvement anchored in quality and social relevance is their main goal.

- *Principle six* is critical to nursing education programs, as the need to partner with an appropriately defined community of interest is in the best interests of both the program and the community. Professional accreditation bodies recognize the value of engaging those within the community of interest in clarifying the problems and seeking workable solutions to real and evolving issues and challenges.

- *Principle seven* underscores the value of the scientific approach to evaluation design and implementation. Evaluation activities should incorporate evidence-based practices that are appropriately aligned to the program being evaluated, the resources at hand, the decisions to be made, and the perceived value of the information being generated to finding answers/solutions to issues raised.

- *Principle eight* suggests that the more knowledgeable and skilled the evaluator(s) is/are, the greater the contribution to the utility of the evaluation process being conducted. The end result of this expertise is better outcomes. The underlying assumption is that the program environment supports the need for expertise and values both the evaluation process and outcomes generated. The value of learning generated from evaluation to programs and institutions is the focal point of principle nine. An established and supported culture of learning within an institution of higher education is not about sustaining what is, but rather about envisioning and reaching for what could and should be given—external and internal accountability and responsibility to society. If one defines learning as change, then evaluation is the vehicle driving change; hence the value and utility of evaluation.

- *The final principle (nine)* relates to accountability of all from inception to completion of the evaluation process. It is the responsibility of all involved in evaluation to be accountable for their actions and to hold others involved accountable.

From Wandersman et al. (2012).

methods. Formative evaluation considers how the evaluation process is conceived and implemented. At the center of summative evaluation are outcomes, judgments, and decisions made as a result of the information generated (Wandersman et al., 2012).

Historically, philosophically, and theoretically, evaluation is rooted in various divergent but often complementary thinking. Few evaluation experts would argue against evaluation being a science grounded in theoretical properties. The evolution of evaluation has evolved into a broadly based applied science in which both applicability and utility are of value to various disciplines. The versatility of evaluation allows stakeholders to respond to calls for accountability, especially in the areas of program productivity and quality, assessment of learning, impact of teaching on learning outcomes, and determination of best educational practices.

For nurse educators, evaluation practices provide answers to professional accreditation standards in the broad areas of effectiveness of program, efficiency of use of resources to promote program quality, and impact of program in meeting internal and external expectations (Boulmetis & Dutwin, 2011). It should be noted, however, that evaluation practices should not be limited to addressing accreditation expectations, as this narrow view of evaluation constrains the depth and breadth of the contributions of evaluation in developing and revising nursing programs on a continuous basis, as established by stakeholders and decision makers.

Given the evolution of evaluation, it is important that nurse educators focus on the following propositions when designing or constructing evaluation models that provide a framework for evaluation activities in their programs. Evaluation should:

- Be of use to those with decision-making authority
- Include an array of both primary (frontline) and secondary (interested parties) stakeholders to capture diverse needs and viewpoints
- Occur within a social-political environment
- Incorporate methodological strategies that generate valid and meaningful results
- Be transparent and consistent with clearly stated goals

EVALUATION MODELS

The majority of evaluation models being employed today are a reflection of one or more theoretical or philosophical orientations noted above. Evaluation models are helpful in providing the framework in which evaluation activities occur. Prior to identifying an evaluation model, evaluators, along with stakeholders, must determine whether the outcomes of the evaluation will actually make a difference to program decisions needing to be made, agree that the evaluation process can be completed in a time frame for the results to be used in the decision process, and question whether the program and/or the decisions needing to be made are of the scope that warrants the time and effort to carry out evaluation (Newcomer, Hatry, & Wholey, 2010). If the perceived need to conduct evaluation does not meet this broad litmus test, then the deliberations as to what evaluation model to use are irrelevant.

If the deliberations result in the need to conduct an evaluation of the program or of some aspects of the program critical to its viability, the next discussion needs to center on what one hopes to achieve from the evaluation process. It is important to ask what information is needed, by whom the information is needed, and what purpose the outcomes of evaluation are to serve. Evaluation is essential to determining the value of the program to stakeholders and to the broader community of interest. Decisions linked to program value or worth include the addition, revision, or deletion of the program. Evaluation models at this level of decision making should be comprehensive and inclusive to be effective in generating adequate information that informs decisions. Evaluation models should be part of any new program design, and not an afterthought once the program has been implemented. The chosen model should stand up to the test of time with modest tweaking. Evaluations with a focus on answering noncyclic questions or specific needs should be less elaborate in design and resource requirements.

Depending on the source you consult, you are likely to discover that there is no set nomenclature for evaluation models. Evaluation models used in higher education are relevant in guiding one's thinking as it relates to how to approach evaluation and what the outcome of the evaluation should achieve. Evaluation models should be chosen for their ability to generate findings that address desired goals. There are some consistencies in evaluation models in use today, as many of the evaluative processes are directed or guided by external expectations. Some of the more commonly used evaluation models and their focus are presented to give you a sense of the options that are available for the purpose of guiding your thinking about evaluation.

GOAL-ORIENTED/FOCUS EVALUATION MODELS

Goal-oriented/focus evaluation models are utilitarian by nature, and they are generally employed to examine change within or across institutions of higher education and their program offerings. This type of model is popular in determining the degree to which a course or program influences student learning. The key to this type of model is efficiency, as the model is most often employed to measure the impact on student learning or on educational outcomes. Decisions related to program impact are designed to compare predetermined goals, outcomes, or objectives to that which has been achieved. The key to goal-oriented thinking requires that the goals be clearly articulated and that consensus be reached prior to conducting an institutional and/or program evaluation (Patton, 2013).

A decision-making evaluation model emphasizes informed judgments as the end result of the evaluation process. Stufflebeam's CIPP model is a good example of a decision-making model that continues to be used extensively. It is therefore important to understand how each element of the model can be interpreted for possible use by evaluators.

- *Context evaluations* assess needs, problems, assets, and opportunities to help decision makers define goals and priorities and to guide the broader group of users to judge goals, priorities, and outcomes.
- *Input evaluations* assess alternative approaches, competing action plans, staffing plans, and budgets for their feasibility and potential cost-effectiveness to meet targeted needs and achieve goals. Decision makers use input evaluations when they choose among competing plans, write grant proposals, allocate resources, assign staff, schedule work, and help others judge an effort's plans and budget.
- *Process evaluations* assess the implementation of plans to help staff carry out activities and later to help the broad group of users judge program performance and interpret outcomes.
- *Product evaluations* identify and assess outcomes—intended and unintended, short- and long-term—to help keep the organization focused on achieving important outcomes and help the broader group of users gauge the effort's success at meeting targeted needs (Stufflebeam, 2004, p. 246).

The CIPP model is flexible in that it can be used to meet both formative and summative evaluation needs when the intent of evaluation is program improvement. Decision-driven models such as the CIPP model tend to center on the effectiveness, quality, and/or impact of the program. In today's higher educational reality, in which scrutiny of program effectiveness is on everyone's mind, the ability to make informed decisions about program effectiveness is essential.

DISCREPANCY EVALUATION MODELING

Discrepancy evaluation modeling is close to decision-making models, as this type of modeling focuses on the ability of programs to meet internal and external standards. Currently, professional accreditation is built on the idea of compliance with standards.

Nurse faculty are expected to provide data as to the program's ability to meet specified standards. Program evaluation plans have been designed around the need to collect, monitor, and interpret program data, based on the standards the accrediting body dictates for compliance purposes. When a discrepancy is noted, faculty need to determine the precipitating factors associated with the discrepancy and present a plan of action to address this discrepancy, along with a timetable for resolution. The challenge in using any type of decision-making approaches is in the identification of who can and should be making decisions related to program integrity. The path followed in making decisions is often convoluted and populated with unexpected or unanticipated hurdles.

GOAL-FREE EVALUATION MODELS

As noted earlier in the chapter, Scriven was the primary advocate for goal-free evaluation models. This approach focuses on measuring what *is* without the context of established goals or expected outcomes that could potentially bias the observations made and the interpretation of findings. The value of this type of evaluation model is determining the degree to which the information collected meets the needs of those using the information (Scriven, 2013). Scriven recognizes five dimensions that need to be included in a goal-free approach to evaluation. These dimensions are *"process, outcomes, cost, comparative advantage,* and *generalizability"* (Scriven, 2004, p. 188). Goal-free evaluation can be conducted either formatively or in a summative fashion, depending on the needs of the program. This model is closest to naturalistic inquiry philosophy. The strength of this approach is that data generated can highlight both intended and unintended consequences of the program. It also negates the need to compare the achievement of expected goals/outcomes to actual achievement of goals/outcomes (Cook, Scriven, Coryn, & Evergreen, 2010).

UTILIZATION-FOCUSED EVALUATION MODEL

The utilization-focused evaluation model is designed around the identification of the information needed, those needing the information (potential users), and the decisions needing to be made. The caveat in this thinking is that users can be fully known, and all information collected is useful to decision makers. It is also important to note that for evaluation findings to be useful to the decision makers, they must be accepting of the findings, and that the seeking of solutions might be beyond what they are willing to explore. Although institutions of higher education have been traditional in their approach to change, the social and political environment is ready for and demanding of organizational change to meet a dynamic, globally focused society. Critical elements identified by Patton (2012) include stakeholder engagement, an understanding of the context in which the program exists, planning, and open communication channels throughout the evaluation process. A utilization-oriented modeling approach can be used, both in the formative and summative approaches to an evaluation project. The steps in using this type of model include the need to establish an evaluation committee, identify the purpose of the evaluation and the roles of the evaluators, develop guidelines for the evaluation process, identify the methods to be employed, implement the evaluation plan, analyze the information collected, and present logically the findings that resonate with the users (Patton, 2012).

OTHER CURRENT EVALUATION MODELS

Relying more on a contextual theoretical underpinning, four other current evaluation models used in education are *success case studies* and *systems-focused, transformative,* and *logic* models. In the *success case study model*, the goal is to compare the successful programs with those that are less successful to identify the variables associated with success. This model tends to generate case-specific contextual information that might or might not be generalized beyond the scope of the programs under study. When one is using a case study model design, it is essential to determine the expressed purpose of the evaluation effort, questions that you wish to answer, the basic assumptions that affect the collection and interpretation of data, clearly defined unit of analysis being used, and a set of criterion that will guide the interpretation of the study results.

System-focused evaluation models are constructed on concepts related to systems thinking, which has been around since the early 1930s. However, system-focused evaluation resonates with nurse educators, as this model is inclusive rather than reductionistic in its approach. The context in which the program operates is important to the evaluation process. Mertens (2009) argued that evaluation models need to be genuine and respectful of the people and culture being evaluated. The ability to holistically examine the relationships between and among all aspects of a program can provide the evaluator with a realistic view of the functionality of a program under study. Critical pieces of a system-focused evaluation include the identification of the boundaries of the system's environment, input, output, process, state, hierarchy, goal-directedness, and information (University of Twente, 2012).

Culturally responsive models that have incorporated Mertens's thinking must incorporate approaches that include appreciation for the cultural backgrounds of the stakeholders. Cultural orientation plays a key role both in determining the value or worth of the data being collected and in making decisions made based on these data. To ensure a high level of visibility, there needs to be a collaborative effort among the evaluator and stakeholders, especially in relation to the culture and politics surrounding the entity being evaluated (Askew, Beverly, & Jay, 2012). For example, the interpretation of evaluation results generated from an evaluation of a nursing program designed to recruit from an educationally disadvantaged population needs to be interpreted within the context of variables such as characteristics of the learner population, community needs, institutional mission and goals, and uniqueness of the educational design.

Another type of contextual model is the *transformative model,* which is grounded in philosophical thinking that addresses social issues as well as building on a scholarly base. Core to a transformative evaluation model is the incorporation of marginalized groups into the evaluation process (Mertens, 2009). The assumption of broadening the circle of participation is grounded in the argument of the value of diverse points of view, especially from the population groups served by the program and/or institution undergoing evaluation. The focus of a transformative model is on objectivity that balances the diversity of experiences with evaluation findings in a way that controls for bias as a result of a lack of understanding regarding the context in which the program lives (Mertens, 2010). Participatory involvement in decisions related to evaluation methods and interpretation of findings is critical to maintaining rigor, credibility, validity, and representative truth.

Mertens (2010) indicated that a transformative evaluation model needs to focus on (a) determining which theoretical tenets best guide a program's approach to evaluating the program; (b) identifying stakeholders and approaches for meaningful engagement in the evaluation process, which in the case of a nursing program might include such characteristics as gender, age, ethnicities, races, languages, economic and family backgrounds, and educational backgrounds; and (c) developing data collection methods that measure findings that will be meaningful to the stakeholders and fuel potential future change. A transformative framework should be able to answer questions related to whether evaluation findings are either emerging or have been stable over a period of time. This type of model also needs to differentiate between evaluation outcomes and program practices in that outcomes might or might not be the result of current practice expectations. As with any evaluation model, it is important to determine the significance of the outcomes to what is of value to stakeholders (Mertens, 2009).

A *logic model* also recognizes the importance of context in that evaluation must consider the environment surrounding the program. This model focuses on input that includes human and institutional resources; processes that highlighted audience needs, collection and summarization of information, and information dissemination; and outputs that spoke to the usefulness of initial outcomes and the intermediate or actual use of evaluation outcomes and the long-term intended outcomes (McLaughlin & Jordan, 2010). The common steps in designing an evaluation using a logic model include the need to describe the program, fully explain how the program is delivered, determine a list of questions that need to be answered, determine how best to collect information to answer the questions posed, describe the existing program resources and the context in which they and the program exist, and implement the evaluation plan (McLaughlin & Jordan, 2010).

Examples of models more utility oriented are the success-focused, meta-analysis, and appreciative inquiry models. *Success-focused evaluation models* are grounded in Patton's (2013) outcome theoretical frame of reference. At the heart of the model's focus is the *so what?* question. The outcome of the evaluation process needs to be interpreted within the framework of impact and change from the perspectives of those who will be using the results. Fundamentals of this framework are inputs, outputs, and outcomes, elements that also define a systems approach. However, Patton is fairly clear on critical features that need to be examined within each of these elements. Inputs include information regarding program resources, findings of a needs assessment, available expertise within and outside the program, physical resources to support the program, and regulatory bodies that guide program implementation. The outputs comprise a determination of the extent of the evaluation to be undertaken, the products being delivered and the size of the population being served, the validity of the observations made, and the results of information collected. The *so what?* question is addressed by the third element of this modeling approach, and it looks at impact or benefit to those who will be using the information generated. It is also critical to evaluate the outcomes to determine whether the right kind of data has been generated to answer the *so what?* question. If not, then adjustments need to be made in the input and output core elements that will generate more useful information for end users (Patton, 2013).

Meta-analysis is most often considered a statistical approach. However, its application to evaluation provides us with a model that allows the synthesis of a variety of evaluation efforts that are directed toward well-defined questions, especially around outcomes targeting best methods. Meta-analysis as a model provides a mechanism that gives evaluation researchers the means to prepare, maintain, and disseminate evaluation outcomes that have been generated through meticulous, systematic collation of information that can be used to shape best practices (Boruch & Petrosino, 2010). There are challenges in using a meta-analysis model, which include the need to be clear about the question being asked, establishing clear rules on what and how to identify and interpret data, and having guidelines for determining validity of data and reporting of results of the analysis. Meta-analysis requires time, talent, and access to a comprehensive and complex database.

Appreciative inquiry is a conceptual model that has limited use in higher education, but that does have conceptual utility, given its focus. This model attempts to ascertain what is working well within a program or organization and to explore how to align resources and functions that support a positive vision for a desired future. Critics of this type of approach to evaluation fear that problems and concerns might be glossed over. Proponents argue that problems are not necessarily ignored, but rather approached from a more positive perspective (Cooperrider & Godwin, 2010). Appreciative inquiry is constructed through the application of four process steps: discovery of or appreciation for what is working well; ability to dream or visualize what the future could be; design or construction of the desired future based on a vision; and achievement of this vision through action, monitoring, and revising as directed by the evaluation results (Cooperrider & Godwin, 2010). Appreciative inquiry has continued to evolve and is used in organizations as a framework, especially in the context of quality improvement that focuses on strengthening best practices. Appreciative inquiry should be designed to be highly inclusive and supportive of the democratic engagement of a diverse group of stakeholders. As this framework emphasizes best practice, it can be a good choice in the early implementation of a new or newly revised program. Again, being able to focus on what is working allows for positively motivated corrections in direction. This type of approach also encourages consensus among primary stakeholders.

Although the approach to thinking about evaluation models is varied, there are some common themes to developing an evaluation model to fit diverse goals. The following checklist summarizes the themes that need to be considered when adopting or adapting an evaluation model:

 1. Identify and engage stakeholders.
 2. Clarify goals of the evaluation.
 3. Assess resources needed for evaluation.
 4. Design the evaluation.
 5. Determine appropriate methods of measurement and procedures.
 6. Develop a work plan, budget, and timeline for evaluation.
 7. Collect the data using agreed-upon methods and procedures.
 8. Process and analyze data.
 9. Interpret and disseminate the results.
10. Take action.

This list corresponds to essential competencies that have been identified (Lee, Altschuld, & Lee, 2012). The critical competencies needed by effective evaluators include the ability to identify and understand the norms and values shaping the program being evaluated, the technical skills to conduct evaluation from a systematic inquiry approach, the analytical skills to understand the context in which the program exists from both a social and political perspective, expertise in managing all the evaluation project elements in a coordinated and timely fashion, communication/interpersonal skills required to keep information and interactions focused on the purpose of each evaluation effort undertaken, and the ability to package the findings in a way that is most meaningful to the primary decision makers (Patton, 2012).

The choice of evaluation models is primarily dependent on which model is believed to be the most useful, the most practical, and the most cost-effective from the perspective of benefits obtained (Alkin, 2011). As many of the models tend to share commonalities, an evaluator might use a combination of models to accomplish desired outcomes (Horne & Sandmann, 2012). Scriven (2013) argued that the discipline of evaluation has generated theory, models, and guidelines that have applicability to various disciplines. What evaluation science brings to the table is a sense of order and rigor for those engaging in evaluation. The main challenge in developing a one-size-fits-all approach to evaluation frameworks or models is the uncertainty of that which is to be evaluated. It is difficult to determine that all will be known about a program under investigation. Due to the increasing environmental complexities, it is impossible to identify specific direct cause-and-effect relationships that make the argument for a single model irrational. Lastly, it is challenging for evaluators to always identify what all stakeholders want as an outcome of evaluation efforts, given likely hidden agendas. Therefore, being able to measure for unknown variables is not feasible (Hermans, Naber, & Easerink, 2012).

EVALUATION RESEARCH METHODOLOGIES

Methodologies differ widely, but there are some critical criteria that must be met for the findings of any evaluation research to be perceived as valid. Wholey (2013) indicated that "performance measurement systems and program evaluation studies can and should be mutually reinforcing," arguing that a single measure can't meet the complex needs of all involved stakeholders (p. 262). The focus of an evaluation project must be clearly stated, as this provides the framework for the process, from developing the design through making conclusions. A clear focus also indicates whether the evaluation project will be formative, summative, or descriptive in nature. The level of analysis needed, as well as the precision in the collection of information, hinges on the focus or purpose of the evaluation to be undertaken (Scriven, 2013). Credibility of the evaluative findings is most reflective of the believability of those providing information. The level of believability relates to bias and relevance of the informant to the issues under study. Reporting of findings and conclusions should be concise and capable of being understood by stakeholders. All evaluation designs must be ethically and legally defensible and respect the rights, responsibilities, and diversity of those involved in the process. The last critical criterion in the design of any evaluation plan is ensuring that the cost of the project proposed is realistic and reflects existing resources (Scriven, 2013). Generalizability is not necessarily an issue in evaluation research unless the purpose of the project is to identify best practices that can be shared widely.

MIXED METHOD APPROACH

Measurement instruments that complement evaluation are plentiful, but they need to be chosen with great skill. Commonly, most evaluators use a mixed method approach in the collection of information. Evaluators need to identify measures that are germane to the study purpose and that show an understanding of the culture and political environment surrounding the program. Measurement instruments must also generate the type of information that will be most meaningful to the stakeholders. To be of worth or value to those making decisions, the data generated have to "speak to them" both in the short- and more long-term decision discussions. One of the ideas that underpins program evaluation is the ability to identify outcomes that were intended from those outcomes that were not intended when making decisions (Howe, 2011, p. 118). Today, much of the evaluation data involve repeated observations that extend over a period of time, so measurements must be stable and perform consistently across data sets.

One of the main arguments that supports the notion that evaluation is not a true science is the assumption that all factors under study are known and can be controlled if the correct research design is chosen and implemented according to its standing protocols. It is an accepted premise that in evaluation research it can be the case that not all factors are known, but they are often discovered within the process; a part of that premise is the concept that the ability to control factors within a human organization is impossible. Mixed methods are helpful in both the collection of existing and new or yet-to-be-discovered information. Stakeholders are essential in the identification of existing data sources and serve as informants in uncovering data that provides meaning and understanding in relation to the program function and outcomes.

USEFULNESS OF DATA COLLECTED

When collecting evaluation data, it is important to weigh the data against the usefulness of the information being collected. The evaluators need to ask such questions as, "Are the data helpful in better understanding the issues under study?" "Can the information be useful as the evaluation process progresses?" "Is the collection and analysis of the information worth the cost?" "Is the information presented from a biased perspective, and, if so, are there other sources of information that offset this bias?" If a program has had prior experiences with evaluations, then it is important to know what the process was like and what information was the most valuable. It is also critical to understand what programmatic changes have been made since the last evaluation and what changes are being contemplated for the future, as change will affect both the collection of information and the interpretation of that information. For example, if new educational programs have been implemented or are being considered, then the proposed evaluation must take into account the impact of those programs from such perspectives as meeting stakeholder needs; physical, fiscal, and human resources; outcomes; relevancy to practice and the job market; potential applicant pools; fit of new or proposed programs with institutional goals; value of programs to community of interest; and impact of graduates on the professional, educational, and social community.

PROCEDURAL STEPS IN PROGRAM EVALUATION

Once the first step (determining the purpose, goals, aims, and decisions to be made) of conducting a program evaluation is done, it is important to identify factors that might affect the ability to obtain evaluation goals. Possible constraints include a restricted budget or time frame; the availability of and access to information; expertise of the evaluator(s); stakeholder support for the evaluation being proposed; and potential, yet-to-be determined environmental challenges.

The next procedural step is to identify the variables that are to be measured. Consistent with research practices, the variables under study need to be articulated in terms specific enough to be able to identify the appropriate collection method. It might be that one or more measures will need to be developed to facilitate data collection. If new data collection methods must be designed, then the time, talent, and energy should be calculated into the overall costs to justify these additional expenditures. One of the critical elements to program evaluation is the ability to measure the concept of "learning," which is essential to an institution's or program's documentation of effectiveness. When considering the culmination of the learning experiences, evaluators employ a summative thinking approach to their choices for measurement methodologies (Loyd & Koenig, 2008). As most nurse educators will be involved with summative evaluation approaches, it is important to choose those measurements that provide useful summative information on learning as it relates to program effectiveness and ultimately to accountability of the program in meeting internal and external expectations (Liu, 2011a).

QUALITATIVE AND QUANTITATIVE MEASUREMENT APPROACHES

Evaluators have a rich array of both qualitative and quantitative measurement approaches available. Common quantitative instruments employed by nurse educators in program evaluation include student performance and achievement tests, including teacher-made tests that are specific to coursework, nationally normed tests, high-stakes tests, document reviews, case logs, performance-focused observations (often employing simulation that incorporate scales or performance checklists), oral examinations, and surveys and questionnaires using a closed-end question approach (Loyd & Koenig, 2008). More common qualitative measures employ participant and nonparticipant observations, case studies that focus more on open-ended, guided discussions, stories that highlight variables being studied, interviews (often with key informants), focus groups, and open-ended surveys or questionnaires.

PORTFOLIOS

Portfolios have become a popular assessment strategy over the last decade. Portfolios have a flexibility that is attractive in both program evaluation and assessment of learning, which is a key element in program evaluation. Portfolios can be constructed to meet the needs of the teacher and the learner. The traditional use of portfolios has been the assessment of the educational maturation of learners as they progress through a program of study. Portfolios are now being paired with outcomes assessment to appraise the learner's progression toward program goal attainment (Karlowicz, 2010). Determination of progression is based on products the learner has produced over her or his course of study. Other, more process-oriented documentation that can go into the construction of a portfolio includes artifacts of a learner's perception of growth and abilities, such as a diary or log. Incorporating metacognitive experiences into the portfolio not only enriches the learning experience but also adds another critical voice (the student's) to evaluation of program outcomes.

Portfolios have made inroads into program evaluation over the last few years. In this capacity, portfolios are more commonly used to judge achievements in relation to organizational mission and goals and to provide evidence associated with professional standards and public accountability. Portfolios provide a great deal of flexibility, depending on how they are constructed. Documentation can be in the form of visual, written, oral, and/or electronic information sources. The construction of a portfolio requires the identification of specific goals that must be addressed by the documentation gathered from various and diverse sources. It also requires a careful selection of evidence that obviously reflects the outcomes. If portfolios are to be used as summative evaluative tools, then there must be a standardization of the evidence included; the documentation must be clearly defined for all learners; assessment criteria are articulated and applied consistently; evaluators should be trained in application of assessment criteria; and interrater reliability must be established (Rhodes, 2012; Senger & Kanthan, 2012).

HIGH-STAKES TESTING

As all nursing programs are embedded in institutions of higher learning, assessment of student learning is focused not only on discipline-specific outcomes, but also on college skill proficiency outcomes. In many cases, the focus of college proficiency outcome assessment has been based on nationally recognized *high-stakes* tests. In taking a value-added approach to learning, these tests tend to be administered at the beginning and end of a student's program of study (Liu, 2011b). However, evaluators continue to raise questions related to validity of these high-stakes testing methods. A major caution in using high-stakes testing as a singular measure of college-level skill proficiency is that these measures do not address the difference in learner populations and institutions. The argument is that, for the purpose of evaluation, there needs to be a systematic approach to interpretation of this type of information, which must be done within a context of other performance variables (Nichols, Meyers, & Burling, 2009). At present there is no one standardized test, or set of tests, that are in place for all institutions, but as the calls for improved student achievement increase, the need grows to develop and test reliable assessment methods that cross disciplines as well as meet discipline-specific outcomes. As these assessment methods are developed, they must address critical measurement issues that include conflicts related to the unit of analysis (student vs. institution) and myriad confounding variables that are difficult to control. There is concern that the use of national tests such as the Collegiate Assessment of Academic Proficiency will be used to make erroneous decisions regarding institutional quality as calls for accountability continue to increase (Banta, 2011).

ALTERNATIVES TO USE OF HIGH-STAKES TESTS

With the need to continue to explore alternatives to the use of high-stakes tests, the Association of American Colleges and Universities (AACU) developed a Valid Assessment of Learning in Undergraduate Education rubric structure to incorporate knowledge beyond what most standardized tests measure. The knowledge elements included in this rubric are "creative writing, critical thinking, information literacy, inquiry and analysis, written and oral communication, problem-solving, quantitative literacy, reading, teamwork, civic knowledge and engagement, ethical reasoning, foundations and skills of lifelong learning, intercultural knowledge and competence, and integrative and applied learning" (AACU, 2010).

A number of universities and programs are incorporating these rubrics into their evaluation processes, especially if they use institutional portfolios as a measure of learning. The essence of each of these elements is woven into their institutional and program/discipline outcomes. The rubric framework is then constructed so that there is continuity from expected learning to actual or measurable learning. Although the portfolio provides a great deal of flexibility, there need to be strategies for dealing with potential reliability and flexibility issues. Interrater reliability is critical, and those asked to judge portfolios must agree not only on how to interpret the assessment values, but on the consistency in assigning these values. Portfolio evaluators need to be trained and monitored to be effective in the use of this type of methodology.

EVALUATION AND ACCOUNTABILITY: ACCREDITATION

In the world of nursing education, accountability is synonymous with accreditation. Accreditation, although extremely time-consuming, does have enormous benefits. Accreditation is usually a voluntary process, although some states mandate that institutions and programs be accredited through established governmental rules and regulations. The accreditation process provides valuable information and data about the ability of a program to meet specified outcomes and standards. It requires faculty and students to be engaged in the process of evaluation, in generating information related to program quality and relevance (Head & Johnson, 2011; Rhodes, 2012).

TYPES OF ACCREDITATION

There are two general types of accreditation critical to education. These are institutional and program accreditation.

Institutional Accreditation

All institutions of higher education hold some type of accreditation (focusing on the whole of the institution), depending on the type and focus of the institution. Currently there are six regional agencies recognized by the U.S. Department of Education and the Council for Higher Education Accreditation, with the authority to accredit public institutions of higher education. Although each regional agency has developed its own accreditation standards, there are common themes that run through those standards. These themes include having the ability to promote learning, an identified mission and goals that lead the operations of the institution, and the ability to demonstrate that the mission and goals are being achieved, assembled and allocated resources to achieve the institution's mission and goals, and evidence that progress is sustainable (Head & Johnson, 2011). Accreditation provides a mechanism for institutions and programs to benchmark their performance against national, regional, and professional standards of expected practice. Accreditation engages faculty and administrators in generating and tracking evaluative information, not only about student performance, but about graduates' relevance in the job market, the value of the program to the public, and the impact of achievements on the citizens and community the program serves.

Like all voluntary accreditation organizations, accreditation agencies are self-regulated, and their accreditation standards are periodically peer-reviewed and updated as appropriate to ensure that institutions are making decisions and changes consistent with their mission and goals. Accreditation processes encourage institutions and programs to look openly at strengths and weaknesses as part of continuous quality improvement.

Nursing Program Accreditation

Although nurse educators participate in institutional accreditation activities based primarily on the contribution their programs and graduates make to the institution's mission and goals, programmatic accreditation requires faculty to focus their main evaluation energies on the programs being offered through their educational unit (Head & Johnson, 2011). At present time, there are two nursing professional accreditation agencies: the Accreditation Commission for Education in Nursing (formerly named National League for Nursing Accrediting Commission) and the Commission on Collegiate Nursing Education. Both agencies are recognized by the U.S. Department of Education, and they operate autonomously as voluntary self-regulatory agencies. Both agencies base their accreditation operations on accepted practices that include the establishment of accreditation standards, a process for the development of materials for those applying to the agency for accreditation status, a systematic system for peer review of nursing units seeking accreditation, a decision process for determination of accreditation status, an established communication route to publicize accreditation actions, and a procedure for systematic review of standards and processes.

Accreditation is an external force for institutional and programmatic evaluation; however, it is seldom the singular vehicle guiding evaluation activities. The majority of institutions of higher education are accountable to state regulations, boards of governors, and other stakeholders. Higher education institutions establish internal systematic evaluation processes that require the participation of all existing programs as well as proposed programs. Depending on the nature of a program, the questions that need to be asked and answered differ. Evaluative questions asked of an established program usually focus on quality, impact, and achievement of outcomes. The focus of an evaluation of a new program is on examining what is working and what improvements need to be made to improve productivity. Information associated with a proposed program centers on program need, innovation, contribution, and potential value that is different from existing programs. Often the introduction of new programs influences existing resources and therefore requires a cost-benefit analysis evaluation approach to identify the gains made with the addition of a new program.

DEVELOPING AND IMPLEMENTING PROGRAM EVALUATION

Whether one is implementing an institutional or program evaluation, the development of a program plan is fundamental. A systematic evaluation plan guides the collection of essential documentation that provides programs and institutions with evidence of compliance with accreditation standards and publicly held expectations. As nursing units are attached to parent educational institutions, the nursing unit's evaluation plan should be designed to be integrated into a broader institutional evaluation plan. Many existing evaluation plans incorporate accreditation standards into their design. It is important to understand when designing an evaluation plan that accreditation standards are integral to the evaluation process, but that they should not be singularly driven by accreditation expectations. Program evaluation plans need to generate valuable information to meet the comprehensive needs of faculty and administrators.

SYSTEMATIC EVALUATION PLAN

The nursing professional accreditation standards assist in the identification of the major dimensions that should be a part of any nursing program evaluation design. These dimensions are mission, governance, faculty and staff, students, resources, curriculum, and evaluation. These evaluative features provide the broad structure on which to begin to shape your evaluation plan. In general, evaluation plans are at least two-dimensional in design. The dimensions serve as one facet, whereas the other part of the design includes expected outcomes, achievements made, and decisions or actions prompted by the differences. In today's reality of accountability, the focus must be on the rationale for existence and how programs work or do not work (Grayson, 2012). Therefore the evaluation plans need to not only identify the dimensions but also reflect how the different dimensions interact in determining the contributions and social value of these contributions to internal and external stakeholders. From a logic model perspective, the vertical axis is populated by the dimensions, whereas the horizontal axis of a two-dimensional approach reflects those components of the program that need to be assessed (Goeschel, Weiss, & Pronovost, 2012).

STEPS IN PROGRAM EVALUATION

Step 1

Conducting program evaluation requires that you have a systematic plan of attack. The first step in this plan should be to determine what you want to accomplish from evaluation activities. It is important that there be agreement on why you are conducting an evaluation and what you hope to gained from such activities (Grayson, 2012). For nursing, one of the major reasons for conducting evaluation is accreditation. However, there is a potential for many other needs for program evaluation based on internal and external social and political factors. When determining what is to be accomplished from evaluation activities, it is important to understand the mission, goals, and outcomes of the parent institution and well as that of the nursing unit. By looking for congruency among these missions, goals, and outcomes across the layers of an organization, you are able to answer questions related to the fit of the nursing unit and program offerings to the parent's institutional mission and goals, and the contribution of the program in the context of societal needs and expectations of the health care system. During this clarification process, the engagement of community and institutional stakeholders is important to ensure that everyone understands the process and has the same outcome expectations. The establishment of goals or outcomes of evaluation might feel counterintuitive to a more grounded approach to theory, but logically it is critical if evaluation is to be meaningful. The major hesitation in establishing outcomes upfront is the concern that faculty and administrators will be held accountable for outcomes perceived to be outside of their control (Patton, 2012).

Steps 2 and 3

The next two steps in designing a program evaluation are the identification of documentation needed and the activities involved in gathering this documentation. Integral to these steps is identification of the type of documentation to be collected, location of the documentation, personnel responsible for document retrieval, timeframe in which the collection is to occur, and the frequency or cycle of repeated collection. Documentation can take many forms, including written, verbal, observational, and electronic. Data retrieved can be either qualitative or quantitative in nature, depending on what information exists. However, data should be able to be validated. Often this validation is accomplished through the use of mixed methodologies and cross-referencing/triangulation. One of the discovery outcomes of data retrieval is the ability to note nonexisting data, or data that do not exist in the format compatible to interpret accurately against established outcomes/goals. The measurements used in the collection of information should be valid, and the processes identified in the collection of information should be systematic and efficient.

Step 4

The logical next step in evaluation planning is the incorporation of processes that will be used to interpret the information collected. These processes should reflect a systematic review and interpretation of information and a summation of findings. The summary of the findings should be presented in a way that supports goals and expected outcomes and is linked to program improvement, accountability, and contributions. If the main purpose of evaluation planning is summative in nature, then examining aggregated information over time is of the most value to stakeholders. When designing an evaluation plan for a proposed or newly implemented program, history would not exist or would be preliminary. This type of preliminary information needs to be interpreted with caution both by evaluators and decision makers.

QUESTIONS TO GUIDE EVALUATION PLAN DESIGN

There are a number of decisions that faculty and administrators must address on a cyclic basis that guide thinking about designing the evaluation plan to ensure that these questions get answered. There is no one acceptable list of questions commonly used by program evaluators. In nursing, many of the questions that might be considered in program evaluation can be generated from the accreditation criteria. These questions often address the areas listed in Exhibit 14.2. Although the questions might seem overwhelming when taken as a collective, they can be distributed across the dimensions suggested above: mission, governance, faculty and staff, students, resources, curriculum, and evaluation. Table 14.1 displays these questions under each dimension, with potential decisions/answers to the questions posed as a clearer visualization for those designing a program evaluation plan. It is important to keep in mind that this table is not an exhaustive list of questions to consider or decisional outcomes to achieve.

EXHIBIT 14.2 Areas That Guide Design of Evaluation Plan

- Expected and unexpected outcomes of the program and their impact on the program
- Balance between the cost of program delivery and the quality of the outcomes achieved
- Impact on mission and goals
- Adequacy of resources
- Appropriate qualifications and credentials for faculty, staff, and unit leader (dean, director, other)
- Existence of numbers and quality of physical and fiscal resources
- Appropriate allocation and use of resources to meet mission goals and needs of existing and potentially new programs
- Ability to implement program in a way that promotes achievement of program outcomes
- Quality and quantity of learning experiences to promote program outcomes
- Program barriers and enablers that positively or negatively affect program effectiveness
- Strategies to facilitate program improvement
- Quality and quantity of learning resources to promote student success
- Quality of graduates
- Alumni ability to perform to expectations
- Contributions of faculty, staff, students, and alumni to the professional and social community
- Value of the program in comparison to similar existing programs

From Commission on Collegiate Nursing Education (2009). *Standards for accreditation of baccalaureate and graduate degree nursing programs*. Retrieved from www.aacn.nche.edu/ccne-accreditation/standards09.pdf

TABLE 14.1 Evaluation Questions by Evaluative Dimensions

Dimensions	Potential Questions to Consider	Potential Decisions
Mission and goals	• Are the mission and goals of the nursing unit consistent with that of the parent institution? • Have professional standards and practice guidelines been incorporated into the goals and outcomes of the nursing unit? Are the standards consistent with community workforce needs and regional health care practices? • Is there an ongoing systematic review process in place to ensure continued accountability?	• Worth/contribution of the nursing unit to the mission and goals of the institution. • Program goals and outcomes are in alignment with professional practice expectations, which indicate program relevance. • Faculty are periodically reviewed for relevance and are accountable to practice for alumni performance.
Governance	• What is the process for faculty and student participation in setting goals, developing policies, and addressing issues related to quality of education and learning experiences?	• Faculty and students take responsibility to provide meaningful input into the academic environment and learning culture that enhance their educational experiences.

(continued)

TABLE 14.1   Evaluation Questions by Evaluative Dimensions (*continued*)

Dimensions	Potential Questions to Consider	Potential Decisions
	• Are educational policies and practices consistent with the learner population, consistently applied, equitable in interpretation and facilitating of student acceptance to and progress through to graduation? Do the policies in place protect individual rights and freedoms?	• The right policies for the right populations are administered at the right time in the right place by the right people. Individual freedoms are protected with appropriate due process mechanisms executed as written.
Faculty and staff	• Are the quantity and quality of the faculty and staff consistent with educational needs and abilities to promote achievement of program goals and student learning outcomes? • Do faculty and staff have the knowledge and skills to contribute to student learning, achievement of student goals, and attainment of nursing and institutional mission and goals through scholarship, practice, and service activities?	• Instructor-to-student ratios within practice guidelines and consistent with best evidence for promoting learning. Faculty and staff hold professional and educational credentials consistent with role expectations, practice guidelines, community partner expectations, university expectations, and student and peer expectations. • Faculty and staff contributions bring value and relevance to the institution, nursing, and professional self. Contributions are consistent with mission and unit goals and facilitate student achievement of outcomes.
Students	• Are student academic support systems in place, accessible, and of the quality needed to support student attainment of academic outcomes and personal goals? • Are support services able to meet the learning needs of students enrolled in programs relying on technology to deliver or enhance the learning experience for students?	• The quality, quantity, and accessibility of academic support facilitate student retention and achievement. • All students are able to meet program outcomes with appropriate leveraging of technological resources and services.
Resources	• Are physical resources and equipment of the quality and quantity to support student attainment of program and learning outcomes?	• Physical resources meet program needs and provide the ability to implement learning experiences that promote achievement of learning outcomes and program goals/mission.

(continued)

Dimensions	Potential Questions to Consider	Potential Decisions
	• Are fiscal resources commensurate with program needs and of the quality to promote achievement of learning outcomes and program goals and mission? • Does a systematic process for review and modification exist to sustain the quality and quantity of resources required to meet mission and goals? Do faculty have a voice in the resource allocation process necessary to ensure resource sustainability?	• Fiscal resources are adequate to meet program mission and goals. They are aligned with institutional fiscal resources and based on goal achievement. • The nursing unit and its faculty and staff are able to acquire resources of the quantity and quality needed to meet the mission and goals of the nursing unit.
Curriculum	• Are the mission, goals, and expected learning outcomes consistent with stakeholders' expectations, professional standards, and best practice guidelines? • Has the curriculum been designed to promote attainment of knowledge and skills commensurate with established learning outcomes across programs? Are learning experiences consistent with and do they complement achievement of learning outcomes. • Are students able to acquire and use the knowledge from their liberal arts foundation in the acquisition of discipline-specific knowledge and skills needed to meet program and course outcomes?	• Program outcomes are consistent with mission and goals. Program is relevant and provides the knowledge and skills consistent with evidence-based best practices. • Students demonstrate the ability to meet course and program learning outcomes. • Demonstrated student behaviors are consistent with institutional and nursing program mission and goals.
Program effectiveness	• What is the overall contribution of value and impact of the program on the professional workforce and the social community? • What factors impede or enhance program effectiveness?	• The performance quality of the graduates meets or exceeds employer expectations. Program costs balance with the ability of graduates to achieve outcomes. Program is effective in meeting goals. • Barriers and enablers have been identified and decisions made to remove or reinforce to support efforts for continuous quality improvement of program.

Once the questions and their expected outcomes have been built into the evaluation plan, it is important to identify what information is needed and how best to gather that information. As discussed earlier in the chapter, the most informative data should be collected in a timely and cost-effective way. Table 14.2 provides examples of possible data sources for answering some of the evaluation questions posed in Table 14.1.

TABLE 14.2 Matching Information Sources to Evaluation Questions

Dimensions	Question Elements	Information Sources/Documentation
Mission and goals	Consistency, contributions, reflect accepted standards of education and practice	• Comparison of institutional mission and goals with nursing units • Comparison of professional standards with program outcomes • Committee documentation of systematic review and actions taken as part of the review process • Verification from practice partners that standards used to develop program outcomes reflect current practice expectations
Governance	Faculty and student involvement in governance, contribution of involvement in promoting institutional and nursing mission and goals	• Listing of faculty and student involvement in governance structure • Determination of level of involvement • Contribution made to policy setting and alignment to implementation of polices • Committee minutes noting policy application to such activities as admission, progression, graduation
Faculty and staff	Qualifications, experience consistent with program needs	• Documentation of credentials, experience consistent with role • Professional contributions consistent with role expectations and educational outcomes that promote learning
Students	Student credentials consistent with academic success	• Admission credentials • Documentation of prior success • Identification of support services and impact on student success • Retention rates and progression to graduation data along with documentation of use of information by appropriate personnel
Resources	Commensurate with program needs to meet program goals	• Documentation of finances in relation to program needs, costs to administer program
Curriculum	Curriculum design facilitates learning	• Documentation of performance, achievement in relation to benchmark performance expectations • Performance evaluations using a 360-degree perspective

(continued)

Dimensions	Question Elements	Information Sources/Documentation
Program effectiveness	Meeting goals, impact of graduates	• Percent graduating on time • Percent employed by specified time • Percent securing appropriate practice credentials • Results of employer surveys documenting ability to meet practice expectations

REPOSITORY OF EVALUATION INFORMATION

A common repository should be created to ensure that information is collected and analyzed on a systematic and cyclic basis. The more complex are the operations of the nursing unit and institution, the more critical it is to establish and preserve evaluative information, especially summative data, to enhance retrieval and distribution to appropriate stakeholders in a timely fashion. As noted earlier in the discussion, evaluation that supports such formative activities as conducting a needs assessment about the possible development of a new program or other initiatives or assessing the implementation of a new program requires specific documentation directed "to implement or not," or "make corrective adjustments midstream." These types of evaluations tend to generate less information, and the need for future retrieval is limited.

The incorporation of electronic informational systems has facilitated not only data-retrieval and storage, but enhanced reporting and dissemination of information in a timely and meaningful fashion for stakeholders, especially for those stakeholders with authority and responsibility for decision making. The design of information systems ranges from fully designed to being customized for a specific institution or program. Start-up costs can be high, as is the time taken for customization and updating the system.

Within informational systems, there should be support tools that facilitate the ability to display information for specific audiences and needs. A couple of tools currently being used in institutions of higher education are the dashboard and report card display mechanisms. These tools allow institutions and programs to share summaries of performance, highlight key traits of performance or factors that are unique to the institution or program, and make comparisons with other national and regional performance indicators. Information shared using tools such as the dashboard or report card can be kept as an internal tracking mechanism or designed for more public use. Dashboards that display more strategic information about institutional operations focus more on decision makers' need to know. Other dashboards focus on performance indicators and are often imbedded within the context of goals and outcomes. Often the designs focus on performance and are created for public informational purposes to highlight institutional or program mission and abilities. Measuring performance and goal attainment can be evidenced by the use of a numeric, alphabetic, or color scheme scale designed to quickly communicated the level of success.

ANALYSIS, REPORTING, AND USE OF EVALUATION INFORMATION

The last implementation steps in evaluation are the analysis, reporting, and use of the information collected. Evaluators are often challenged in distributing the information to the right stakeholders at the right time, as the information required by the stakeholders might need to be collected, or existing data might have to be analyzed differently to meet emerging needs. As an evaluator you will most likely have to assist stakeholders in interpreting information in a way that is most useful in meeting individual needs.

In today's environment, many institutions and programs are being required to provide information associated with costs (Powell, Gilleland, & Pearson, 2012). Program evaluation plans often include processes that allow administrators to determine program costs in relation to program outcomes. Two types of approaches frequently used are cost-effectiveness and cost-benefit analysis. Cost-effectiveness analysis relates the costs of a program to the key outcomes or benefits of the program. In cost-benefit analysis, the process goes one step farther, comparing costs with the dollar value of all (or most) of the program's benefits (Cellini & Kee, 2010, p. 493). As funding continues to be closely tied to institutional and program outcomes, cost analysis will be integral to evaluation.

BUILDING A CULTURE OF EVALUATION

Building and sustaining a culture in which evaluation plays an important role is critical to sustain evaluation activities in the life of the institution and the various disciplines and programs housed within it. Institutions and programs need to build an environment in which decisions are based on valid information, collected using accepted research practices. Weiner (2009) identified elements that need to be in place to support evaluation in an institution (Exhibit 14.3).

EXHIBIT 14.3 Elements to Support an Institution's Evaluation Activities

1. Clear goals
2. Commonly shared use of evaluation terminology across disciplines and campuses
3. Faculty ownership of evaluation and assessment activities
4. Continuous faculty development activities related to evaluation practices
5. Top-down support for evaluation activities that includes budgeting and planning at the institutional and unit levels
6. Established goals and outcomes that can be measured
7. Evaluation plan that can be and is implemented and participated in by faculty, staff, administration, students, and other primary stakeholders
8. Systematic and cyclic institution plan for program reviews
9. Ongoing evaluation of institutional effectiveness in relation to its mission and goals
10. Support of initiatives that promote evaluation efforts
11. Means of recognizing and celebrating evaluation efforts and successes

From Weiner (2009).

Mayne (2008) suggested that a strong culture of evaluation is sustained by valuing self-reflection and self-examination. The information obtained through these processes facilitates the monitoring of organizations, as well as incorporating information into their decisional approach to dealing with challenges. A strong evaluative culture engages in learning from the evidence generated and encourages experimentation and innovation as ways to improve performance and strengthen a program. The greatest gain from self-examination is more internally focused.

Ndoye and Parker (2010) examined the challenges to the establishment of an assessment culture. Informants indicated that faculty involvement, resources, and the systematic use of information affected the ability to sustain such a culture. Another key to the establishment and sustainability of a culture of assessment and evaluation is having one or more people in the environment who has the skills needed to support evaluation practices. These skills include knowledge of evaluation and assessment, ability to ask the appropriate questions that will drive the process, management skills to coordinate and ensure that the evaluation plan is systematically and consistently implemented as designed, ability to know when and how to make adjustments to the plan, and skills to communicate findings to stakeholders by making connections between findings and expected outcomes.

SUMMARY

Evaluation is critical to institutions and programs, with the pressures from accreditation requirements; state mandates; funding and allocation priorities within a continually shrinking budget; and pressures from students, families, and employers. Evaluation science has grown in sophistication to keep abreast of these pressures. Program evaluation plans are more complex and consume more time and expense for nursing programs today than in the past, and this trend is likely to continue. However, with the aid of technology and experienced evaluators, evaluation activities can be more effective and efficient. As nurse educators not only do we know what information is needed, but we are also learning how best to use evaluative information to maintain the quality and integrity of our programs. Making decisions based on valid evidence ensures that we continue to provide sustainable relevant educational programming through a continuous quality improvement process, program evaluation.

REFERENCES

Alkin, M. C., & Christie, C. A. (2004). An evaluation theory tree. In M. C. Alkin (Ed.), *Evaluation roots: Tracing theorists' views and influences* (pp. 12–65). Thousand Oaks, CA: Sage Publications.

Alkin, M. C. (2011). *Evaluation essentials: From A to Z*. New York, NY: The Guilford Press.

Askew, K., Beverly, M. G., & Jay, M. L. (2012). Aligning collaboration and culturally responsive evaluation approaches. *Evaluation and Program Planning, 35*, 552–557.

Association of American Colleges and Universities. (2010). VALUE: Valid assessment of learning in undergraduate education. Retrieved from http://www.aacu.org/value/rubrics/pdf/AllRubrics.pdf

Banta, T. W. (2011). Will we just stand by and watch this happen? *Assessment Update, 23*. Retrieved from http://www.assessmentupdate.com/sample-articles/will-we-just-stand-by.aspx

Boruch, R. F., & Petrosino, A. (2010). Meta-analysis, systematic reviews, and research syntheses. In J. S. Wholey, H. P. Hatry, & K. E. Newcomer (Eds.), *Handbook of practical program evaluation* (pp. 531–554). San Francisco, CA: Jossey-Bass.

Boulmetis, J., & Dutwin, P. (2011). *The ABC's of evaluation: Timeless techniques for program and project managers*. San Francisco, CA: Jossey-Bass.

Cellini, S. R., & Kee, J. E. (2010). Cost-effectiveness and cost-benefit analysis. In J. S. Wholey, H. P. Hatry, & K. E. Newcomer (Eds.), *Handbook of practical program evaluation* (pp. 493–530). San Francisco, CA: Jossey-Bass.

Chen, H. Y. (2013). The roots and growth of theory-driven evaluation: An integrated perspective for assessing viability, effectuality, and transferability. In M. C. Alkin (Ed.), *Evaluation roots: A wider perspective of theorists' views and influences* (pp. 113–129). Thousand Oaks, CA: Sage Publications.

Christie, C. A., & Alkin, M. C. (2013). An evaluation theory tree. In M. C. Alkin (Ed.), *Evaluation roots: A wider perspective of theorists' views and influences* (pp. 11–58). Thousand Oaks, CA: Sage Publications.

Commission on Collegiate Nursing Education. (2009). *Standards for Accreditation of Baccalaureate and Graduate Degree Nursing Programs*. Retrieved from http://www.aacn.nche.edu/ccne-accreditation/standards09.pdf

Cook, T. D., Scriven, M., Coryn, C. L. S., & Evergreen, S. D. H. (2010). Contemporary thinking about causation in evaluation: A dialogue with Tom Cook and Michael Scriven. *American Journal of Education, 31*, 105–117. doi:10.1177/1098214009354918

Cooperrider, D. L., & Godwin, L. N. (2010, August 26). Positive organization development: Innovation-inspired change in an economy and ecology of strengths [Draft]. Retrieved from http://www.appreciativeinquiry.case.edu/intro/POD_8—26-10.pdf

Goeschel, C. A., Weiss, W. M., & Pronovost, P. J. (2012). Using a logic model to design and evaluate quality and patient safety improvement programs. *International Journal for Quality in Health-care, 24*, 330–337. doi:10.1093/intqhc/mzs029

Grayson, T. E. (2012). Approaches to evaluation in higher education. In C. Secolsky & D. B. Denison (Eds.), *Handbook on measurement, assessment, and evaluation in higher education* (pp. 455–458). New York, NY & London: Routledge, Taylor, & Francis Group.

Head, R. B., & Johnson, M. S. (2011). Accreditation and its influence on institutional effectiveness. *New Directions for Community Colleges, 153*, 37–52. doi:10.1002/cc.435

Hermans, L. M., Naber, A. C., & Easerink, B. (2012). Theory-based evaluation: Challenges to this approach. *Evaluation and Program Planning, 35*, 427–438.

Horne, E. M., & Sandmann, L. R. (2012). Current trends in systematic program evaluation: An integrative literature review. *Journal of Nursing Education, 51*, 570–581. doi:10.3928/01484834-20120820-06

Howe, K. R. (2011). Mixed methods, mixed causes. In N. K. Denzin & M. D. Giardina (Eds.), *Qualitative inquiry and global crises* (pp. 118). Walnut Creek, CA: Left Coast Press, Inc.

Karlowicz, K. A. (2010). Development and testing of a portfolio evaluation scoring tool. *Journal of Nursing Education, 49*, 78–86. doi:10.3928/01484834-20090918-07

Lee, Y., Altschuld, J. W., & Lee, L. (2012). Essential competencies for program evaluators in a diverse cultural context. *Evaluation and Program Planning, 35*, 439–444.

Liu, O. L. (2011a). Value-added assessment in higher education: A comparison of two methods. *Higher Education, 61*, 445–461. doi:10.1007/s10734-010-9340-8

Liu, O. L. (2011b). Outcomes assessment in higher education: Challenges and futures research in the context of voluntary system of accountability. *Educational Measurement: Issues and Practice, 30*(3), 2–9. doi:10.1111/j.1745-3992.2011.00206.x

Loyd, G. E., & Koenig, H. M. (2008). Assessment of learning outcomes: Summative evaluations. *International Anesthesiology Clinics, 46*, 97–111. doi:10.1097/AIA.0b013e31818623cd

Madaus, G. F. (2013). Ralph W. Tyler's contribution to program evaluation. In M. C. Alkin (Ed.), *Evaluation roots: A wider perspective of theorists' views and influences* (pp. 157–164). Thousand Oaks, CA: Sage Publications.

Mayne, J. (2008). *Building an evaluative culture for effective evaluation and results management.* ILAC Working Paper 8, Rome, Institutional Learning and Change Initiative. Retrieved from www.cgiar-ilac.org/files/publications/working_papers/ILAC_Working

McLaughlin, J. A., & Jordan, G. B. (2010). Using logic models. In J. S. Wholey, H. P. Hatry, & K. E. Newcomer (Eds.), *Handbook of practical program evaluation* (pp. 55–80). San Francisco, CA: Jossey-Bass.

Mertens, D. M. (2009). *Transformative research and evaluation.* New York, NY: The Guildford Publications, Inc.

Mertens, D. M. (2010). *Research and evaluation in education and psychology: Integrating diversity with quantitative, qualitative, and mixed methods.* Thousand Oaks, CA: Sage Publications.

Ndoye, A., & Parker, M. A. (2010). Creating and sustaining a culture of assessment. *Planning for Higher Education, 38*, 28–39.

Newcomer, K. E., Hatry, H. P., & Wholey, J. S. (2010). Planning and designing useful evaluations. In J. S. Wholey, H. P. Hatry, & K. E. Newcomer (Eds.), *Handbook of practical program evaluation* (pp. 5–29). San Francisco, CA: Jossey-Bass.

Nichols, P. D., Meyers, J. L., & Burling, K. S. (2009). A framework for evaluating and planning assessments intended to improve student achievement. *Educational Measurement: Issues and Practice, 28*(3), 14–23. doi:10.1111/j.1745-3992.2009.00150.x

Patton, M. Q. (2008). *Utilization-focused evaluation.* Thousand Oaks, CA: Sage Publications.

Patton, M. Q. (2012). *Essentials of utilization-focused evaluation.* Thousand Oaks, CA: Sage Publications.

Patton, M. Q. (2013). The roots of utilization-focused evaluation. In M. C. Alkin (Ed.), *Evaluation roots: A wider perspective of theorists' views and influences* (pp. 293–303). Thousand Oaks, CA: Sage Publications.

Powell, B. A., Gilleland, D. S., & Pearson, L. C. (2012). Expenditures, efficiency, and effectiveness in U.S. undergraduate higher education: A national benchmark model. *The Journal of Higher Education, 83*(1), 102–127. doi:10.1353/jhe.2012.0005

Rhodes, T. L. (2012). Show me the learning: Value, accreditation, and the quality of the degree. *Planning for Higher Education, 40*(3), 36–42.

Scriven, M. (1991). Pros and cons about goal-free evaluation. *American Journal of Evaluation, 12*(1), 55–62. doi:10.1177/109821409101200108

Scriven, M. (2004). Reflections. In M. C. Alkin (Ed.), *Evaluation roots: Tracing theorists' views and influences* (pp. 183–195). Thousand Oaks, CA: Sage Publications.

Scriven, M. (2013). Conceptual revolution in evaluation: Past, present, and future. In M.C. Alkin (Ed.), *Evaluation roots: A wider perspective of theorists' views and influences* (pp. 167–179). Thousand Oaks, CA: Sage Publications.

Senger, J., & Kanthan, R. (2012). Student evaluations: Synchronous tripod of learning portfolio assessment-self-assessment, peer-assessment, instructor assessment. *Creative Education, 3*(1), 155–163.

Stufflebeam, D. L. (1971). *The relevance of the CIPP evaluation model for educational accountability.* Paper presented at the 1971 Annual Meeting of the American Association of School Administrators. Paper retrieved from http://www.eric.ed.gov:8/PDFS/ED062385.pdf

Stufflebeam, D. L. (2004). The 21st-century CIPP model: Origins, development, and use. In M. C Alkin (Ed.), *Evaluation roots: Tracing theorists' views and influences* (pp. 245–266). Thousand Oaks, CA: Sage Publications.

Stufflebeam, D. L. (2013). The CIPP evaluation model: Status, origin, development, use and theory. In M. C. Alkin (Ed.), *Evaluation roots: A wider perspective of theorists' views and influences* (pp. 243–260). Thousand Oaks, CA: Sage Publications.

University of Twente. (2012, December 18). *System theory [communication].* Retrieved from http://www.utwente.nl/cw/throrieenoverzicht/theory%20Clusters/Communication%20 Processes/Sytem_Theory.doc

Wandersman, A., Snell-Johns, J., Lentz, B. E., Fetterman, D. M., Keener, D. C., Livet, M., ... Flaspoher, P. (2012). The principles of empowerment evaluation. In D. M. Fetterman, A. Wandersman, & R. A. Millett (Eds.), *Empowerment evaluation principles in practice* (pp. 27–41). New York, NY: The Guilford Press.

Weiner, W. F. (2009). Establishing a culture of assessment. *Academe, 95*(4), 28–32.

Weiss, C. (1991). Evaluation research in the political context: Sixteen years and four administrators later. In M. W. McLaughlin & D. C. Phillips (Eds.), *Evaluation and education: At quarter century* (90th Yearbook of the National Society for the Study of Education; Part II, pp. 213). Chicago, IL: University of Chicago Press.

Wholey, J. S. (2013). Using evaluation to improve program performance and results. In M. C. Alkin (Ed.), *Evaluation roots: A wider perspective of theorists' views and influences* (pp. 261–266). Thousand Oaks, CA: Sage Publications.

15

Evidence-Based Teaching in Nursing

MARILYN H. OERMANN

Evidence-based teaching is the use of research findings and other evidence to guide educational decisions and practices. Available evidence should be used when developing the curriculum and courses, selecting teaching methods and approaches to use with students, planning clinical learning activities, and assessing students' learning and performance. Yet many nurse educators rarely search for evidence when they make educational decisions. They update their courses by incorporating new evidence about the content, but they might not seek evidence on how those courses are best designed, taught, and evaluated. How much practice do students need to retain their motor skills? What are best practices with debriefing? What characteristics of online courses are critical to learning and retention? These are the types of questions that every educator should be raising no matter what course or level of learner they are teaching.

Teachers can then search the literature for research studies and other evidence to answer these questions and guide their educational practices. By reviewing the literature, the teacher can also learn about the experiences of other educators, to build on those rather than to start anew. This chapter describes evidence-based teaching in nursing, the need for better research in nursing education, and a process for engaging in evidence-based teaching.

EVIDENCE-BASED TEACHING IN NURSING: WHAT IS IT?

Evidence-based teaching is the use of research findings and other knowledge to guide educational practices in nursing. Cannon and Boswell (2012) defined evidence-based teaching as a dynamic and holistic system using educational principles validated by evidence to support and promote learning in a variety of settings (pp. 8–9). Nursing, medicine, education, and other fields have a body of knowledge that can be used to inform practice as a nurse, physician, or teacher—this knowledge provides the evidence to guide what we do. In evidence-based teaching, nurse educators use knowledge about how students learn, how best to promote their learning and performance, effective teaching and assessment methods, and other practices to guide what they do as educators.

Definitions of evidence-based nursing provide a framework for conceptualizing evidence-based teaching in nursing. Many of these definitions view evidence-based nursing as the integration of research evidence with clinical expertise and the values and preferences of the patient. Scott and McSherry (2009) analyzed 83 articles to identify the key concepts associated with evidence-based nursing. Based on their analysis, they defined evidence-based nursing as an ongoing process by which evidence, nursing theory, and the nurse's clinical expertise are evaluated critically and considered in conjunction with patient involvement, with the goal of providing optimal nursing care to the patient (p. 1089). This analysis and resulting definition are useful for conceptualizing evidence-based teaching in nursing: it is the integration of the best research evidence with theories and concepts about learning, teaching, assessment, and other areas related to nursing education, the teacher's expertise, and the learner's preferences and goals.

In an online survey of 295 nurse educators from 86 programs, faculty members reported using quantitative and qualitative research findings as evidence for their teaching, and they also considered conference information, course evaluations, student feedback from class, and students' comments as other evidence (Patterson & Klein, 2012). Conference proceedings and other sources of expert opinion are considered low levels of evidence. The personal beliefs of the teacher were the most frequent facilitator of evidence-based teaching (Patterson & Klein).

NURSING EDUCATION RESEARCH AND EVIDENCE-BASED TEACHING

We need rigorous research in nursing education to generate evidence that can be used to guide teaching. Early on, many researchers explored nursing education topics, but over the years the focus of research has shifted to the study of clinical problems, with limited funding available for nursing education. Although the emphasis of nursing research is no longer on education, nursing education studies continue to be done (Yucha, Schneider, Smyer, Kowalski, & Stowers, 2011). Many of these studies, though, are conducted with small samples of students in one setting only, with investigator-developed tools that have not been validated. Many are pilot studies, and, although valuable, they need to be followed up and replicated. One of the issues in nursing education is that few studies are replicated across schools of nursing and across students (Oermann, 2009). The lack of funding has made it difficult to conduct large, multisite educational studies in nursing (Oermann, Hallmark, Haus, Kardong-Edgren, McColgan, & Rogers, 2012). Addressing these shortcomings is critical, though, to generalizing the findings and determining whether the educational practice can be used with different students and settings.

Yucha et al. (2011) found that most nursing education studies in their sample were done with a single group, either as cross-sectional or posttest only studies ($n = 74$, 55.6%). Less than 20% ($n = 25$, 18.8%) were single-group pre- and posttest. Studies in both nursing and medicine often compare the outcomes of a new educational approach using the learners' baseline as their own control. These studies are relatively easy to conduct as part of a typical teaching situation, and they can be done with minimal or no funding. Although they might support the use of a new method, some experts have suggested they contribute little to advancing the science of education because they do not inform the development of the next course, curriculum, or tool (Cook, 2012; Cook, Bordage, & Schmidt, 2008).

Nurse educators develop many educational innovations and new initiatives, but without research to document their effectiveness and outcomes, it is not known whether the new approaches are better than the prior ones. Providing an evidence base for nursing education is not only important to advance the science of nursing education. Nursing education is expensive, and better studies would guide teachers and administrators in schools of nursing to develop cost-effective and higher-quality education (Broome, 2009). Yucha and colleagues (2011) suggested that the methodological quality of nursing education studies could be improved if the researchers used objective measures of the outcomes, used instruments that were valid and reliable, employed more experimental designs, and included the impact of educational approaches on patient outcomes. Although the effects of education on patient outcomes are important to study, some researchers in medical education have cautioned that they should not be the main focus of medical education research (Cook & West, 2013). The same is true when evaluating the impact of educational interventions in nursing: the focus needs to remain on the students and their learning and development.

Levin (2004) developed a model of educational research that provides a framework for understanding the current state of nursing education research. *Stage 1* includes preliminary ideas, hypotheses, observations, and pilot studies. *Stage 2* involves controlled laboratory experiments and interventions tested in the classroom, as well as observational studies of master teachers. *Stage 3* studies are randomized control trials of educational interventions comparing a new approach to the standard one. Levin emphasized that in Stage 3 the interventions are assigned randomly to different groups of learners and educational situations, which are both realistic and controlled. With rigorous studies, effective interventions can be tested across settings (*Stage 4*). Most nursing education studies are at Stages 1 and 2. However, with rigorous studies at Stages 1 and 2 that are replicated in various schools of nursing and settings, research findings can be synthesized to create an evidence base for nursing education (Oermann, 2009).

PHASES OF EVIDENCE-BASED TEACHING

Evidence-based teaching includes four phases: (1) questioning educational practices and identifying the need for evidence to guide teaching, (2) searching for research studies and other evidence on educational practices, (3) evaluating the quality of the evidence, and (4) deciding whether the findings are applicable to one's own program, courses, students, and context in which one is teaching (Oermann, 2007, 2009). Similar to evidence-based practice in nursing and other fields, the teacher also considers theories and concepts about learning and teaching, and the teacher's own philosophy of nursing education and expertise as an educator. Students also need to have input as to their preferences for learning and their personal goals to be met in the course. The evidence alone does not dictate what methods and practices to use. It is up to the teacher to integrate the evidence with these other considerations, as the teacher understands the students and context in which the education takes place.

QUESTION EDUCATIONAL PRACTICES AND IDENTIFY NEED FOR EVIDENCE

The first phase in evidence-based teaching is for nurse educators to recognize that it is their responsibility to reflect on their educational practices and question whether there is a better way of teaching students (Oermann, 2007, 2009). Reflection and questioning our practices as teachers are defining characteristics of a professional, and they are critical to thinking about changes in education that could lead to improved learning and performance.

The questions can be general questions about an educational practice or intervention being considered. These are descriptive questions that guide a search of the literature for information about the practice, but not necessarily about whether it is superior to another practice in terms of outcomes. Examples of these general questions are: How can podcasts be used for instruction in nursing courses? What are strategies for incorporating audience response systems that allow the teacher to ask questions and gather students' responses in large group lectures? What are best practices in debriefing in simulation-based learning? These general questions are valuable too, because they allow the teacher to learn about the experiences of other nurse educators. With this type of question, the teacher can search the literature and other resources to learn more about the educational practice and build on those experiences.

Another type of question leads to a search for evidence to support an educational practice or intervention. With this type of question the teacher is searching for studies on the outcomes of various practices to make a decision as to the best approach to use. Examples of this type of question include the following: Is there a difference in knowledge retention between face-to-face lectures and segmented podcasts (podcasts divided into segments)? What are the effects of audience response systems on learning outcomes in nursing education? Does scripted versus nonscripted debriefing and/or simulator realism affect performance of nurses in simulated cardiopulmonary arrests? In nursing education, this type of question is often more difficult to answer than it would be in other disciplines, as the research might not have been done, and the evidence is not available, or the studies are of such poor quality that the findings cannot be used for making educational decisions.

SEARCH FOR EVIDENCE ON EDUCATIONAL PRACTICES

In the second phase, teachers search the literature for studies on the topic and for other articles and resources to answer their questions. This research requires knowledge of bibliographic databases to search, search skills, and awareness of other resources, such as websites that report evidence on educational practices.

Although there are many *bibliographic databases* that contain reports of studies that might be relevant to teaching in nursing, three databases are recommended for a search in nursing education:.

1. MEDLINE®, which has more than 20 million references to biomedical and life sciences journal articles, including nursing education (United States National Library of Medicine, 2013). MEDLINE is searched through PubMed®, available at www.ncbi. nlm.nih.gov/pubmed.
2. Cumulative Index to Nursing and Allied Health Literature (CINAHL), the database covering nursing and allied health literature (EBSCO Industries, Inc., 2012).
3. Education Resources Information Center (ERIC) database, from the Institute of Education Sciences of the United States Department of Education (n.d.), which indexes education research and also conference proceedings and other reports that might provide evidence about a teaching practice

For some questions, other bibliographic databases such as PsycINFO®, which covers studies and other peer-reviewed literature in the behavioral sciences and mental health (American Psychological Association, 2013), might be relevant, depending on the topic.

It is important to search multiple databases because different journals are indexed in them, and thus a broad search of the literature provides a better evidence base. An example can be seen in a search for evidence on audience response systems. A search in PubMed using the phrase "audience response system" revealed three times as many articles as in the CINAHL database, and only some of these articles overlapped. If searching only one database, the nurse educator might miss some relevant studies.

The questions asked about the topic or educational practice guide the search for studies. Nurse educators need to be proficient in *searching the literature*. They should be knowledgeable about the databases and the literature in them, as well as about how they are organized. Educators also need skills in selecting keywords for a search, for example, Medical Subject Headings (MeSH) terms in PubMed and subject headings in CINAHL, and combining search terms. Those skills are critical to locate relevant educational studies. Exhibit 15.1 lists strategies nurse educators can use to prepare themselves to conduct a search for evidence on teaching.

EXHIBIT 15.1 Strategies Nurse Educators Can Use to Prepare Themselves to Conduct a Search

Ask the Right Question

Learn how to ask clear questions to guide a search.

Develop a PICO(TS)[a] as applicable.

Write a focused question based on the PICO(TS).

Plan search strategies in advance.

Locate the thesaurus, if one is available, in each of the databases to be used in the search.

Identify subject headings and text word terms for your topic or to answer your question.

Find a few sample articles and confirm or alter the search terms.

Select the Right Database

Select relevant databases to search and use multiple databases.

Become familiar with different bibliographic databases including the Cumulative Index to Nursing and Allied Health Literature (CINAHL), PubMed, Education Resources Information Center (ERIC), PsycINFO, and others, depending on the subject.

Review the types of literature indexed in each of the databases.

Learn how each database is organized.

Learn to use the databases by completing the tutorial with each database and then practicing.

Learn how to broaden and narrow a search, use filters, combine searches, conduct advanced searches, and use other search strategies in each database.

Review sample records and different views of each record to be familiar with them.

Critically Evaluate the Search Terms and Process Based on Citations Returned

Be prepared to adjust or change search terms or strategies and/or databases used to match needs.

Refer to Exhibit 15.2 for specifics on evaluating the nursing education studies retrieved in the search.

Organize Citations and Information Returned

Learn how to save items, create collections, and manage collections in databases as appropriate.

Learn how to save and manage searches in bibliographic management software.

Develop a system for recording results of searches; review available resources such as PRISMA (Preferred Reporting Items for Systematic Reviews and Meta-Analyses) flow diagram (www.prisma-statement.org/statement.htm).

Use PRISMA checklist and flow diagram if conducting systematic review or meta-analysis.

PICO(TS), Population or problem, intervention, comparison, outcomes, timing (if applicable), and setting (if applicable).

Teachers also should be aware of *other resources*, such as websites that report evidence on educational practices. For example, the Best Evidence Medical Education (BEME) Collaboration is an international group with the aim of developing evidence-based education in medicine and other health professions. Researchers conduct systematic reviews to provide the best available evidence for teaching in the health fields and to disseminate the findings of their reviews at their website and in journals (Best Evidence Medical Education [BEME], 2013b). Nurse educators can search for evidence reviews related to their topic or question at the BEME website (www.bemecollaboration.org/Published+Reviews/). Although these reviews are not specific to nursing education, many of the reviews are applicable to teaching in nursing. Teachers can also search websites of nursing education organizations for summaries of evidence and reports of relevant studies.

Systematic Reviews

For areas of education that have been well studied, the teacher should begin by searching for a systematic review in which experts critically appraise and synthesize the findings of multiple studies on a particular educational topic to identify best practices. These reviews include an assessment of the original studies; in evidence-based practice, such studies are referred to as *appraised resources*.

One type of systematic review is a meta-analysis, which uses quantitative methods to synthesize the findings from individual research studies. Meta-analyses typically calculate effect sizes, which determine whether the differences between groups are significant and the magnitude of these differences, when considering the studies as a whole (Oermann, 2009). For example, Cook et al. (2010) conducted a meta-analysis of research on instructional design variations to improve Internet-based learning in health professions education. From a review of 2,705 articles, they identified 51 eligible studies. By analyzing findings across these studies, they found that interactivity, practice exercises, repetition, and feedback were associated with improved learning outcomes. There was, however, inconsistency in findings across studies.

With a systematic review, the researchers use an organized method of searching for studies; decide which studies to include in the review, based on specific criteria; appraise the quality of each study; and synthesize the findings. The protocol for conducting the review ensures that each study in the review is critiqued similarly, and a standardized process is used. For example, reviews done by BEME follow a protocol that includes the description of the background of the topic, review questions and objectives, search sources and strategies, selection criteria for studies to review, procedures for extracting data, and synthesis of the evidence, among other areas (BEME, 2013a).

Literature Reviews

With a literature review, the author selects studies to review based on specific criteria, evaluates the studies, and integrates the findings. A literature review is an examination of the literature from the author's perspective. The benefit of systematic reviews and meta-analyses is that only studies that meet certain criteria are included, and the reviews follow an established protocol (Oermann, 2009). An issue with literature reviews is that they are frequently summaries of the findings of studies, with little analysis of their quality and the impact of that quality on the results.

When a systematic review has not been done, however, a comprehensive literature review can be valuable in a search for evidence. For example, Dahlke, Baumbusch, Affleck, and Kwon (2012) conducted a review of the literature on clinical teachers' perceptions of their role and factors that facilitate and constrain their teaching in undergraduate nursing programs. They reviewed 15 articles published in English and identified themes related to teachers' perceptions of their role, characteristics of effective clinical teaching, and the influence of the clinical and academic context on their role. Clinical teachers recognized the importance of being effective as educators and competent as clinicians.

Individual Studies

When systematic and literature reviews are not available, the teacher needs to review individual studies and critique their quality. With systematic reviews, the researchers assess the methodological quality of studies included in the review. However, when teachers are reviewing the literature themselves, they need to critically appraise each study to determine whether the findings are valid, whether they answer the educational questions raised earlier in the process, and whether they will be useful to the teacher considering own students and context. The study validity depends on whether the research methods are rigorous enough for the findings to be as "close to the truth as possible" (Melnyk, Fineout-Overholt, Stillwell, & Williamson, 2010, p. 52). For example, were students randomly assigned to the teaching intervention and control groups, and were valid and reliable tools used to measure outcomes? Flaws in the study design, the lack of a control or comparison group, use of measurement tools without established validity and reliability, issues with the procedures used for data collection (e.g., the teacher distributing surveys to own students), errors in the statistical analysis, and so forth weaken the findings and limit their use.

The teacher also evaluates whether the results answer the questions identified for the review, support the educational practice or intervention, and are applicable to own students and setting. The study might have been well-designed, but a small sample size in one school of nursing limits generalizing the findings to other groups of learners and settings. Exhibit 15.2 provides a general guide for analyzing nursing education research literature. Table 15.1 provides a form for recording a review of studies with a sample excerpt from a review.

EXHIBIT 15.2 Guide for Analyzing Nursing Education Research Literature

Title

Does it clearly describe the educational study reported in the paper? Is it informative?

Abstract

Does it emphasize the study's purpose, method, major findings, and conclusions?

Is this a quantitative, qualitative, or mixed methods study in nursing education?

Introduction

Does it state the problem in nursing education and why it is important to learn more about it?

Does the introduction provide the background and rationale for the study?

What is the purpose of the study, and is it clear and understandable?

If a conceptual or theoretical framework is presented, does it relate to the purpose and describe the concepts underlying the study and their relationships?

(continued)

Exhibit 15.2 Guide for Analyzing Nursing Education Research Literature (*continued*)

Literature Review

Is the literature critically reviewed?

Are strengths and weaknesses of prior studies included in the review?

Does the review support the reason for conducting the study and identify gaps in our understanding of how best to promote student learning, teach students, develop nursing programs, and so forth?

Is the literature review up-to-date, that is, most articles in the last 5 years?

Are primary sources used?

Research Questions

Are the research questions clear, specific, and stated appropriately?

Are variables defined if appropriate?

Design

Is the design consistent with the questions?

What type of design is used?

What are strengths and weaknesses of the design?

Sample

What criteria were used to select the sample?

Is the sample size adequate?

Is the sample representative of learners, teachers, nursing programs, and so forth?

Instruments

Are the instruments and other measures described, and are they appropriate?

Are they valid and reliable?

Data Collection Procedure

Is the procedure clearly described?

Are methods for collecting and analyzing qualitative data appropriate for the type of study?

Findings

Are the findings interpreted correctly including any statistical analyses?

Are the statistics appropriate for analyzing the data?

Are the findings presented clearly and in relation to the study questions or hypotheses?

Are the findings presented logically?

Are tables and figures easy to read, and do they support the text?

Are the statistics in the tables and figures and the statistics in the text consistent?

Discussion

Is the discussion related to the literature, and does it include how the study builds on earlier research in nursing education (and higher education if relevant)?

Are the limitations identified, and could they have been resolved?

Can the findings be generalized and, if so, to what populations?

Are there implications for teaching, assessment, program development, and so forth, and are they relevant?

Are the conclusions based on the study results and accurate?

Strengths and Weaknesses

Overall, what are the study's major strengths and weaknesses?

Adapted from Oermann and Hays (2010). Copyright 2010. Reproduced with the permission of Springer Publishing Company, LLC.

TABLE 15.1 Form for Recording Evidence Review of Nursing Education Studies

Components of Review	Evidence Summary
Question to be answered	What are the effects of audience response systems on learning outcomes in nursing education?
Search terms	Audience response system
	Audience response system and nursing
	(limits: English language, human, 2000–present)
Databases searched	PubMed, CINAHL, ERIC
Number of relevant citations	10
Research study and level of evidence[a]	Vana, Silva, Muzyka, & Hirani (2011).
	The aim was to evaluate whether a lecture format using multiple-choice PowerPoint slides and an audience response system was more effective than a lecture format using only multiple-choice PowerPoint slides in comprehension and retention of pharmacological knowledge among 78 baccalaureate nursing students. The study also assessed whether Clickers positively affected students' satisfaction. There were no significant differences in test scores between the groups. In the group using Clickers, 92.3% recommended use in future courses.
	Level 2b

[a]Kirkpatrick's Four-Level Evaluation Model

EVALUATE THE QUALITY OF THE EVIDENCE

There are many systems for rating the quality of the evidence that can be applied to nursing education. In traditional rating systems, evidence from systematic reviews and meta-analyses are at the highest level. These are followed by randomized controlled trials (of which there are few in nursing education); then cohort studies (e.g., two groups or cohorts of students, one of which receives the educational intervention, whereas the other does not); case control and descriptive studies; and last, expert opinion, the lowest level. The stronger the evidence, the more likely that it is valid and relevant for a particular educational situation.

As an example, a meta-analysis explored the effectiveness of feedback, information on performance from an instructor, a peer, or a computer, either during or after a simulation activity, in facilitating procedural skills learning (Hatala, Cook, Zendejas, Hamstra, & Brydges, 2013). There were 31 articles included in the review. The results suggested that there was a moderate benefit of feedback; feedback at the end of the simulation activity appeared to be more effective than concurrent feedback for novice learners; and multiple sources of feedback, including instructor feedback, were superior to any single source of feedback. In another study with a quasi-experimental design, researchers examined the effects of using unfolding case studies and situated peer coaching for providing nursing students with individualized feedback for learning skills in the laboratory (Himes & Ravert, 2012). Pre- and postintervention data were collected to evaluate changes in student ratings of the course. Students were positive about the personalized feedback associated with peer coaching, among other outcomes. The results from the meta-analysis provide stronger evidence on feedback during skill learning, sources of feedback, and when to deliver it than the single study.

Other models have been developed for evaluating evidence from educational studies that are appropriate for use in nursing education. Levin's model of educational research, described earlier, can be used for this purpose (Levin, 2004). With this model, the lowest level of evidence would be pilot and observational studies. These are followed by controlled experiments in the classroom, laboratory, and clinical setting, and observational studies of master teachers, and then randomized controlled trials of educational interventions, the highest level.

Kirkpatrick's Four-Level Evaluation Model has also been used to appraise educational evidence (Kirkpatrick, 1998). The levels of this evaluation model consist of the following:

1. Learners' reaction: How well did the students like the learning process?
2. Learning: What did they learn (i.e., the extent to which the learners gained knowledge and skills)?
3. Changes in behavior: What changes in behavior resulted from the learning process (i.e., changes in the learner's capability to perform newly learned skills)?
4. Results: What are the tangible results of the learning process in terms of reduced cost, improved quality, efficiency, and so forth?

Kirkpatrick's Model can be used for assessing the level of outcomes of an educational study, and it is appropriate for nursing education research. Studies that examine learners' perceptions of and satisfaction with an educational practice or intervention, curriculum, course, teaching or assessment method, learning activity, and so forth, are at the lowest level. At the next level are studies that measure changes in learner attitudes; knowledge (e.g., acquisition of concepts, principles, and cognitive skills); and psychomotor skills, as a result of the education. The next two levels of studies have outcomes relating to changes in behaviors, such as ability to transfer learning to the clinical setting, followed by changes in the organization and patient outcomes as a result of the educational practice or intervention (Exhibit 15.3).

Although Kirkpatrick's Model is used for appraising educational evidence, including reviews by the BEME Collaboration, Yardley and Dornan (2012) suggested this model was appropriate for relatively simple educational interventions and programs with short-term endpoints, but the levels were not suitable for complex educational interventions with long-term outcomes, in which process evaluation was as important as the learning outcomes. Concerns they have with using these levels for appraising educational evidence are that teachers are not included, and the model does not

EXHIBIT 15.3 Appraisal of Educational Evidence Using Kirkpatrick's Four-Level Evaluation Model

- Level 1 Participation in educational experiences: outcomes of the study include learners' views on the learning experience, teaching method, aspects of the instruction, quality of the teaching
- Level 2a Change in learners' attitudes or perceptions: outcomes of the study relate to changes in the attitudes or perceptions of learners or between groups of learners about the educational practice or intervention
- Level 2b Change in learners' knowledge and/or skills: outcomes of the study relate to the acquisition of concepts, principles, cognitive skills, problem-solving ability, psychomotor skills
- Level 3 Change in behaviors: outcomes of the study document the transfer of learning to the clinical setting, workplace, and other settings, or the willingness of learners to apply new knowledge and skills to clinical practice
- Level 4a Change in professional practice: outcomes of the study include changes in the organization or delivery of care related to the educational practice or intervention
- Level 4b Benefits to patients: outcomes of the study include improvement in patient outcomes as a direct result of the educational practice or intervention

From Issenberg, McGaghie, Petrusa, Gordon, and Scalese (2005); Yardley and Dornan (2012).

allow for the rich variety of outcomes with both qualitative and quantitative educational studies (Yardley & Dorman). This is important, as many nursing education studies use qualitative methods and explore educational practices that are complex with many variables.

Yardley and Dorman (2012) suggested that, for experimental studies, the critical appraisal tools of evidence-based practice can be applied to education evidence. For other studies evaluation of the quality of the evidence can be based on global judgments of trustworthiness, such as with the following BEME scale:

1. No clear conclusions can be drawn; not significant.
2. Results ambiguous, but there appears to be a trend.
3. Conclusions can probably be based on the results.
4. Results are clear and very likely to be true.
5. Results are unequivocal (Hammick, Dornan, & Steinert, 2010; Yardley & Dorman, 2012).

This scale of 1 to 5 could be used for rating the strength of the findings of a nursing education study.

DECIDE WHETHER FINDINGS ARE APPLICABLE TO OWN PROGRAM, COURSES, STUDENTS, AND CONTEXT

The fourth phase of evidence-based teaching is as important as the earlier phases: deciding whether the findings are ready for implementation based on the evidence and, if so, whether they are applicable to one's own teaching situation. Teachers should assess if the findings are relevant to their students, program, courses, and the context in which they teach. The key in making this decision is whether the characteristics of the students, nurse educators, and other aspects of the nursing program are similar to the research that has been done. The findings from a systematic review of studies with students in prelicensure nursing programs might not be applicable for teaching nurses and other staff. Studies done in a small school of nursing might not be transferable to a large school with a diverse student population.

As a next step, if a new educational practice is used, studies should be planned to evaluate its effectiveness. Is the new practice better than the previous approach? Did it improve learning and performance? What outcomes changed as a result of this new practice or educational intervention? The goal is to design studies that measure outcomes other than satisfaction with the new teaching approach and that provide strong evidence that can be used to guide future decisions about teaching in nursing.

SUMMARY

Evidence-based teaching is the use of research findings and other evidence to guide educational decisions and practices. Available evidence should be used when developing the curriculum and courses, selecting teaching methods and approaches to use with students, planning clinical learning activities, and assessing students' learning and performance. This evidence is generated from rigorous pedagogical research; for findings to be useful to nurse educators, they must be valid and the result of well-designed studies. Most of the studies in nursing education are done with small samples in one setting only. These need to be replicated and include diverse samples of learners, teachers, and programs to determine whether the educational practice is applicable across settings and with varied student groups.

Evidence-based teaching includes four phases: (1) questioning educational practices and identifying the need for evidence to guide teaching, (2) searching for research studies and other evidence on educational practices, (3) evaluating the quality of the evidence, and (4) deciding whether the findings are applicable to one's own program, courses, students, and the context in which one is teaching. Teachers also consider theories and concepts about learning and teaching, their own philosophy of nursing education, and their expertise as educators. The learner needs to have input and consideration as to preferences for learning and personal goals to be met in the course. The evidence alone does not dictate the educational practices to use. It is up to the teacher to integrate the evidence with these other considerations.

The first phase in evidence-based teaching is for nurse educators to reflect on their educational practices and to question whether there is a better way of teaching students. In the second phase, teachers search the literature for studies done on the topic and other articles and resources to answer their questions. This phase requires knowledge of databases to search, ability to conduct a search, and knowledge of other resources, such as websites that report evidence on educational practices. Although there are many databases that contain reports of studies that might be relevant to teaching in nursing, three databases are recommended for a search in nursing education: (a) MEDLINE (via PubMed), (b) CINAHL, and (c) ERIC.

For areas of education that have been well studied, the teacher should begin by searching for a systematic review in which experts evaluate and synthesize the findings of multiple studies on a particular educational topic to arrive at conclusions about best practices. When systematic reviews are not available, the teacher should search for literature reviews. If reviews have not been done, the next step is to locate individual studies and critique their quality. Typically, a few studies on an educational practice will not be sufficient to make a major educational change.

There are many systems for rating the quality of the evidence that can be applied to nursing education, such as Levin's model of educational research, Kirkpatrick's Four-Level Evaluation Model, and a scale for making a global judgment, such as the BEME scale of 1 to 5. The review provided evidence about the educational practice or intervention, but the fourth phase is equally important: deciding whether the findings are ready for implementation based on the evidence and, if so, whether they are relevant for the teacher's own students, program, courses, and context.

REFERENCES

American Psychological Association. (2013). *PsycINFO®*. Retrieved from http://www.apa.org/pubs/databases/psycinfo/index.aspx.

Best Evidence Medical Education. (2013a). A guide to writing and submitting a BEME review protocol. Retrieved from http://www.bemecollaboration.org/Step+5+Protocol+Preparation/.

Best Evidence Medical Education. (2013b). *The BEME Collaboration*. Retrieved from http://www.bemecollaboration.org/About+BEME/

Broome, M. E. (2009). Building the science for nursing education: Vision or improbable dream. *Nursing Outlook, 57*(4), 177–179. doi:10.1016/j.outlook.2009.05.005

Cannon, S., & Boswell, C. (2012). *Evidence-based teaching in nursing*. Sudbury, MA: Jones & Bartlett Learning.

Cook, D. A. (2012). If you teach them, they will learn: Why medical education needs comparative effectiveness research. *Advances in Health Science Education, 17*, 305–310. doi:10.1007/s10459-012-9381-0

Cook, D. A., Bordage, G., & Schmidt, H. G. (2008). Description, justification, and clarification: A framework for classifying the purposes of research in medical education. *Medical Education, 42*(2), 128–133.

Cook, D. A., Levinson, A. J., Garside, S., Dupras, D. M., Erwin, P. J., & Montori, V. M. (2010). Instructional design variations in internet-based learning for health professions education: A systematic review and meta-analysis. *Academic Medicine, 85*, 909–922. doi:10.1097/ACM.0b013e3181d6c319

Cook, D. A., & West, C. P. (2013). Perspective: Reconsidering the focus on "outcomes research" in medical education: A cautionary note. *Academic Medicine, 88*, 162–167. doi:10.1097/ACM.0b013e31827c3d78

Dahlke, S., Baumbusch, J., Affleck, F., & Kwon, J. Y. (2012). The clinical instructor role in nursing education: A structured literature review. *Journal of Nursing Education, 51*, 692–696. doi:10.3928/01484834-20121022-01

EBSCO Industries, Inc. (2012). Cumulative Index to Nursing and Allied Health Literature. Retrieved from http://www.ebscohost.com/biomedical-libraries/the-cinahl-database

Hammick, M., Dornan, T., & Steinert, Y. (2010). Conducting a best evidence systematic review. Part 1: From idea to data coding. BEME Guide No. 13. *Medical Teacher, 32*(1), 3–15. doi:10.3109/01421590903414245

Hatala, R., Cook, D. A., Zendejas, B., Hamstra, S. J., & Brydges, R. (2013). Feedback for simulation-based procedural skills training: A meta-analysis and critical narrative synthesis. *Advances in Health Sciences Education: Theory and Practice, 32*(1), 3–15. doi:10.3109/01421590903414245

Himes, D. O., & Ravert, P. K. (2012). Situated peer coaching and unfolding cases in the fundamentals skills laboratory. *International Journal of Nursing Education Scholarship, 9*. doi:10.1515/1548-923X.2335

Institute of Education Sciences, U.S. Department of Education. (n.d.). About the ERIC program. Retrieved from http://www.eric.ed.gov/ERICWebPortal/resources/html/about/about_eric.html

Issenberg, S. B., McGaghie, W. C., Petrusa, E. R., Gordon, D. L., & Scalese, R. J. (2005). Features and uses of high-fidelity medical simulations that lead to effective learning–a BEME systematic review. *Medical Teacher, 27*(1), 10–28.

Kirkpatrick, D. L. (1998). *Evaluating training programs: The four levels* (2nd ed.). San Francisco, CA: Berrett-Koehler.

Levin, J. R. (2004). Random thoughts on the (in)credibility of educational psychology intervention research. *Educational Psychologist, 39*, 173–184

Melnyk, B. M., Fineout-Overholt, E., Stillwell, S. B., & Williamson, K. M. (2010). The seven steps of evidence-based practice. *American Journal of Nursing, 110*(1), 51–53. doi:10.1097/01. NAJ.0000366056.06605.d2

Oermann, M. H. (2007). Approaches to gathering evidence for educational practices in nursing. *Journal of Continuing Education in Nursing, 38*, 250–257.

Oermann, M. H. (2009). Evidence-based programs and teaching/evaluation methods: Needed to achieve excellence in nursing education. In M. Adams & T. Valiga (Eds.), *Achieving Excellence in Nursing Education* (pp. 63–76). New York, NY: National League for Nursing.

Oermann, M. H., Hallmark, B. F., Haus, C., Kardong-Edgren, S. E., McColgan, J. K., & Rogers, N. (2012). Conducting multisite research studies in nursing education: Brief practice of CPR skills as exemplar. *Journal of Nursing Education, 51*, 23–28. doi:10.3928/01484834-20111130-05

Oermann, M. H., & Hays, J. (2010). *Writing for publication in nursing* (2nd ed.). New York, NY: Springer Publishing Company.

Patterson, B. J., & Klein, J. M. (2012). Evidence for teaching: What are faculty using? *Nursing Education Perspectives, 33*, 240–245.

Scott, K., & McSherry, R. (2009). Evidence-based nursing: Clarifying the concepts for nurses in practice. *Journal of Clinical Nursing, 18*, 1085–1095. doi:10.1111/j.1365-2702.2008.02588.x

United States National Library of Medicine. (2013). Fact sheet. MEDLINE, PubMed, and PMC (PubMed Central): How are they different? Retrieved from http://www.nlm.nih.gov/pubs/factsheets/dif_med_pub.html

Vana, K. D., Silva, G. E., Muzyka, D., & Hirani, L. M. (2011). Effectiveness of an audience response system in teaching pharmacology to baccalaureate nursing students. *Computers Informatics Nursing, 29* (6 Suppl), TC105-13. doi:10.1097/NCN.0b013e3182285d71

Yardley, S., & Dornan, T. (2012). Kirkpatrick's levels and education "evidence". *Medical Education, 46*(1), 97–106. doi:10.1111/j.1365-2923.2011.04076.x

Yucha, C. B., Schneider, B. S. P, Smyer, T., Kowalski, S., & Stowers, E. (2011). Methodological quality and scientific impact of quantitative nursing education research over 18 months. *Nursing Education Perspectives, 32*, 362–368. doi:10.5480/1536-5026-32.6.362

16

Becoming a Scholar in Nursing Education

MARILYN H. OERMANN

The role of the nurse educator includes more than teaching, assessing learning, and developing courses: it also includes scholarship and contributing to the development of nursing education as a science. Research in nursing education is essential, but scholarship is more than studies about students, teachers, and programs: scholarship can be conceptualized broadly as inquiry about learning and teaching. Scholars in nursing education question and search for new ideas; they debate and think beyond how it has "always been done." For the teacher's work to be considered as scholarship, it needs to be public, peer-reviewed and critiqued, and shared with others so they can build on that work. This chapter examines scholarship in nursing education and developing one's role as a scholar. Because of the importance of dissemination to scholarship, the chapter includes a description of the process of writing for publication and other strategies for dissemination. Assessment of teaching, by students and peers, and the scholarship of teaching are also discussed, including development of a teaching portfolio to document teaching excellence and scholarship. This chapter builds on Chapter 1, which examined career development as a nurse educator.

SCHOLARSHIP OF TEACHING IN NURSING

Scholarship is essential to nursing education because without it our educational practices cannot develop further. It is through research and other forms of scholarship that teachers make contributions to the science, the body of knowledge, of nursing education. There are many different views about the scholarship of teaching. Scholarship in nursing education can be conceptualized broadly as inquiry about learning and teaching. That inquiry can involve developing new concepts about learning, systematic reflection on learning and teaching that becomes public, the discovery of new knowledge and evidence on educational practices, and translating and using research findings to guide teaching. Kanuka (2011) defined the scholarship of teaching and learning as teachers seeking evidence for what works and making those findings widely available through various dissemination methods. The scholarship of teaching is a way of approaching knowledge generation, testing, and dissemination about teaching, which is relevant to any field of study (Emerson & Records, 2008, p. 360).

BOYER'S FORMS OF SCHOLARSHIP

Views about the scholarship of teaching in nursing education have been influenced significantly by Boyer (1990) and Glassick, Huber, and Maeroff (1997), who provided a broader view of scholarship than only formal research. Boyer believed that scholarship also involved searching for connections, building bridges between theory and practice, and communicating one's knowledge to learners. He identified four separate but overlapping forms of scholarship:

1. Scholarship of discovery: conducting original research that expands current knowledge and understanding in a field
2. Scholarship of integration: developing connections across disciplines and synthesizing research done by others, essential for evidence-based teaching
3. Scholarship of application: applying knowledge to practice and translating research findings into practical interventions that solve problems
4. Scholarship of teaching: inquiry that focuses on student learning that results from our educational practices (Boyer, 1990)

CONCEPTUALIZATIONS OF SCHOLARSHIP OF TEACHING IN NURSING

Conceptualizations of the scholarship of teaching in nursing are not well developed. Some nurse educators view the scholarship of teaching as parallel to the scholarship of discovery, that is, research (Glanville & Houde, 2004). However, that view negates the creative work of nurse educators in developing innovations and new approaches to teaching. For example, the development of an interactive, virtual environment for learning community health nursing concepts is scholarship, but it is not traditional research with the aim of discovering new knowledge.

A second perspective is that the scholarship of teaching in nursing is excellence in teaching, but being an outstanding teacher does not mean the nurse educator is a scholar. Glanville and Houde (2004) suggested that expert teachers may not reflect on their teaching or view teaching and learning as "matters for inquiry and communication" (p. 9). The scholarship of teaching is more than excellence as a teacher.

Another perspective is that scholarship of teaching in nursing is applying theory and research to one's own educational practices (Glanville & Houde, 2004). Although this may lead to evidence-based teaching, there need to be products of one's scholarship, such as an article in a peer-reviewed journal, a presentation at a professional conference, or a description of an educational innovation.

Thoun (2009) expressed concerns that Boyer's framework did not reflect the richness and breadth of contributions of scholarship in nursing. She proposed three patterns of scholarship for nursing. The first is emergent scholarship that involves generating research and new knowledge. The second pattern of scholarship is educational and administrative scholarship, the inquiry of teaching, learning, and administrative processes (Thoun). That type also includes evaluation of teaching methods and educational technologies, curriculum development, and leadership in teaching and administration of nursing education programs. The third type, professional scholarship, is the inquiry of practice, resulting in new insights and understanding about clinical practice.

The scholarship of teaching in nursing needs to embrace the many forms that scholarship can take. This includes:

1. Conducting original research about teaching, with a focus on students and their learning
2. Evaluation studies of educational practices and teaching methods

3. Systematic and other types of reviews that synthesize knowledge and provide evidence for educational practices and decisions
4. Development and application of concepts and theories to guide teaching and assessment, which lead to dissemination
5. Development of educational innovations and new initiatives with outcomes evaluated
6. Development of new programs, courses, teaching methods, instructional materials, and assessment methods, among others, that are systematically evaluated

The scholarship of teaching in nursing can take any of these forms, but it is not the same as excellence in teaching, evidenced by outstanding student evaluations. It also is not the same as scholarly teaching, which is teaching grounded in sound principles and reflecting well-designed strategies of course design, transmission, interaction with learners, and assessment (Shulman, 2000). Scholarship involves inquiry and reflection, the development of products as a result of the scholarly work, and their dissemination. Once these products are made public, peers can assess their quality and value (Grigsby & Thorndyke, 2011). The most common product of the teacher's scholarship is a journal article about education, but examples of other products are book chapters; books; essays on teaching; editorials; descriptions of teaching methods and materials, learning activities of students, educational innovations, a program or course, assessment strategies, and tools; a simulation scenario; and media and technology for teaching (McGaghie & Webster, 2009).

SCHOLARSHIP OF TEACHING: CRITERIA TO BE MET

Shulman (2000) proposed that all forms of scholarship have to meet three criteria. First, the work needs to be public for others to consider and review it. Second, all forms of scholarship must be subject to peer review and critique. Third, the scholarly work must be shared with other nurse educators, so they, in turn, can build on that work. Educational studies disseminated beyond a school of nursing can be replicated, and findings can be accumulated. Innovations and new initiatives shared with others can be used to spread ideas throughout the nursing education community. Dissemination is critical to build evidence for teaching in nursing.

BECOMING A SCHOLAR IN NURSING EDUCATION

Meeting these three criteria transforms the teacher's work as an educator into scholarship. Teachers can begin this process by reflecting on their educational practices and experiences, discussing their ideas and reflections on teaching with other educators in their schools of nursing or other settings, and sharing their work with colleagues for critique. This process of reflection and critique can lead to new practices, which are then evaluated and disseminated.

Weston and McAlpine (2001) described a continuum of growth of teachers toward the scholarship of teaching. In Phase 1, teachers develop personal knowledge about their own educational practices and their impact on students' learning. In Phase 2, teachers dialogue with colleagues about learning and teaching and engage in conversations that demonstrate their knowledge. Phase 3 is growth in the scholarship of teaching, in which teachers develop knowledge about education that has significance and impact on the field (Weston & McAlpine). Table 16.1 applies these phases to nurse educators.

TABLE 16.1 Progression Toward Scholarship of Teaching

Phase 1: Develop Personal Knowledge About Own Teaching	Phase 2: Share Ideas and Practices About Teaching and Learning With Colleagues	Phase 3: Develop Scholarship of Teaching
Reflect on own teaching	Engage in conversations about teaching and learning with others	Integrate nursing education research and evidence in teaching
Learn about own educational practices and impact on student learning	Develop expertise in an area of nursing education and be recognized for that in your school or other setting	Conduct studies, evaluate teaching innovations and practices, and develop products of own scholarship of teaching
Read nursing education literature	Attend nursing education conferences and discuss ideas about learning and teaching with colleagues	Publish papers in peer-reviewed journals, present scholarly work at conferences, and disseminate work through other venues
Learn about theories to guide teaching	Expand understanding of concepts and theories to guide teaching	Become an expert in an area of nursing education and know the research done on that topic
Conduct self-assessments of the quality of teaching and seek peer evaluations	Provide leadership in teaching at the course or program level, serve on educational committees	Provide leadership at the national level in advancing knowledge in an area of nursing education
	Mentor novice teachers	Mentor others on research and developing their scholarship of teaching

From Weston and McAlpine (2001).

Nurse educators as scholars are creative and open to new ideas. They reflect on their educational practices, develop new approaches, and study their outcomes. They engage in conversations and debates with colleagues about learning and teaching. Scholars critically question ideas that are taken for granted, are brave enough to suggest unpopular ideas, and are resilient (Stockhausen & Turale, 2011). Strategies nurse educators can use to develop as scholars are presented in Exhibit 16.1.

DISSEMINATING YOUR SCHOLARSHIP

One of the issues related to the scholarship of teaching in nursing is that too few nurse educators share their work. There are many lost opportunities to spread new ideas and innovations: nurse educators in one setting develop an educational innovation and evaluate its effectiveness, but they never share that work with others. The reality is that the contributions of nurse educators are limited if they do not share their innovations with others (Clark & Webster, 2012). There are many venues for teachers

EXHIBIT 16.1 Strategies to Become a Scholar in Nursing Education

1. Complete a self-assessment. Do you have attributes of a scholar: creativity, an inquiring mind, openness to new ideas, integrity, willingness to critically question and reflect on own educational practices, confidence in being questioned about own ideas and products of scholarly work, collegial, resilient, respectful of the scholarly process, and prepared to develop scholarship and grow as a scholar?[a] Set a goal to develop attributes you do not currently possess.

2. Identify an area of nursing education to learn more about and on which to focus your scholarship. Ask yourself what are you curious about in terms of teaching and learning. What problems and issues have you encountered with student learning? What do you want to know more about in terms of learning and teaching?

3. Discuss your questions and ideas for an area of scholarship with colleagues, and use their critique and feedback to refine them.

4. Do a quick search of the literature to answer your questions and learn more about your potential area of scholarship. What do we know about the topic, and what questions remain unanswered? Discuss your findings and continued thinking with colleagues. Consult with experts in the area of scholarship you are considering and confirm the gaps in knowledge that you identified from your literature review.

5. Select your area of scholarship and be open to modifying it as you engage in your scholarly work.

6. Become known as an expert in that area of nursing education and share your expertise with colleagues.

7. Identify your products of scholarship and strategies for disseminating them, for example, writing an abstract for submission to a nursing education conference about a clinical evaluation tool you developed, preparing a manuscript on the use of multiple patient simulations in your leadership course, etc. In planning dissemination strategies, consider your time and resources.

8. Search for funding if planning a pilot study or evaluation.

9. Disseminate widely, including presentations and publications.

10. Attend nursing education conferences and interact with other nursing education scholars there. Share your work and ideas with them.

11. Be realistic in terms of the time you have available for your scholarly work. Set goals with dates for completion that are attainable.

[a] Stockhausen and Turale (2011).

to disseminate the products of their scholarship to make them public and accessible for critique and use by others. They can present their scholarship at conferences, both nursing education and others; describe their work in newsletters; post summaries of their studies, projects, and innovations on relevant websites and the school of nursing intranet; report at faculty meetings, which provide an opportunity for critique; and disseminate their scholarly work through publications. Articles published in peer-reviewed journals provide the widest dissemination, spreading the ideas to other educators for consideration and use in their own teaching. When research findings are published, these results can be synthesized to generate evidence for teaching, as discussed in Chapter 15.

Publications in peer-reviewed journals are a requirement for promotion and tenure in many schools of nursing—this is another reason for teachers to disseminate their scholarship through publications. Nurse educators need to be aware of the criteria for contract renewal, promotion, and tenure in their school of nursing and the importance given to journal publications. In some settings, databased articles (papers that report the findings of research studies) published in peer-reviewed journals, also called refereed, are considered more important in these decisions than descriptive articles, chapters, and books about teaching and other educational topics. Peer-reviewed journals, for example, *Journal of Nursing Education*, *Journal of Continuing Education in Nursing*, *Nursing Education Perspectives*, *Nurse Education Today*, and *International Journal of Nursing Education Scholarship*, among others, have experts (peers) who critically evaluate manuscripts submitted to the journal, ensuring their quality.

PLANNING PHASE OF WRITING FOR PUBLICATION

In planning the dissemination of the teacher's scholarship, the first step is to identify the purpose of the manuscript (Oermann & Hays, 2010). The term *manuscript* is the unpublished paper; once published it is referred to as an article. The purpose of the manuscript might be to share new ideas and concepts about learning and teaching in nursing; describe a nursing program or course; present a research study and findings, or the results of an evaluation of an educational innovation; and report other educational topics. The purpose guides the development of the manuscript, and it should be stated early in the paper.

As part of the planning phase, the teacher reviews the literature to build on what has already been published. The two databases most valuable for this purpose are MEDLINE®, searched through PubMed, and the Cumulative Index to Nursing and Allied Health Literature (CINAHL®). Similar to searching for evidence for teaching, if those databases provide limited citations, then the teacher should also search the Education Resources Information Center (ERIC) database. A review of the literature might reveal that the teacher's ideas and topic for dissemination have been reported by others. Then the key is identifying how the scholarly work builds on those ideas and provides new knowledge for readers.

Typically, reviewing the literature for the prior 5-year period is sufficient, unless few citations are located; in that case the teacher should extend the time period for the search. Citations can be saved by using bibliographic management software, which allows the teacher to create citations and reference lists formatted in the appropriate style. Many nurse educators are familiar with the reference style of the American Psychological Association (APA, 2010), but not all journals use APA style. Some journals use a numbered citation format, such as the *AMA Manual of Style* (American Medical Association [AMA], 2007) or the *Uniform Requirements for Manuscripts Submitted to Biomedical Journals* (International Committee of Medical Journal Editors, 2013). The journal's author guidelines specify the style to use when preparing references.

Prior to beginning to write the paper, the teacher selects possible journals for submission of the manuscript. One consideration is whether readers of the journal would be interested in the topic. For example, if the manuscript reports the findings of a study on concept maps, potential readers would be nursing faculty members, and a journal intended for academic nurse educators would be more appropriate than one for staff educators. In contrast, a paper on multiple simulations would be of interest to nurse educators in schools of nursing and clinical settings, expanding the number of possible journals. It is also important to determine whether the journal publishes the type of manuscript being planned. Some journals publish mainly research in nursing education, whereas others do not.

There are hundreds of possible journals in which nurse educators can publish their scholarship. To search for appropriate journals, teachers can use directories of nursing and other journals available on the web such as the *Nurse Author & Editor* Journals Directory (nurseauthoreditor.com/library.asp), or search PubMed and CINAHL for journals that publish similar types of papers. Teachers should select about five possible journals for submission, rank-order them, and prepare their papers to be consistent with the journal format and author guidelines, available at the journal's website, which provide details about how to prepare the paper. The teacher can send a short query e-mail to the editors of the potential journals to determine their interest, although doing so is not essential. Though a manuscript can be sent to only one journal at a time, query e-mails can be sent to multiple editors. If the manuscript is rejected by a journal, the teacher at that point can revise the paper and submit it to the next journal on the rank-order list.

WRITING PHASE OF WRITING FOR PUBLICATION

The second phase is focused on writing the manuscript. This begins with an outline to guide writing the first draft and to ensure including the essential content to reflect the purpose of the paper. The outline also allows the teacher to plan the approximate number of pages to write for each content area and to avoid preparing a manuscript that is too short or too long. Although journals have different limits on the number of pages for a manuscript, the desired length is often between 15 and 18 double-spaced pages.

Using the outline, the teacher then writes the first draft. The goal of the first draft is to write quickly and without concern about grammar and writing style (Oermann & Hays, 2010). It is critical in this phase to include the citations as the content is developed. When the content is drafted sufficiently, the teacher revises the grammar, punctuation, writing style, and format. In preparing the final version of the paper, the teacher should explicitly follow the author guidelines in terms of format.

PEER REVIEW PHASE OF WRITING FOR PUBLICATION

Peer review of the manuscript is conducted by content area experts who serve as reviewers for the journal. The peer-review process ensures that papers published in the journal are of high quality and have accurate and up-to-date content; peers also critique the research methods if the paper reports a nursing education study (Oermann, 2010; Oermann & Hays, 2010). In most nursing journals, peer review is considered a blind review: the author does not know who reviewed the paper, and the reviewers are unaware of the author's identity, removing potential bias. Typically, reviewers rate the quality of the manuscript on a form and provide a narrative summary of their critique of the paper. An example of a review form is in Table 16.2. The narrative summary is usually returned to the author with the editor's comments and decision about acceptance.

The editor may accept the manuscript without or with revision, ask the teacher to revise and resubmit the paper for another review, or reject it. In revising the manuscript, the teacher should make the suggested revisions or provide a rationale for not

TABLE 16.2 Example of Form for Peer Review of Manuscript

Yes	No	Comments
——	——	Does the paper present new findings or ideas about nursing education?
		Is the content:
——	——	timely/relevant?
——	——	logically and clearly developed?
——	——	sophisticated enough for our readers?
——	——	innovative?
——	——	Introduction: Is the purpose of the paper clear?
——	——	Methods (*research paper*)
——	——	Are the sample and sampling method adequate?
——	——	Are the instruments reliable and valid?
——	——	Are statistical tests appropriate?
——	——	Methods (*other types of papers*)
——	——	Were the objectives clearly identified?
——	——	Were the outcomes evaluated adequately?
——	——	Do conclusions and implications go beyond what findings support?
——	——	Are the references current?
——	——	Does the content include implications for teaching in nursing? other implications for nursing education?
——	——	Was the paper interesting to read?

Recommendation:

( ) **Accept for publication without revision**

( ) **Accept for publication after satisfactory revision**

( ) **Review again after major revision**

( ) **Reject**

Please circle the number that best indicates the overall quality of this manuscript:

1	2	3	4	5	6
Outstanding	Excellent	Good	Acceptable	Uncertain of acceptability	Unacceptable

Comments/Suggestions: _____

making them (Oermann, 2010). A summary sheet of the revisions proposed and made should accompany the manuscript (Exhibit 16.2). For rejected manuscripts, the teacher should consider the feedback from the reviewers, modify the paper as appropriate, and submit it to the next journal on the list established earlier.

PRESENTATIONS AT CONFERENCES AND OTHER DISSEMINATION METHODS

For scholarship not ready for dissemination in peer-reviewed journals, the teacher should plan to disseminate her or his scholarly work via other venues, such as presenting it at nursing education and other conferences. The teacher can begin by presenting

EXHIBIT 16.2 Sample Summary of Manuscript Revisions

Ms. Ref. No.: 1034

Original Title: Differences in Performance of Nursing Students Trained With Computer-Based CPR Course With Voice Advisory Manikin and Instructor-Led Course With Traditional Manikin

Revisions Proposed and Made

REVIEWER 1:

Was there a conceptual framework for this study?

 Ericsson's deliberate practice model. See lines 42–43 and 219 and citation 26

Please make sure you have more than two sentences in a paragraph.

 Revised throughout paper

Shorten the title. Need to be concise.

 We have shortened the title to: Comparison of Two Instructional Modalities for Nursing Student CPR Skill Acquisition.

Literature Review: describe outcomes in your Aims...what are you measuring?

 We added the outcomes in the aims statement: see abstract lines 3–4; text lines 37–41.

 The outcomes also are identified in lines 111–117.

Line 34: define beginning nursing students.

 Revised line 6 in the abstract to omit "beginning" because these details about the students are not essential in the abstract. In the Methods we added information about the schools: "Twelve schools of nursing from across the United States, including six associate degree programs and six bachelor of science programs ..." (see lines 48–50).

Line 57: what is meant by the "quality of CPR"?

 We added an explanation. See lines 4–6

Line 62: need reference for psychomotor and technical skills lost.

 We removed the sentence in original line 62 because we have this finding with a citation earlier in the paper (see line 19).

Line 64: what is the feedback received?

 We added examples of the feedback: "Use of a voice advisory manikin (VAM) can improve CPR skills by providing continuous verbal feedback, for example, 'do not compress so fast' and 'ventilate more slowly,' during training." See lines 11–13.

Line 71: delete the word "Some"

 Done

Line 75: what are their evaluations? define, otherwise appears like bias statement.

 Deleted this statement: it was not essential to our paper.

Line 86–88: Provide reference for statements in this paragraph.

 Added (lines 33–34): "The researchers speculated that their findings indicated a lack of initial skill acquisition rather than retention."[23]

Line 90: What are the measurable outcomes? Include in the aim.

 We added the outcomes in the aims statement. See Abstract lines 3–4.

 See also text lines 37–41.

(continued)

Exhibit 16.2 Sample Summary of Manuscript Revisions (*continued*)

REVIEWER 2:

Title—too long.

Title revised to Comparison of Two Instructional Modalities for Nursing Student CPR Skill Acquisition

34 Define "beginning" nurse

Revised line 6 in the abstract to omit "beginning" because these details about the students are not essential in the abstract. In the Methods we added information about the schools. See lines 48–50.

41 Results: were they significant? Include in abstract

The results were significant, and we added this to the abstract.

92 Year group of nurses?

We removed the term "prelicensure nursing students" for clarity among readers who are non-nurses. See lines 48–50.

116 How was sport defined?

Removed sport reference from manuscript and tables.

150 How did you adjust for this in the data analysis?

See revised data analysis section to explain this (see lines 127–137).

255 Needs some evidence to support these points, e.g., reference to self-directed learning, etc.

Sentences (lines 219–220) were revised; two references were added.

266 Or was it their preferred learning style?

Paragraph removed for clarity.

---

a paper at local, state, and regional conferences and then progress to national and international ones. Organizations such as the National League for Nursing (NLN), Sigma Theta Tau International, and the regional nursing research societies, for example, Midwest Nursing Research Society, sponsor education summits and conferences at which teachers can present their work. These venues also provide an opportunity to engage in discussions about teaching and scholarship, critical to developing as a scholar in nursing education. Many of the organizations listed in Appendix D.4 sponsor conferences where teachers can present their educational research and other types of scholarly work.

Other dissemination strategies include writing about scholarly work in newsletters, in other non–peer-reviewed publications such as nursing magazines, and as letters to the editor, among others. Reports at faculty and committee meetings and sharing ideas through informal discussions provide other strategies for making scholarship public for review and critique by peers.

ASSESSMENT OF TEACHING AND SCHOLARSHIP OF TEACHING

The NLN's Core Competencies of Nurse Educators (2012), which were discussed in Chapter 1, describe the essential knowledge, skills, and attitudes of a teacher in nursing. Appendix D.3 presents sample activities of the teacher for each of the core competencies. These competencies are consistent with research findings on qualities of effective teaching in nursing and higher education. For effective teaching, the nurse educator needs to

1. Be an expert in the content area
2. Be clinically competent if teaching in the laboratory, simulation, and the practice setting

3. Have expert teaching skills
4. Develop positive interpersonal relationships with learners as a group and individually
5. Possess attributes such as enthusiasm, patience, friendliness, integrity, perseverance, and willingness to admit mistakes, among others (Oermann & Gaberson, 2014)

In most settings in which nurse educators work, the quality of their teaching; scholarship; service to the nursing program, college or university, community, and profession; and clinical practice, if relevant, are assessed to provide feedback to the teacher (formative evaluation) and for annual performance reviews and personnel decisions such as contract renewal, promotion, and tenure (summative evaluation). This assessment is done by students during and at the end of a course; by peers; by formal committees such as the appointment, promotion, and review committee; and by administrators to whom the teacher reports. In health care settings, though there are differences in the formal committees responsible for evaluation, the quality of the teaching is evaluated by learners, peers, and administrators. Most important is that teachers periodically reflect on and assess the quality of their own teaching and scholarship.

STUDENT RATINGS

Student evaluations of teaching are one source of information about the teacher's effectiveness, but not the only one. Evidence suggests that students can make valid and reliable interpretations about the quality of teaching from their perspectives. Their evaluations focus on the teacher's effectiveness, rather than on the course itself (Benton & Cashin, 2012). Students can assess teaching methods used in the course, whether the evaluation by the teacher was fair, the degree of interest the teacher exhibited in students and their learning, and the teacher's enthusiasm. It is unlikely, however, that students can assess the quality of the content of a course, for example, accuracy and depth of the teacher's knowledge, because they are not expert enough in the subject matter to assess this. Student ratings and comments provide feedback to the teacher on improving teaching. Research suggests that discussing ratings with a peer or consultant, combined with students' feedback, is more useful for improving teaching than feedback alone (Benton & Cashin, 2012; Hampton & Reiser, 2004).

Most nursing programs have standard forms for the evaluation of teaching by students. There may be one form for assessing the quality of teaching in courses, a separate form for student rating of clinical teaching effectiveness, or a general tool that is used for all courses in the nursing program. Exhibit 16.3 lists typical areas assessed by students when evaluating teaching effectiveness.

EXHIBIT 16.3 Typical Areas Assessed on Student Evaluation of Teaching Forms

> **Teaching Skills**
> - Organized course well
> - Gave clear explanations
> - Used examples, illustrations, and other methods to promote understanding of content
> - Was well prepared for class
> - Was enthusiastic about content and teaching
> - Stimulated students' interest in subject
> - Motivated students to do best work
> - Used learning activities, readings, and assignments that facilitated understanding of course content

(continued)

Exhibit 16.3 Typical Areas Assessed on Student Evaluation of Teaching Forms (*continued*)

Interactions With Students Individually and in Groups

- Encouraged student participation and discussion
- Showed respect for students' views and opinions
- Was readily available to students

Breadth of Coverage of Subject Matter

- Demonstrated knowledge of course content
- Presented different views and perspectives as appropriate

Assessment and Grading Practices

- Communicated student responsibilities clearly
- Explained course assignments, assessment methods, and grading procedures
- Was fair in assessment and grading
- Provided prompt and valuable feedback

Overall Course Evaluation

- Course difficulty (e.g., rated on scale of *too difficult* to *too elementary*)
- Workload in course (e.g., rated on scale of *too heavy* to *too light*)
- Course pace (e.g., rated on scale of *too fast* to *too slow*)
- Extent of learning in course (e.g., rated on scale of *a great deal* to *nothing new*)
- Overall course rating (e.g., rated on scale of *excellent* to *poor*)

Overall Teacher Evaluation

- Overall quality of the teaching (e.g., rated on scale of *excellent* to *poor*)

Clinical Teaching Items

Did the teacher:

1. Encourage students to ask questions and express diverse views in the clinical setting?
2. Encourage application of theoretical knowledge to clinical practice?
3. Provide feedback on student strengths and weaknesses related to clinical performance?
4. Develop positive relationships with students in the clinical setting?
5. Inform students of their professional responsibilities?
6. Facilitate student collaboration with members of health care teams?
7. Facilitate learning in the clinical setting?
8. Strive to be available in the clinical setting to assist students?

Was the instructor an effective clinical teacher?

Adapted from Oermann and Gaberson (2014). Copyright 2014. Reproduced with the permission of Springer Publishing Company, LLC.

PEER REVIEW

Peer review is another source of information for the assessment of teaching, but peers can also evaluate the teacher's scholarship. Peers can observe teaching performance and provide feedback to the nurse educator about areas to be improved;

these observations are intended for formative evaluation, because there are many variables that can influence the reliability of observing teaching in the classroom or clinical setting (Oermann & Gaberson, 2014). Peers can review course and instructional materials, teaching methods and strategies developed for learners, online learning activities, tests, and other documents developed for teaching. That type of review can be done for formative evaluation, to provide feedback to the teacher, or for summative evaluation, as part of an annual performance review and reviews for reappointment, promotion, and tenure.

In terms of the scholarship of teaching, peers can discuss the teacher's scholarly works, review products of scholarship, critique educational grants, review manuscripts, and assess the teacher's overall scholarly performance. This assessment can be used for formative purposes, to give feedback for continued development of the teacher's scholarship, or for summative purposes, such as in annual reviews and for making decisions about promotion (Oermann & Gaberson, 2014).

TEACHING PORTFOLIO

A teaching portfolio or dossier is a collection of materials selected by nurse educators to document the quality of their teaching, illustrate their creativity in teaching, present innovative teaching and assessment methods they have developed for their courses, and provide documentation of their overall teaching effectiveness. Teaching portfolios can be used to improve teaching (formative evaluation), providing an organized collection of documents for review and critique by others. Or, they may be submitted to the administrator to whom the faculty member reports and to committees such as the appointment, promotion, and review committee for formal peer review (summative evaluation). Types of documents typically included in the portfolio are listed in Exhibit 16.4. These provide a source of data for assessment by others of the nurse educator's expertise in teaching.

EXHIBIT 16.4 Types of Documents Included in Teaching Portfolio

- Philosophy of teaching and goals for teaching
- Syllabi
- Sample teaching methods and materials, student learning activities and assignments, assessment methods, evaluation tools, others
- Innovations in teaching and descriptions of their success
- Descriptions of technologies developed for teaching and their successful application
- Descriptions of and documents related to new courses and programs developed in school of nursing (with individual contributions described if work was done by a team)
- Accreditation and comprehensive program reports
- Publications of educational studies, teaching and assessment methods, innovations, new initiatives, and others on teaching and learning
- Presentations related to teaching and learning
- Educational grants
- Teaching awards and other recognition of teaching effectiveness
- Peer evaluations of teaching

Glanville and Houde (2004) suggested that teaching portfolios can also be used to document the scholarship of teaching. Faculty members can include in their portfolios descriptions of their innovations in teaching and how they improved student learning; can explain creative strategies they developed for teaching and assessment; can describe their contributions on committees, on teams, and in organizations related to nursing education; and can summarize their dissemination of their scholarship beyond what is listed on the curriculum vitae. Portfolios allow educators to make their scholarship public and share it with others for peer review.

CAREER DEVELOPMENT

Chapter 1 explored the nurse educator role and career development in that role. As teachers gain experience and develop their expertise, they can be recognized through the NLN's Academic Nurse Educator Certification Program. To be certified, nurse educators need to successfully pass an examination that assesses their knowledge about learning, methods for facilitating learning and development of the learner, assessment and evaluation, curriculum development and evaluation, quality improvement in the nurse educator role, and the scholarship of teaching, service, and leadership (NLN, 2012). Further information about the NLN Certification program and examination is provided in Appendices D.1 and D.2.

The importance of faculty development in nursing education was discussed in Chapter 1. In developing as a scholar, however, the teacher might need additional preparation and mentoring. Teachers need to set short- and long-term career goals for their scholarship and identify areas in which they need further learning and skills development. For some nurse educators, additional course work might be required; for others continuing education programs and workshops such as those offered by the NLN, the American Association of Colleges of Nursing, other organizations, and schools of nursing will be adequate to meet their learning needs. Some of the organizations listed in Appendix D.4 provide educational programs that would enable teachers to gain skills essential to advance their scholarship. It is also valuable to bookmark websites that could serve as resources for teaching and scholarship. As an example, the IDEA (Individual Development and Educational Assessment) Center provides papers and resources for faculty evaluation, reflection, and improvement, which can be downloaded at no charge.

SUMMARY

Scholarship in nursing education can be conceptualized broadly as inquiry about learning and teaching. That inquiry can involve the discovery of new knowledge and evidence on educational practices, translating and using research findings to guide teaching, and developing new concepts about teaching and learning in nursing. Boyer (1990) believed that scholarship was more than formal research and also involved searching for connections, building bridges between theory and practice, and communicating one's knowledge to learners.

The scholarship of teaching in nursing needs to embrace the many forms that scholarship can take. These include conducting original research about teaching and learning; evaluation studies; reviews that synthesize knowledge and provide evidence for teaching; development and application of concepts and theories to guide teaching; development of educational innovations and new initiatives; and development of new programs, courses, teaching methods, instructional materials, and others, that are systematically evaluated and disseminated.

To transform the teacher's work as an educator into scholarship, all forms of scholarship need to be public, peer-reviewed and critiqued, and shared with other educators so they, in turn, can build on that work. There are many venues for teachers to disseminate the products of their scholarship to make them public and accessible for critique and use by others. They can present their scholarship at conferences, at faculty meetings, and through other venues. Articles published in peer-reviewed journals, however, provide the widest dissemination. A section in the chapter presented the phases of writing for publication and important principles for disseminating scholarship through publications.

In most settings in which nurse educators work, the quality of their teaching, scholarship, service, and clinical practice, if relevant, are assessed by students, peers, administrators, and formal committees. This evaluation, including the use of teaching portfolios, was discussed in the chapter. However, the most important evaluation is that done by teachers themselves: nurse educators need to periodically reflect on and assess the quality of their own teaching and scholarship. With this self-assessment, combined with feedback from others, teachers can identify areas in which they need further development and mentoring, set short- and long-term career goals, find resources to help them with their career development, expand their teaching competencies, and advance their scholarship of teaching.

REFERENCES

American Medical Association. (2007). *AMA manual of style: A guide for authors and editors* (10th ed.). New York, NY: Oxford Press.

American Psychological Association. (2010). *Publication manual of the American Psychological Association* (6th ed.). Washington, DC: Author.

Benton, S. L., & Cashin, W. E. (2012). *Student ratings of teaching: A summary of research and literature. Idea paper #50*. Manhattan, KS: The IDEA Center. Retrieved from http://www.theideacenter.org/sites/default/files/idea-paper_50.pdf

Boyer, E. (1990). *Scholarship reconsidered: Priorities of the professoriate*. San Francisco, CA: Jossey-Bass.

Clark, E., & Webster, B. (2012). Innovation and its contribution to the scholarship of learning and teaching. *Nurse Education Today, 32*, 729–731. doi:10.1016/j.nedt.2012.06.001

Emerson, R. J., & Records, K. (2008). Today's challenge, tomorrow's excellence: The practice of evidence-based education. *Journal of Nursing Education, 47*, 359–370.

Glanville, I., & Houde, S. (2004). The scholarship of teaching: Implications for nursing faculty. *Journal of Professional Nursing, 20*, 7–14.

Glassick, C. E., Huber, M. T., & Maeroff, G. I. (1997). *Scholarship assessed: Evaluation of the professoriate*. San Francisco, CA: Jossey-Bass.

Grigsby, R. K., & Thorndyke, L. (2011). Perspective: Recognizing and rewarding clinical scholarship. *Academic Medicine, 86*, 127–131. doi:10.1097/ACM.0b013e3181ffae5e

Hampton, S. E., & Reiser, R. A. (2004). Effects of a theory-based feedback and consultation process on instruction and learning in college classrooms. *Research in Higher Education, 45*, 497–527.

International Committee of Medical Journal Editors. (2013). *Uniform requirements for manuscripts submitted to biomedical journals*. Retrieved from http://www.icmje.org/urm_main.html

Kanuka, H. (2011). Keeping the scholarship in the scholarship of teaching and learning. *International Journal for the Scholarship of Teaching and Learning, 5*(1). Retrieved from http://academics.georgiasouthern.edu/ijsotl/v5n1/invited_essays/PDFs/_Kanuka.pdf

McGaghie, W. C., & Webster, A. (2009). Scholarship, publication, and career advancement in health professions education: AMEE Guide No. 43. *Medical Teacher, 31*, 574–590.

National League for Nursing Certification Commission Certification Test Development Committee. (2012). *The scope of practice for academic nurse educators: 2012 revision*. New York, NY: National League for Nursing.

Oermann, M. H. (2010). Writing for publication in nursing: What every nurse educator needs to know. In L. Caputi (Ed.), *Teaching nursing: The art and science* (2nd ed., pp. 146–166). Glen Ellyn, IL: College of DuPage.

Oermann, M. H., & Gaberson, K. B. (2014). *Evaluation and testing in nursing education* (4th ed.). New York, NY: Springer Publishing Company.

Oermann, M. H., & Hays, J. (2011). *Writing for publication in nursing* (2nd ed.). New York, NY: Springer Publishing Company.

Shulman, L. S. (2000). From Minsk to Pinsk: Why a scholarship of teaching and learning? *Journal of Scholarship in Teaching and Learning, 1*(1), 48–53.

Stockhausen, L., & Turale, S. (2011). An explorative study of Australian nursing scholars and contemporary scholarship. *Journal of Nursing Scholarship, 43,* 89–96. doi:10.1111/j.1547-5069.2010.01378.x

Thoun, D. S. (2009). Toward an appreciation of nursing scholarship: Recognizing our traditions, contributions, and presence. *Journal of Nursing Education, 48,* 552–556. doi:10.3928/01484834-20090716-01

Weston, C. B., & McAlpine, L. (2001). Making explicit the development toward the scholarship of teaching. *New Directions for Teaching and Learning, 86,* 89–97.

Appendix A: Examples of Teaching Materials and Other Documents for a Laboratory Module

APPENDIX A.1: HOW TO SET UP A LABORATORY: EXAMPLE
CENTRAL VENOUS ACCESS DEVICES (CVAD) LABORATORY

Supplies (location)

- Triple lumen central line 7.0 Fr/20 cm (room 5 shelf 5)
- Empty 250 mL, 500 mL, or 1,000 mL NS bag for each manikin with spike port intact (room 5 drying rack)
- Spike and drip chamber cut from old primary or secondary tubing (room 5 drying rack)
- Needleless access devices (room 5 shelf 5)
- Blue slide clamps for catheter lines (room 5 shelf 5)
- Catheter clamp and clamp fastener for each manikin—soft white rubber piece and hard blue plastic piece that fits over it to keep central line from pulling out when students use the line (room 5 shelf 5)
- 10 mL or 20 mL luer lock syringe (room 5 shelf 26)
- Bag of saline (room 5 shelf 12)
- Labels for "clotted" line (room 5 shelf 5)
- 10 cm × 12 cm transparent bio-occlusive dressing and simulated protective disk (room 5 shelf 5)
- Manikin lubricant (room 5 cleaning cabinet)
- Hemostats (room 5 shelf 2)
- Cyanoacrylate adhesive or hot wax (room 5 cleaning cabinet)
- Snap fasteners, one per central line (room 5 shelf 5)
- Sewing supplies or suture material (room 5 shelf 3)

Procedure

1. If snap buttons haven't already been applied to manikin chest wall, secure the male side of the snap button to the manikin chest approximately 1 inch away from the access hole in the front chest wall to allow room for the simulated protective disk; use cyanoacrylate adhesive or hot wax to secure the button.

(continued)

2. Secure the female side of the snap button to the back of the central line port using strong sewing thread or suture material.

3. Put a needleless valve connector and blue slide clamp on each catheter line and label one line as "clotted" (can switch which line is clotted from manikin to manikin).

4. Open the manikin chest and thread the central line through the access hole (either on the left or the right side, depending on the manikin); snap the button together.

5. Attach white catheter clamp around the central line inside the chest close to the opening and cover with the blue clamp fastener (helps decrease play on the line as old dressing is removed).

6. Spike the empty Normal Saline IV bag with the cut drip chamber.

7. Thread the central line into the IV bag reservoir through the cut drip chamber; may need to use the hemostats to slightly widen the tubing and lubricate the line to feed into the bag.

8. Secure the reservoir bag inside the chest opening and put the chest plate back on.

9. Fill the 10 mL or 20 mL syringe with saline and flush each line (may pull back first to vacuum some air out of the reservoir bag and minimize air in the line).

10. No sooner than an hour before the lab, put the transparent bio-occlusive dressing and simulated protective disk on each central line (dries out if on too long, difficult to remove).

CVAD, central venous access device; cm, centimeter; Fr, French; IV, intravenous; mL, milliliter; NS, normal saline.

Copyright Education-Innovation-Simulation Learning Environment, School of Nursing, The University of North Carolina at Chapel Hill, 2013. Reprinted by permission, 2013.

APPENDIX A.2: LABORATORY SUPPLY AND EQUIPMENT SETUP AND BREAKDOWN GUIDE FOR TEACHER: EXAMPLE CVAD LABORATORY

Prior to Lab

1. At each student bedside table (plus one for the educator's table), set out:
   a. Two student packets with CVAD dressing, lipid filter, and PLUM™ tubing (all new and unopened)
   b. Two bags of fake PN with labels matching PN recipe sheet
   c. A patient mask for manikin (one mask placed on manikin to simulate placing one on patient—can be used repeatedly)
   d. Two scantrons per bed for the quiz (educator does not need one)
   e. Patient folder with two sets of CVAD orders (set = PO, MAR, and PN recipe sheet)
   f. Each med drawer (one drawer for two students) with:
      • Two vials of Heparin 100 U/mL
      • One vial of a distractor heparin, either 1,000 or 10,000 U/mL
      • Two 22 g needles
      • Two empty 10 mL syringes, individually peel-packed
      • Two peel packs of 10 mL prefilled syringes with two syringes per pack (make sure there is 10 mL of fluid, air in each, and each syringe has a cap)

2. Have the quiz version you are giving ready to pass out once you start.

3. Check the chest reservoir to be sure it is empty.

4. Put a fake patch and a transparent dressing on each manikin (can leave the last one on from the laboratory before if teaching the same day).

5. Set up Chester Chest™ with two prefilled syringes (one wasted down to 5 mL saline), a labeled syringe with 3 mL heparin, vacutainer tubes, and needleless access devices to demonstrate drawing blood and changing a device.

6. Set out hemostats and blue toothless hemostats to pass around to show the difference.

7. Have extra transparent dressings to replace in student kits, extra heparin for the medication drawers, extra Chloraprep™ and alcohol swabs for kits, in case they are needed (store in the CVAD teaching box).

8. Have the storage box used to reclaim tubing, filters, and prefilled syringes (and caps with all of them) prominently placed in room.

9. If teaching multiple laboratory sessions in one day, may need to check and empty the chest reservoirs between laboratory sessions to prevent leakage.

Between Labs and at End of Labs

1. Leave completed quiz scantrons in the quiz folder, not the scantron binder.

2. If you have wet linen, drape it over the linen hamper to dry.

3. Between labs:

    a. Unspike the PN—capping it again—and return the used tubing, lipid filters, and all syringes (and caps) to the reclaiming box—students can do this.

    b. Have students **DISPOSE** of the used needle in the sharps container.

    c. Have students put heparin vials back in the medication drawers and put PO/MAR/PN sheets back in patient folder on bedside table.

4. If you have time between laboratories, refill the prefilled syringes and re-peel pack in twos and leave in room for future use. Otherwise do at the end of the day.

5. Reset for the next laboratory as outlined above if the room won't be used for a different laboratory in between the CVAD laboratories, EXCEPT don't put a transparent dressing over the site if room is not in use again that day.

6. If the last laboratory of the day:

    a. Have students peel off the old dressing, but saving the patch (they can leave it on the site for safekeeping)—go behind them and CHECK!!

    b. Empty the chest reservoir bags.

    c. Drain the tubing—don't need to rinse—and empty out the lipid filter (use an empty 10-mL syringe)—they can be taken to room 5 (staging area) to dry and be repackaged.

    d. Refill and repack prefilled syringes and leave in room for practice laboratory and evaluation.

CVAD, central venous access device; MAR, medication administration record; mL, milliliter; PO, per os (by mouth); PN, parenteral nutrition; U, unit.

APPENDIX A.3: LABORATORY LESSON PLAN: EXAMPLE CVAD LABORATORY

Laboratory Schedule*

Time	Skill
5 minutes	Short question and answer
10 minutes	Quiz

(continued)

Laboratory Schedule

15 minutes	Demonstrate and discuss types of CVADs on Chester Chest™
	Discuss potential complications
	Demonstrate and discuss nursing care for discontinuing a central line on manikin
10 minutes	Demonstrate and discuss changing needle-less access devices
	Students practice on manikins
10 minutes	Demonstrate and discuss drawing blood from a CVAD on manikin or Chester Chest™
40 minutes	Work through combined skills from evaluation form
	Demonstrate and discuss (use round table technique with students preparing their PN and flushes at the same time):
	• Selection of PN, medication checks, recipe checks
	• Preparation of CVAD flushes (NS and heparin) with medication checks and medication lookup for heparin
	• Priming PN using IV tubing and micron filter
	Demonstrate CVAD flush for PN, CVAD flush of unused line, and CVAD dressing change at bedside with students observing
	Demonstrate troubleshooting on manikin after connecting PN
15 minutes	**BREAK**
65 minutes	Students practice skills, starting with all supplies prepared and in room

*This laboratory schedule is a guide. You can re-arrange your schedule after the quiz based on your needs. Please try to adhere to the scheduled time allotted for each skill.

Throw away any used or previously recycled tubing after the laboratory. Drain the new tubing and the micron filters used by the students for reuse later.

CVAD, central venous access device; IV, intravenous; NS, normal saline; PN, parenteral nutrition.

APPENDIX A.4: LABORATORY TEACHING BOX SUPPLY LIST (LIST PLACED IN TEACHING BOX): EXAMPLE CVAD LABORATORY

Item	Location
Textbook	In room
Chester Chest™ with fake blood to demo lab collection and device change	In room
CVAD kit per student (micron filter, primary tubing, dressing kit)	Supply cart; room 5 above shelves 1–3
Fake PN, 2 bags per bed	Supply cart; room 5 shelf 5
Alcohol wipes	Overbed table (extras in bedside table), room 5 shelf 1
Exam gloves	Supply cart; room 5 shelf 4
Provider's Order/MAR/PN order form	Patient chart; S drive
Teaching demonstration set per lab (micron filter, primary tubing, dressing kit)	Teaching box; room 5 shelf 5, shelf 14
Transparent bio-occlusive dressings	Teaching box; room 5 shelf 5
Simulated protective disk	Teaching box; room 5 shelf 5
Heparin vials, various strengths	Teaching box; room 5 shelf 12
10 mL prefilled normal saline luer lock syringes	Teaching box; room 5 shelf 11
10 mL luer lock syringes	Teaching box; room 5 shelf 26
18–22 gauge needles, 1–1.5"	Teaching box; room 5 shelf 11
Needleless access devices	Teaching box; room 5 shelf 5
Various lab tubes	Teaching box; room 5 shelf 27
Hemostats and toothless clamps demo	Teaching box; room 5 shelf 2
Huber needle demo	Teaching box; room 5 shelf 5
Replacement alcohol swabs and cleaning swabs	Teaching box; room 5 shelf 5

Manikins in bed with triple lumen catheters in place, transparent bio-occlusive dressings with protective disks on, and reservoir bags attached

CVAD, central venous access device; MAR, medication administration record; mL, milliliter; PN, parenteral nutrition.

APPENDIX A.5: STANDARDIZED LEARNING MODULE OVERVIEW: EXAMPLE CVAD LABORATORY

Central Venous Access Devices

Key Concepts and Procedures

Preparation

1. Wear your name tag and bring your student identification card.
2. Bring your Laboratory Module, CVAD Key Concepts and Procedures.

(continued)

3. Come prepared for a 10-item quiz at the start of laboratory on the Key Concepts listed in the module.

4. Come prepared to practice the skills in this module by having completed the outlined reading and assignments.

5. Come prepared to demonstrate the proper use of body mechanics and universal precautions throughout laboratory and evaluation.

6. Supplies should be saved for practice and may be required for use in subsequent laboratories and/or evaluations—DO NOT discard any materials until after your evaluation! Take care of the supplies, but do use them for practice. If you have questions, please ask laboratory staff.

7. Gather your supplies and clean up your work area before leaving the laboratory.

There are no supply bag items to bring to laboratory today. You will receive your supplies in lab.

Objectives

At the completion of this module, the student should be able to:

1. Differentiate between short-term and long-term access devices.

2. Identify the potential complications of a central line for the client.

3. Describe the precautions to prevent air embolus.

4. Describe the signs and symptoms of central line infections.

5. Describe the precautions to prevent infection of central lines.

6. Demonstrate the procedure for flushing a CVAD.

7. Demonstrate the procedure for changing needleless access devices.

8. Describe proper technique for drawing blood from a CVAD.

9. Describe proper nursing care after removal of a CVAD.

10. Demonstrate a CVAD dressing change and site care.

11. Demonstrate procedure for administering PN.

Required Readings/Audiovisuals

Books

Potter, P. A., Perry, A. G., Stockert, P. A., & Hall, A. M. (2013). *Fundamentals of nursing* (8th ed.). St. Louis, MO: Elsevier.

Chapter 40: Medication Administration; Chapter 41: Fluid, Electrolyte, and Acid-Base Balance; Chapter 44: Nutrition

Journals

Infusion Nurses Society. (2006). STANDARDS: Infusion therapy. *Journal of Infusion Nursing, 29* (Suppl 1), S75–S76.

Internet Sites

Infusion Nurses Society http://www.ins1.org

Topic	Assignments
Medication Administration Review	Potter, Perry, Stockert, & Hall (p. 584)
Parenteral Nutrition/Total Parenteral Nutrition (PN/TPN)	Potter, Perry, Stockert, & Hall (p. 1019) (Box 44-11 only), 1021–1024

Demonstrate proper technique for administering PN/TPN.	Infusion Nurses Society. (2006). STANDARDS: Infusion therapy. *Journal of Infusion Nursing, 29* (Suppl 1), S75–S76. Infusion Nurses Society: http://www.ins1.org

CVAD, central venous access device; PN, parenteral nutrition.

APPENDIX A.6: LEARNING MODULE CONTENT: EXAMPLE CVAD LABORATORY

Medication Administration Review **(Potter, Perry, Stockert, & Hall, pp. 584, 590)**

The SIX RIGHTS of Medication Administration are:

1. Right Client
2. Right Drug
3. Right Dose
4. Right Route
5. Right Time (current time to give, based on administration time schedule in order)
6. Right Documentation

(Potter, Perry, Stockert, & Hall, 2013)

The THREE MED CHECKS for Parenteral Medication Administration are:

1. When taking a medication bag from the client's drawer, medication cart, medication refrigerator or the Pyxis.
2. After initially verifying the medication bag/checking contents in the medication room.
3. Before spiking and priming the bag at the client's bedside.

The TWO CLIENT IDENTIFICATION (ID) CHECKS for Medication Administration are:

1. Compare the MAR to the client's ID bracelet, checking name.
2. Compare the MAR to the client's ID bracelet, checking medical record number.

A third identifier can be used:

3. Ask the client to state his/her name (Potter et al., 2013).

PARENTERAL NUTRITION (PN) Potter, Perry, Stockert, & Hall, p. 1019 (only Box 44-11, Indications for Enteral and Parenteral Nutrition), pp. 1021–1024 (Parenteral Nutrition and Preventing Complications)

Key Concepts

- PN may also be referred to as Total Parental Nutrition (TPN).
- When the GI tract cannot be used for the ingestion, digestion, and absorption of essential nutrients, parenteral (meaning intravenous) nutrition (PN) may be used.
- PN is administered through an indwelling central venous catheter (resting in either the subclavian or the superior vena cava central vein) that may be inserted peripherally or centrally. Examples of each will be shown in lab.
- Peripherally inserted central catheters (PICC) are inserted percutaneously in the arm and threaded up to the central vein.

(continued)

- Centrally inserted catheters are either inserted percutaneously directly into the central vein, or are implanted or tunneled up to the central vein.
- In order to promote safe care of the client receiving PN:
  - nutritional requirements have to be regularly assessed via laboratory tests,
  - the CVAD has to be meticulously managed,
  - the client has to be carefully monitored for clinical complications. (Potter, et al., 2013)

Nutrition:
- The purpose of PN is to promote healing and avoid malnutrition by the administration of a nutritionally adequate formula that includes dextrose, electrolytes, and other nutrients such as amino acids, fat emulsions, vitamins, and trace elements.

[...]

Administration:
- PN is a medication and must be checked as such, using the six rights of medication administration, 3 med checks, and 2 client identity checks in addition to general checks for intravenous fluid administration.

[...]

Complications:
- Principles of asepsis must be maintained when preparing PN infusions, accessing the central line, and changing needleless access devices to ensure safe delivery of PN.

[...]

Procedure

Checks agency's protocol for flushing central lines
Compliance with protocol promotes safe, accurate procedure

Checks order:
- Ensures complete Provider's Order—signature, date, time, order legible
- Verifies MAR against Provider's Order using 5 rights of medication administration—client, drug, dose, route, time
- Checks for client allergies on Provider's Order and MAR (*promotes client safety*)

Order must be legally written and properly transcribed to implement

Determines if any assessments need to be completed before administering PN (lab values)
Obtaining necessary assessment data promotes safe, accurate procedure

Performs hand hygiene at appropriate intervals throughout the skill
Reduces risk of cross-contamination

Prepares medication for one client at a time:
- Selects correct PN for correct client at correct time, confirming correct dose and route, and comparing medication to MAR—first med check (assesses clarity, expiration date, etc.)
- Verifies PN bag label against PN order sheet ("recipe checks" the contents)
- Completes second med check by comparing PN bag to MAR, checking client, medication, dose, route, and time

Use strict guidelines to prevent medication errors

Prepares supplies for procedure:
- Using aseptic technique, prepares one 5 mL NS flush in 10 mL syringe per unused line:
  1. Opens prefilled 10 mL NS syringe package
  2. Removes cap and sets aside

3. Expels air and any unneeded fluid (wastes down to 5 mL)

4. Checks to ensure correct dose of NS remains in syringes

5. Recaps syringe

Appropriate sterility promotes client safety

- Gathers supplies and equipment needed for PN administration: bag of PN, IV tubing, micron filter, alcohol wipes, flush (*avoids repeated trips*)

Prepares client for procedure:

- Introduces self to client (*clients have a right to know their caregiver*)
- Identifies client using two client checks—compares MAR to client ID band, checking name and medical record number; may ask client to state name (*promotes accurate, safe care*)
- Checks for allergies with client (*promotes client safety*)
- Explains procedure and answers questions (*clients have a right to know about their care*)

Prepares PN for administration:

- Completes third med check by comparing PN to MAR, checking client, medication, dose, route, and time (*use strict guidelines to prevent medication errors*)
- Primes tubing according to procedure for preparing a new bag and tubing, attaching filter to end of tubing and luer-locking filter on before hanging new PN bag on IV pole (*in practice, threads tubing through pump and hangs PN bag on pole; appropriate sterility promotes client safety*)
- Times and dates tubing according to agency policy (*promotes client safety*)
- Sets PN rate on pump

Prepares work area for procedure:

- Raises bed to working height (*promotes sterility of procedure and nurse safety*)
- Dons clean gloves (*reduces risk of cross-contamination*)
- Inspects CVAD site for type of catheter, patency of all lumens, signs and symptoms of phlebitis, infiltration, or infection, and checks integrity of sutures (*promotes appropriate care and timely interventions*)

Aseptically initiates PN infusion:

- Monitors for asepsis during procedure; if device/port becomes contaminated, cleanses again with a new alcohol wipe (*appropriate sterility promotes client safety*)
- Does not flush a lumen that is labeled "clotted" (*flushing a clotted line could push the clot into the bloodstream, causing an embolus*)

1. Vigorously cleanses the selected port with an alcohol swab for 15 sec

2. Luer-locks 10 mL NS syringe to port (*flush ports before use to ensure patency and minimize risk of medication incompatibility*)

3. Opens/releases catheter slide clamp (*slide clamps act as a backup to the needleless access device and should be activated whenever the line is not in use and no syringe is attached*)

4. Aspirates for blood return, then flushes port, ensuring no air is introduced into the catheter and checking for obstructions to flow—DOES NOT PUSH AGAINST PRESSURE

5. Closes/activates catheter slide clamp

6. Luer-locks PN tubing to the port

7. Releases all roller clamps or slide clamps on tubing and on catheter lumen

8. Turns on the IV pump at the prescribed rate and assesses to ensure fluid begins to flow

Ensures nurse, client, and environmental safety:

- Disposes of used supplies appropriately
- Removes gloves without contaminating self

(continued)

- Leaves client with bed low and locked, side rails up x2, call bell in reach
- Performs hand hygiene at appropriate intervals throughout skill (ex: before handling medications, before and after client care)

Reduces risk of cross-contamination and promotes safety

Documents date, time, procedure, client tolerance, and PN on appropriate forms (sixth right of medication administration)

Promotes communication and accurate, timely care

Rechecks client at appropriate intervals as needed to assess response to PN

Promotes accurate, timely care

CVAD, central venous access device; GI, gastrointestinal; MAR, medication administration record; mL, milliliter; NS, normal saline; PN, parenteral nutrition.

Copyright Education-Innovation-Simulation Learning Environment, School of Nursing, The University of North Carolina at Chapel Hill, 2013. Reprinted by permission, 2013.

APPENDIX A.7: PROVIDER'S ORDER SHEET: EXAMPLE CVAD LABORATORY

Carrington General Hospital
Computer Provider Order Entry

Patient Name:

Patient MRN:

Patient DOB:

Patient Room #:

Allergies: No Known Allergies   Weight: 48 kg

Order	Start Date/Time	Order	Stop Date/Time
#0001	To/da/yy 0800	Flush unused ports of central line with 5 mL 0.9% NS Follow with 3 mL 100 Units/mL heparin Three times a day	
#0002	To/da/yy 0800	PN as ordered at 42 mL/hr via central line (See parental nutrition order form)	
#0003	To/da/yy 0800	Central line dressing change and site care Every 7 days Note: Start today	

Signed Electronically: John Q. Public, MD   Provider #12345 Pager# 987-6543

Ordered at:

Transcribed by: (Initials, Title, Date)

Checked by: (Initials, Title, Date)

This is not a part of the permanent chart. Working document only. Do not send to Medical Records.

CVAD, central venous access device; DOB, date of birth; hr, hour; kg, kilogram; MD, medical doctor, mL, milliliter; MRN, medical record number; NS, normal saline; RN, registered nurse.

APPENDIX A.8: MEDICATION ADMINISTRATION RECORD: EXAMPLE CVAD LABORATORY

Carrington General Hospital	Name
School of Nursing, NC 27599	MRN
	DOB
	Room #

Admitting DX: Malnutrition s/p Chemotherapy

Pt. Weight: 48 kg

Allergies: No Known Allergies

OMITTED MEDICATION CODE

N = NPO, V = NAUSEA/VOMITING, R = REFUSED, H = HELD, O = OFF UNIT, C = SEE CHART

START	STOP	MEDICATION	0700-1900	1900-0700
		Flush unused ports of central line with 5mL 0.9% NS	0800 1600	2400
		Follow with 3 mL 100 Units/mL Heparin		
		Three times a day		
		PN as ordered at 42 mL/hr via central line	0800	
		(See Parental Nutrition order form)		
		Central line dressing change and site care	0800	
		Every 7 days		
		Note: Start today		

(continued)

	PRN Meds	Reassess Code
		E–med effective
		A–additional meds needed
		M–MD notified

Injection Site Code:

Site #1–Left Deltoid	Site #5–Left Upper Quad	Site #9–Left Ventrogluteal
Site #2–Right Deltoid		Site #10–Right Ventrogluteal
Site #3–Left Vastus Lateralus	Site #6–Left Lower Quad	Site #11–Left Dorsogluteal
Site #4–Right Vastus Lateralus		Site #12–Right Dorsoglutal
	Site #7–Right Upper Quad	
	Site #8–Right Lower Quad	

Initials   Legal Signature/Title

For Educational Use Only—Not For Actual Patient Care

CVAD, central venous access device; DOB, date of birth; DX, diagnosis; hr, hour; kg, kilogram; MD, medical doctor; mL, milliliter; MRN, medical record number; NS, normal saline; PRN, Pro re nata (as needed); Pt., patient; PN, parenteral nutrition; RN, registered nurse.

Copyright Education-Innovation-Simulation Learning Environment, School of Nursing, The University of North Carolina at Chapel Hill, 2013. Reprinted by permission, 2013.

APPENDIX A.9: PARENTERAL NUTRITION ORDER FORM: EXAMPLE CVAD LABORATORY

Carrington General Hospital	Name
Adult Parenteral Nutrition Order Form	MRN
Daily order must arrive in Pharmacy by 2 AM to receive PN	DOB
	Room #

To begin at 08:00 AM (Date) _____ Route of infusion: ☒Central ☐ Peripheral

I. ALLERGIES: No Known Allergies Weight: 48kg

II. INDICATE TOTAL DAILY AMOUNT OF BASE MIXTURE (CONTAINS NO ADDED ELECTROLYTES—SEE SECTION III)

1018 milliliters/day* at an infusion rate of 42 mL/hr**

PER 1,000 mL:	☒Standard Central	☐ Standard Peripheral	☐ Other
Amino Acids 10% (mL)***	500	300	Amino Acids 10%*** mL/day:
(g)	50	30	Amino Acids 15% mL/day:
Dextrose 70% (mL)	300	86	Dextrose 70% mL/day:
(g)	210	60	(2.4 kcal/mL)
(kcal)	714	204	
Intravenous Fat Emulsion 20% (mL)	150	250	Intravenous Fat Emulsion 20% mL/day:

(kcal)	300	500	(2.0 kcal/mL)
Non-Protein kcals	1,014	704	☐ Infuse Intravenous Fat Emulsion by piggyback mL/hr:
% lipid calories	30	71	

III. INDICATE ELECTROLYTES TO BE ADDED TO BASE MIXTURE (USE ANY COMBINATION)

STANDARD CENTRAL ELECTROLYTES PER DAY:

(1 vial per 1,000 mL of Central PN recommended)

STANDARD PERIPHERAL ELECTROLYTES PER DAY:

(1 vial per 1,000 mL of Peripheral PN recommended)

Standard Electrolytes			☒ OTHER ELECTROLYTES PER DAY			
	Central	Peripheral	P	as sodium	21	mmole
	1 vial	1 vial		(3mmole P provides 4 mEq Na)		
Phosphate (mmole)	15	6		as potassium (3mmole P provides 4.4 mEq K)		mmole
Electrolyte Package:			N	as chloride	70	mEq
Na (mEq)	45	33	a	as acetate	30	mEq
K (mEq)	40	20	K	as chloride	50	mEq
Mg (mEq)	8	5		as acetate		mEq
Ca (mEq)	5	5	Mg	as sulfate	16	mEq
Cl (mEq)	33	30	Ca	as gluconate	7	mEq
Acetate (mEq)	41	25				

IV. The following are added per daily volume unless otherwise indicated.

Heparin 1 unit/mL	☒ Do not add
Multiple vitamins	☐ Do not add
Trace elements	☐ Do not add
Vitamin K I mg	☒ Do not add

V. Miscellaneous additives per daily volume.

Regular Human insulin units: NONE

Other: Vitamin K 250 mcg

Signed Electronically: John Q. Public, MD Pager Number 987-6543 Ordered (date) at 0200

For Educational Use Only—Not For Actual Patient Care

CVAD, central venous access device; DOB, date of birth; DX, diagnosis; g, gram; hr, hour; kcal, kilocalorie; kcal/mL, kilocalorie/milliliter; kg, kilogram; MD, medical doctor; mcg, microgram; mEq, milliequivalent; mg, milligram; mL, milliliter; mmole, millimole; MRN, Medical Record Number; NS, normal saline; PRN, Pro re nata (as needed); PN, parenteral nutrition; RN, registered nurse.

APPENDIX A.10: SKILL EVALUATION CHECKLIST: EXAMPLE PARENTERAL NUTRITION VIA CVAD

Evaluation Criteria: miss any 1 bullet in a 1-star item (*), have to redo

miss any 2 bullets out of 2-star items (**), have to redo

miss any 3 bullets out of 3-star items (***), have to redo

Administering PN	✓/-		
	Eval	Redo 1	Redo 2
Checks order:			
• Ensures complete provider order (*)			
• Verifies MAR against provider's orders using 5 rights of medication administration (*)			
• Checks for allergies on Provider's Order and MAR (*)			
Performs hand hygiene at appropriate intervals throughout skill (***)			
Prepares medication for one client at a time:			
• Completes two med checks using 5 rights of medication administration (*)			
• Completes ingredient check, comparing PN label to "Adult Parenteral Nutrition Order Form" on client chart (*)			
Prepares supplies for procedure:			
1. Using aseptic technique, prepares one 10 mL syringe with 5 mL sterile NS (*)			
2. Gathers supplies and takes to room (***)			
Prepares client for procedure:			
• Introduces self to client (***)			
• Identifies client using 2 client checks (*)			
• Checks for allergies (*)			
• Explains procedure and answers questions (***)			
Prepares PN for administration:			
1. Completes 3rd medication check for PN using 5 rights of medication administration (*)			
2. Using aseptic technique, connects tubing to filter, attaches PN, appropriately primes tubing, and hangs on IV pole (*)			
Prepares work area for procedure:			
• Raises bed to working height (**)			
• Dons clean gloves (**)			
• Inspects catheter and insertion site and checks integrity of sutures (***)			

Aseptically initiates PN infusion (note if port is contaminated during procedure, must cleanse again with alcohol and allow to dry)			
1. Does not flush a line that is labeled "clotted" (*)			
2. Vigorously cleanses the appropriate port with alcohol for 15 seconds and allows to dry (*)			
3. Luer locks NS syringe to port (*)			
4. Opens slide clamp and aspirates for blood return, then gently infuses flush (*)			
5. Closes slide clamp and disconnects syringe (*)			
6. Luer locks PN tubing to port (*)			
7. Opens slide clamps on central line and tubing (*)			
8. States ordered flow rate to program pump for PN infusion (*)			
Ensures nurse, client, and environmental safety:			
• Disposes of supplies appropriately (***)			
• Removes gloves without contaminating self (**)			
• Leaves bed low and locked, side rails up x2, call bell in reach (***)			
• Performs hand hygiene at appropriate intervals throughout skill (before handling medications, before and after client care, etc.) (***)			
Documents procedure: date, time, PN, condition of site, and client's response (6th right of medication administration) (***)			

	DATE	EVALUATOR NAME	SCORE (circle one)
Evaluation			PN: Pass (10) Redo
Redo 1			PN: Pass (5) Redo
Redo 2			PN: Pass (0) Redo

IV, intravenous; MAR, medication administration record; NS, normal saline; PN, parenteral nutrition.

Copyright Education-Innovation-Simulation Learning Environment, School of Nursing, The University of North Carolina at Chapel Hill, 2013. Reprinted by permission, 2013.

REFERENCES

Infusion Nurses Society. (2006). STANDARDS: Infusion therapy. *Journal of Infusion Nursing, 29* (Suppl. 1), S75–S76. Retrieved from http://ovidsp.tx.ovid.com/AN=00129804-200601001-0007

Potter, P. A., Perry, A. G., Stockert, P. A., & Hall, A. M. (2013). *Fundamentals of nursing* (8th ed.). St. Louis, MO: Elsevier.

Appendix B: Clinical Teaching Activities and Resources for Students

APPENDIX B.1: SAMPLE INTERACTIVE EXERCISE FOR CLINICAL ORIENTATION

Minimal supplies are needed for this exercise, and it is an excellent way to engage students during orientation to the clinical setting. Equipment needed includes: a large glass jar or vessel, one bag of large-sized shells, one bag of medium-sized shells, one bag of small shells, and a small bag of sand. Before beginning the exercise, have only the large glass jar in view for students. Ask for four volunteers from the group.

The clinical teacher produces the first bag of large shells and asks a student volunteer to arrange them inside the glass jar. After the student has completed this exercise, the group is asked, "Is the vessel full?" The likely answer will be "no." The faculty member then produces the second bag of medium-sized shells and asks the second student volunteer to arrange these inside the same jar. This student may need to get creative by first removing some of the larger shells, adding the medium size shells into the container, and then replacing/rearranging the large shells again. On completion, the clinical group is again asked, "Is the vessel full?" Usually, by now, the students have become wise to this question and state "no." Sequentially, the faculty member produces the third bag of small shells and has the third volunteer add these to the jar, then the bag of sand is produced and the fourth student volunteer adds the sand. Each time after the student volunteer has completed his/her task, the student group is asked whether the jar is full. They will likely continue to state that the jar is not full, as they could still add water or other materials.

Students are then asked to brainstorm about what they learned from this exercise, and the relationship that this interactive exercise has to their clinical practice and group functioning. Many valuable analogies can be made using this exercise. The following are only a few key points that students and/or teacher might raise based on the "shell exercise."

- Keep your "big shells," or your nursing priorities, in place. If the small shells were deposited into the jar first, the big shells would not have fit. Similarly, the nurse who gets sidetracked with repeated tasks may lose sight of the "big picture" and nursing priorities are unlikely to be met.

- Students may point out the importance of teamwork, as various student volunteers were required to work together to fill the vessel. They may also point out creative thinking toward patient goals and having to be flexible as a nurse, just as some of the large shells had to be temporarily removed and then replaced in the jar in order to make room for some of the smaller items.

- Students may articulate that the well-rounded nurse (in other words, the full jar) is made up of many different qualities, such as knowledge, technical skill, caring, the ability to educate the patient and family, patient advocacy, communication skills, and so forth. An observation may be made that the jar was not full when it contained only large, or only large- and medium-sized shells, but that a *variety* of shells were needed for it to be full. Similarly, the nurse needs knowledge and a variety of competencies to make a difference to patients and their care.

- Students might raise the issue of reflection on one's professional practice and the importance of consciously reflecting on one's professional growth at regular intervals, just as the clinical group reflected on whether the jar was full during regular points within the shell exercise.

- Students may comment on the aesthetically pleasing end result of a jar filled with an array of shells and sand, and faculty members may draw an analogy to the beauty of developing the art and science of nursing.

APPENDIX B.2: SAMPLE CLINICAL SETTING ORIENTATION TREASURE HUNT

Fire stations

Crash carts

Alarms/codes

Biohazardous waste management system

Staff bathroom

Report room

Pneumatic tube system

Patient refreshments

Ice machine, cups, plastic utensils, straws

Bladder scanner

Skin care supplies

Mechanical lifts

Sliding board for patient transfer

Medications and supplies associated with medication administration

Isolation supplies

Laundry hampers

Where to dispose:

  Soiled transfer sheets

  Used equipment for cleaning

  Used patient meal trays

Quick references:

  Nursing policies

  Accepted abbreviations

  Mission statement of agency

  Other site-specific information

Medical records: provider orders, history, progress notes, diagnostics and lab reports, consultations, etc.

Medical record system, charting (confirm students have log-in information)

Pharmacology references

Patient education references

In an empty patient room, find:

Gloves

Computer for charting

Call bell

Familiarize yourself with bed operations

Sink, toilet, shower

Sharps containers

Thermometers

Suction and oxygen equipment

Portable blood pressure (BP) machines, manual BP cuff	Saline flushes
Pulse oximeter	Saline/water for irrigation
Linens: sheets, towels, patient gowns, nonslip footwear	Nasogastric and other tubes
	Primary and secondary intravenous tubing
Sequential compression devices	Suction catheters
Lift equipment and transfer sheets	Catheter sets
Glucometers	Personal care items (shampoo, toothpaste, etc.)
Medication system	Oxygen tubing/nasal cannula etc.
Glucometer docking port	Tape
	Dressing change supplies
	Urinals
	Specimen containers

APPENDIX B.3: ORGANIZATIONAL TOOL FOR NURSING STUDENTS: CLINICAL TIMELINE EXAMPLE 1

Time	Clinical Activity
0800–0830	Meet in patient resource room. Preconference with your fellow students and clinical teacher.
0830–0845	Introduce yourself to the staff nurse as well as the nursing assistant. Communicate what you will and will not be involved in during the clinical experience with respect to patient care. Be specific in what time you will be leaving the unit and obtain a patient update from the staff nurse.
0845–0930	Introduce yourself to the patient, establish priorities, revisit your time sequence plan for the day, check the chart for any new orders, check the medication records for any new medications or changes to previously ordered medications. Obtain baseline patient assessments and document accordingly. Brief morning care, nutrition, intake, and output.
0930–1300	Medications, skills, nursing rounds, therapies, and treatments (e.g., deep breathing and coughing, ambulation, turning and positioning, toileting, pain management, patient education, glucometer readings, hygiene). Linen changes, attend to room environment. Keep documentation in e-chart current. Review medical records to learn more about patient, plan of care, and modifications of treatment plan. Attend team/family conferences. Enter patient documentation as you go—remember this is the only way other members of the healthcare team can have access to the information you have gathered. Report to your student buddy and the staff nurse prior to your morning break and lunch. Have your e-charting cosigned by the clinical teacher prior to [time].
1300–1400	Nursing rounds and/or postconference, shift wrap up, report off (handoff) to the staff. Do not start new procedures during this time.

APPENDIX B.4: ORGANIZATIONAL TOOL FOR NURSING STUDENTS: CLINICAL TIMELINE EXAMPLE 2

Time	Nursing Activity	Meds	Comments/Notes
0700	Report and preconference		
0800	Obtain patient's vital signs (VS) and document		After getting report:
	Safety equipment check		Chart for new orders
	E-chart: (1) brief assessment, (2) activities and interventions, (3) intake (oral/IV), (4) output if applicable, (5) vascular access device if applicable, (6) pain assessment, (7) neurological assessment if applicable		Review MAR
			Check overnight VS and physical assessment
0900	Patient physical assessment and documentation		
	E-chart: (1) intake and output, (2) vascular access device, (3) activities and interventions, (4) pain		
1000	Patient rounds[a]		
	E-chart: (1) intake and output, (2) vascular access device, (3) activities and interventions, (4) pain		
1100	Patient rounds[a]		
	E-chart: (1) intake and output, (2) vascular access device, (3) activities and interventions, (4) pain		
1200	Patient rounds[a]		Prior to leaving unit:
	Obtain patient's VS and document		Make sure all documentation is current
	Neurological check if applicable		Chart, MAR check!
	E-chart: (1) intake and output, (2) vascular access device, (3) activities and interventions, (4) pain, (5) VS		Safety check!
			Report to your buddy and registered nurses (handoff)

MAR, medication administration record.

[a]Use the CARE acronym for patient rounds:

C = Comfort. Is the patient comfortable? Is the patient experiencing any pain?

A = Access. Does the patient have access to the call bell, telephone, food/drink, bed controls, and other necessities?

R = Restroom. Does the patient need to use the bathroom or need other assistance?

E = Environment. Check the environment for clutter, privacy, room controls, noise level, and the effect that this environment is having on the patient.

Adapted from Baird, K. 2008. *Raising the bar on service excellence: The healthcare leader's guide to putting passion into practice.* Fort Atkinson, WI: Golden Lamp Press.

Appendix C: Caputi's Alternative Approach to Clinical Evaluation

Teaching and evaluating student learning and performance in the clinical setting is one of the most challenging aspects of nursing education. However, no matter the setting or unique challenges the setting presents, there is one important principle that oversees clinical evaluation—is the student performing at a passing level related to the student learning outcomes? Therefore, when developing and implementing a clinical evaluation tool, it is important to consider all learning outcomes, not just those that relate to physical contact with the patient (Caputi, 2010a).

It can be difficult to ensure students are engaging in student learning outcomes that are not readily observable. Because teachers need to ensure safe patient care is delivered by all students, many learning outcomes may not be evaluated completely. Evaluation of such learning outcomes may result from assessing care plans, typically written by students and graded by faculty away from the clinical setting following the actual experience. A major purpose of the clinical experience is to provide learning in actual patient contexts. Removing the evaluation of student performance to outside that context is less than desirable. Students are no longer able to return to the setting to collect further information to answer questions teachers may pose, and teachers are no longer in the setting to verify information.

To remedy these and other weaknesses in clinical education, Caputi's perspective requires evaluating students in the clinical setting with a clinical evaluation tool (CET) that is both valid and reliable (Caputi, 2010b). Clinical teachers provide guidance to assist students to think like a nurse as they demonstrate achievement of all student learning outcomes reflected on the CET. However, to provide one-to-one guidance on all learning outcomes for all students in the clinical setting is difficult.

A new perspective is one that examines student learning outcomes performed in the clinical setting with student activities tied directly to the behaviors on the CET. These behaviors reflect the course student learning outcomes and competencies. If a course has both a theory component and a clinical component, the same student learning outcomes and competencies are applied to both learning environments. Once those student learning outcomes and competencies are written, they become the CET. Using them as the CET ensures consistency between theory and clinical.

For example, many courses require students to demonstrate knowledge about and performance of learning outcomes related to major areas such as safety, evidence-based practice, caring, informatics, teamwork/collaboration, clinical reasoning, and others. If the theory component of a course expects a particular level of behavior about these major concepts as expressed through student learning outcomes and competencies, then the student's ability to apply these same behaviors during clinical is desirable. Unfortunately, what tends to happen is clinical teachers guide learning and assessment of psychomotor and technological skills, then rely on other means of documentation for the other concepts—such as a written care plan or reflection journal. This can be remedied with a CET that has activities tied to the CET behaviors. This provides a valid tool because the activities evaluated are related directly to the competencies on the CET. To ensure inter-rater reliability of the activity, grading rubrics are used.

For example, a course has a student learning outcome of: Engage in clinical reasoning to make patient-centered care decisions with expected behaviors (competencies) of:

a. Use clinical reasoning to make management decisions to ensure accurate and safe care in all nursing actions, including addressing anticipated changes in the patient's condition.
b. Use clinical reasoning when implementing all steps of the nursing process while integrating best-available evidence in the care of adult patients with complex health issues.
c. Anticipate risks, and predict and manage potential complications when caring for adult patients with complex health issues.
d. Prioritize patient care.

How will the faculty determine if each student has satisfactorily completed all four competencies for this student learning outcome? Caputi's approach is to include activities students are required to complete during the clinical experience. The faculty members teaching the course now have an established focus of expectations for each of these competencies—the same focus and expectations for all students. This helps to ensure reliability. Because the activities are specifically aligned with the competencies, the tool becomes valid in that it is evaluating what the course is teaching. The following example demonstrates this approach: the learning activities align with each of these four competencies.

Course Student Learning Outcome: Engage in clinical reasoning to make patient-centered care decisions

Competencies demonstrating the Course Student Learning Outcome has been achieved:

a. Use clinical reasoning/clinical judgment to make management decisions to ensure accurate and safe care in all nursing actions, including addressing anticipated changes in the patient's condition.
b. Use clinical reasoning/clinical judgment when implementing all steps of the nursing process while integrating best available evidence in the care of adult patients with complex health issues.

Tool: Apply and analyze Clinical Reasoning (Uses Tanner's [2006] steps of the Clinical Reasoning model)

Choose two events that occurred during the experience in the clinical setting that required you to engage in clinical reasoning.

For each event, complete the following tool to guide your thinking.

Overview of the Problem:

Background:

Noticing:

Interpreting:

Responding:

Reflection-in-Action

Reflection-on-Action

Explain the following:

1. How did you use the above model?
2. How did the model assist in you in arriving at decisions?
3. What available evidence did you use when completing the "responding" section of the tool?
4. Do you use another approach for thinking? Explain.

Grading Rubric for Applying Critical Thinking

Performance Criteria	S	NI	U
Clear and accurate answers to all questions on tool.	Clearly and accurately answers all questions on tool.	Clearly and accurately answers some but not all questions on tool.	Unable to clearly and accurately answer all questions on tool.

NI, needs improvement; S, satisfactory; U, unsatisfactory.

c. Anticipate risks, and predict and manage potential complications when caring for adult patients with complex health issues.

Tool: Predict and Manage Potential Complications
For each patient answer these questions:

1. What are you on alert for today with this patient?
2. What are the important assessments to make?
3. What complications may occur? What could go wrong?
4. What interventions will prevent complications?
5. How will you prioritize implementation of nursing interventions? Explain.
6. What actions will you take for each complication should it occur?

Grading Rubric to Predict and Manage Potential Complications

Performance Criteria	S	NI	U
Able to identify the potential complications.	Clearly identifies potential complications.	Description of potential complications for this patient is scant.	Unable to identify potential complications.
Able to identify the important assessment data to monitor for this patient.	Clearly identifies the important assessment data to monitor for this patient.	Description of the important assessment data to monitor for this patient is scant.	Unable to identify the important assessment data to monitor for this patient.

(continued)

Performance Criteria	S	NI	U
Able to identify all factors influencing the most important data to monitor.	Clearly identifies all factors influencing the most important data to monitor.	Description of all factors influencing the most important data to monitor is scant.	Unable to identify the most important data to monitor.
Able to prioritize planned interventions.	Clearly identifies ways to prioritize planned interventions.	Superficially discusses ways to prioritize planned interventions.	Unable to prioritize planned interventions.
Able to plan actions to take if complications occur.	Clearly identifies actions to take if complications occur.	Superficially discusses actions to take if complications occur.	Unable to discuss actions to take if complications occur.

NI, needs improvement; S, satisfactory; U, unsatisfactory.

d. Prioritize patient care.

Tool: Prioritizing Patient Needs

Refer to your concept map for patient care. Categorize the identified patient needs using the following criteria (National Council State Boards of Nursing [NCSBN], n.d.). Explain your rationale.

1. First-order priority need—immediate threat to health, safety, or survival.
2. Second-order priority need—actual problem for which immediate help has been requested by the patient or family.
3. Third-order priority need—actual or potential issue of which the patient or family is not aware.
4. Fourth-order priority need—actual or potential issue that is anticipated in the future and for which help will be needed.

First-Priority Needs With Rationale

_____

_____

Second-Priority Needs With Rationale

_____

_____

Third-Priority Needs With Rationale

_____

_____

Fourth-Priority Needs With Rationale

_____

_____

Grading Rubric for Prioritizing Patient Needs

Performance Criteria	S	NI	U
Prioritizes patient needs	Prioritization of needs is correct.	Prioritization is correct in some but not all identified patient needs.	Unable to accurately prioritize patient needs.
Provides rationales	Rationales are clear and accurate.	Rationales are superficial and are not clearly explained.	Unable to provide any correct rationales.

NI, needs improvement; S, satisfactory; U, unsatisfactory.

SUMMARY

In summary, the purpose of this approach for evaluation of students' behaviors or competencies in the clinical setting is to provide a more objective evaluation tool. With this approach students are required to complete specific activities that demonstrate their ability to meet the expected outcomes of the clinical course. By using these tools and grading rubrics, faculty are less reliant on subjective evaluations based totally on observation. Faculty may not be able to make all the necessary observations of each student because of the demands to oversee student care to ensure patient safety. The burden of proof of meeting the expected behaviors is now on the student rather than on the faculty's opportunity, or lack thereof, to observe every student performing every expected behavior on the clinical evaluation tool.

REFERENCES

Caputi, L. (2010a). Evaluating student in the clinical setting. In L. Caputi, (Ed.), *Teaching nursing: The art and science* (pp. 152–174). Glen Ellyn, IL: College of DuPage Press.

Caputi, L. (2010b). Transforming clinical education: The Caputi clinical activities portfolio®. In L. Caputi, (Ed.), *Teaching nursing: The art and science* (pp. 216–255). Glen Ellyn, IL: College of DuPage Press.

National Council State Boards of Nursing. (n.d.). *Transition to practice: Outline of NCSBN's Transition to Practice.* Chicago, IL: Author. Retrieved from https://www.ncsbn.org/1603.htm

Tanner, C. (2006). Thinking like a nurse: A research-based model of clinical judgment in nursing. *Journal of Nursing Education, 45*(6), 204–211.

Appendix D: Resources for Nurse Educators

APPENDIX D.1: CERTIFICATION FOR NURSE EDUCATORS

Mission of Certification Program

The National League for Nursing's Academic Nurse Educator Certification Program "recognize[s] excellence in the advanced specialty role of the academic nurse educator."

Goals of Certification:

- Distinguish academic nursing education as a specialty area of practice and an advanced practice role.
- Recognize the academic nurse educator's specialized knowledge, skills, and abilities and excellence in practice.
- Strengthen the use of the core competencies of nurse educator practice.
- Contribute to nurse educators' professional development.

From National League for Nursing. (2011). *Certification for nurse educators*. Retrieved from www.nln.org/certification/index.htm

APPENDIX D.2: CERTIFIED NURSE EDUCATOR^{CM} EXAMINATION CONTENT AREAS AND PERCENT OF TEST ITEMS

Facilitate Learning, 22%
Facilitate Learner Development and Socialization, 14%
Use Assessment and Evaluation Strategies, 17%
Participate in Curriculum Design and Evaluation of Program Outcomes, 17%
Pursue Continuous Quality Improvement in the Academic Nurse Educator Role, 9%
Engage in Scholarship, Service, and Leadership, 21%

From National League for Nursing. (2012). *Certified nurse educator (CNE) 2012–2013 candidate handbook* (p. 5). Retrieved from www.nln.org/certification/handbook/cne.pdf

APPENDIX D.3: CORE COMPETENCIES OF NURSE EDUCATORS AND SAMPLE ACTIVITIES FOR EACH COMPETENCY

Competency	Sample Activities
Facilitate learning	Develop innovative teaching-learning activities
	Base teaching strategies on educational theory and evidence
	Use information technologies in teaching
Facilitate learner development and socialization	Assist students to develop as nurses and integrate expected values and behaviors
	Identify individual learning styles and needs for culturally diverse, at-risk, or physically challenged learners
	Assist learners to engage in thoughtful constructive self- or peer evaluation
Use assessment and evaluation strategies	Create appropriate assessment instruments to evaluate learner outcomes
	Design tools for assessing clinical practice
	Provide input for the development of program policies related to admission, progression, or graduation
Participate in curriculum design and evaluation of program outcomes	Design curricula that reflect trends while preparing graduates to function in the health care environment
	Develop or revise courses reflecting theoretical framework of curriculum
	Support educational goals through community partnerships
Pursue continuous quality improvement in the nurse educator role	Develop and maintain competence in the nurse educator role (e.g., by attending conferences, seminars, workshops)
	Mentor and support faculty colleagues in the role of academic nurse educator
	Use feedback from peers, learners, and others for improvement
Function as a change agent and leader	Provide leadership in the nursing program or other organization
	Work on a special panel or in a think tank for an educational issue
	Represent nursing education on an interdisciplinary work group
Engage in scholarship	Develop an area of expertise within the academic educator role
	Implement scholarly activities
	Share expertise with colleagues (e.g., through publications and presentations)

Competency	Sample Activities
Function within the educational environment	Collaborate with other disciplines to enhance the academic environment
	Participate in committee work on the departmental or institutional level
	Develops collaborations and partnerships within the academic institution and with clinical agencies

Adapted from Wittmann-Price, R. A., Godshall, M., & Wilson, L. (2013). *Certified nursing educator (CNE) manual* (2nd ed., pp. 15–16). New York, NY: Springer Publishing Company. Reprinted by permission, 2013.

APPENDIX D.4: SELECTED NURSING AND HIGHER EDUCATION ORGANIZATIONS

American Academy of Nursing	Serves the public and nursing profession by advancing health policy and practice. Academy's members, known as Fellows, are nursing's most accomplished leaders in education, practice, administration, and research.	www.aannet.org/about-the-academy
American Association of Colleges of Nursing	Represents baccalaureate and higher-degree nursing programs. Promotes quality nursing education. Offers faculty development programs and webinars. Collects data about nursing education programs, faculty, and students, and analyzes trends in nursing education. Publishes position papers.	www.aacn.nche.edu
American Association of Community Colleges	Provides advocacy for community colleges at the national level. Works closely with states on policy.	www.aacc.nche.edu
American Association of University Professors	Focuses on advancing academic freedom and shared governance. Defines fundamental professional values and standards for higher education and faculty.	www.aaup.org

(continued)

American Association of University Women	Promotes equity and education for women and girls. Advocates for fundamental educational, social, economic, and political issues.	www.aauw.org
American Council on Education	Represents presidents of accredited, degree-granting institutions (2- and 4-year colleges, private and public universities, and nonprofit schools) in the United States. Focuses on higher education challenges, with the goal to improve access and better prepare students.	www.acenet.edu/Pages/default.aspx
Association of American Colleges and Universities	Focuses on promoting high-quality undergraduate liberal education. Website contains links to resources on liberal education, general education, curriculum, faculty work, assessment, diversity, and others.	www.aacu.org/about/index.cfm
Association of Black Nursing Faculty, Inc.	Provides a group for Black professional nurses with similar interests and concerns to promote health-related issues and nursing education. Assists members in professional development and provides continuing education.	www.abnf.net/index.html
Association of Community Health Nursing Educators	Focuses on promoting excellence in community and public health nursing education, research, and practice.	www.achne.org/i4a/pages/index.cfm?pageid=1
EDUCAUSE	Advances higher education through use of information technology. Focuses on issues and emerging trends and technologies affecting higher education.	www.educause.edu
Multimedia Educational Resource for Learning and Online Teaching (MERLOT)	Includes repository of resources and information for faculty development and to download for use in teaching. Publishes *Journal of Online Learning and Teaching*.	www.merlot.org

National League for Nursing	Promotes excellence in nursing education at all levels. Offers faculty development programs, webinars, and annual educational conference. Sponsors certification program for nurse educators (CNE). Publishes position papers on nursing education and has a grant program for nursing education research.	www.nln.org
National Organization for Associate Degree Nursing (N-OADN)	Is dedicated to enhancing the quality of Associate Degree (AD) nursing. Advocates for AD nursing and promotes academic progression of AD nursing graduates in furthering their education.	https://www.noadn.org
National Organization of Nurse Practitioner Faculties	Focuses on promoting quality nurse practitioner (NP) education at national and international levels. Leading organization for NP faculty in US and globally.	www.nonpf.com
National Student Nurses Association	Serves as organization for nursing students with goal of enhancing their professional development and promoting transition into the profession.	www.nsna.org
POD Network	Focuses on faculty, instructional, and organizational development in higher education.	www.podnetwork.org
Sigma Theta Tau International Honor Society of Nursing	Supports learning and professional development of nurses worldwide. Membership is by invitation to baccalaureate and graduate nursing students with excellence in scholarship and to nurse leaders with exceptional achievements in nursing. Offers conferences for sharing research and publishes *Journal of Nursing Scholarship*, among other resources.	www.nursingsociety.org

Index